Hematology for Students

Hematology for Students

Edited by

Archie A. MacKinney, Jr., MD
Alumni Professor of Medicine, Emeritus
University of Wisconsin Medical School
Madison, Wisconsin

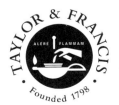

TAYLOR & FRANCIS
ALERE FLAMMAM
Founded 1798

USA   Publishing Office:

TAYLOR & FRANCIS
A member of the Taylor & Francis Group
29 West 35th Street
New York, NY 10001
Tel: (212) 216-7800
Fax: (212) 564-7854

Distribution
Center:

TAYLOR & FRANCIS
A member of the Taylor & Francis Group
7625 Empire Drive
Florence, KY 41042
Tel: 1-800-634-7064
Fax: 1-800-248-4724

UK

TAYLOR & FRANCIS
A member of the Taylor & Francis Group
27 Church Road
Hove
E. Sussex, BN3 2FA
Tel: +44 (0) 1273 207411
Fax: +44 (0) 1273 205612

HEMATOLOGY FOR STUDENTS

1 2 3 4 5 6 7 8 9 0

Printed by Sheridan Books, Ann Arbor, MI, 2002.

The paper in this publication meets the requirements of the ANSI Standard Z39.48-1984 (Permanence of Paper).

Brithish Library of Congress Cataloging-in-Publication Data

A CIP catalog record for this book is available from the British Library.

ISBN 90-5702-646-5

About the Author

Archie A. MacKinney, Jr., MD, is alumni professor of medicine, emeritus, University of Wisconsin-Madison Medical School. He received his M.D. from the University of Rochester School of Medicine, New York, and his bachelor's degree from Wheaton College, Illinois, where he graduated summa cum laude. In addition to his extensive hospital appointments, he has supervised the second-year hematology course at the University of Wisconsin-Madison Medical School for twenty-eight years.

Table of Contents

Contributors

Edwin A. Azen, MD
Professor of Medicine and Medical Genetics
University of Wisconsin Medical School
Madison, Wisconsin

Timothy Cripe, MD
Assistant Professor of Pediatrics
University of Wisconsin Medical School
Madison, Wisconsin

Robert E. Exten, MD
Private Practice
Masselon, Ohio

Jonathon L. Finlay, MD, ChB
Professor of Pediatrics
New York University Medical Center
New York, New York

Donald R. Harkness, MD
Love Professor of Medicine, Emeritus
University of Wisconsin Medical School
Madison, Wisconsin

Archie A. MacKinney, Jr., MD
Alumni Professor of Medicine, Emeritus
University of Wisconsin Medical School
Madison, Wisconsin

Naveen Manchanda, MD
Instructor in Medicine
University of Illinois Medical School—
Champaign/Urbana
Urbana, Illinois

Deane F. Mosher, MD
Schilling Professor of Medicine
University of Wisconsin Medical School
Madison, Wisconsin

Robert F. Schilling, MD
Washburn Professor of Medicine, Emeritus
University of Wisconsin Medical School
Madison, Wisconsin

Bradford S. Schwartz, MD
Professor of Medicine
Dean of Medical School
University of Illinois—Champaign/Urbana
Urbana, Illinois

Nasrollah Shahidi, MD
Professor of Pediatrics, Emeritus
University of Wisconsin Medical School
Madison, Wisconsin

Elizabeth Silverman, MD
Professor of Medicine
University of Wisconsin Medical School
Madison, Wisconsin

Karl Voelkerding, MD
Associate Professor of Pathology and
Laboratory Medicine
University of Wisconsin Medical School
Madison, Wisconsin

Eliot C. Williams, MD, PhD
Associate Professor of Medicine
University of Wisconsin Medical School
Madison, Wisconsin

Robert D. Woodson, MD
Professor of Medicine
University of Wisconsin Medical School
Madison, Wisconsin

Acknowledgments

I extend my heartfelt thanks to my colleagues in hematology, whose dedication to medical student teaching made this text possible. The test has been polished and tempered by hundreds of students, fellows, and practitioners who have studied it. Bob Zelm and Joan Kozel did the artwork. Marci Salmon and Kathy Holland did the transcription. Drs. Dean Mosher, Elizabeth Silverman and Robert Woodson made many editorial improvements. Dr. Elizabeth Silverman has been an invaluable co-worker and sounding board for the teaching of hematology. Dr. Robert Schilling has been the master teacher of us all at University of Wisconsin Medical School.

Preface

Blood is the most easily sampled tissue. As such, those working with diseases of the blood have historically had an advantage in identifying the causes of disease and assessing its treatment. There are many important medical discoveries involving diseases of the blood and blood-forming tissue. The first genetic disease to be associated with an alteration in the amino acid sequence of a protein was sickle cell anemia; the first nutritional disease to be associated with malabsorption of a vitamin was pernicious anemia; the first neoplastic disease to be associated with an acquired alteration of the karyotype was chronic myelogenous leukemia; one of the first neoplastic diseases in which cures were possible with chemotherapy was acute lymphocytic of childhood. In addition, blood diseases can be caused by enzyme defects. For example, hemolytic anemia is due to an abnormality of glucose-6-phosphate dehydrogenase.

This book begins with an overview of the hematopoietic system. The red cell occupies the next five chapters moving through iron metabolism, DNA synthesis, and cell destruction. Each general pathophysiologic process leading to shortened red cell life (e.g., abnormal membranes, enzyme defects, and hemoglobin disorders) is given a chapter. Following this first section are two chapters on blood banking and red cell bodies, and three chapters on the pathophysiology of each of the principal kinds of leukocytes. Finally, the book concludes with three chapters on the roles of platelets, blood coagulation factors, and blood vessels in the maintenance and repair of vascular space.

Because there are so many diseases of the blood and blood-forming tissues, we have been selective in the ones emphasized here. Some, such as iron deficiency anemia, are ones that every physician will encounter, and you therefore must know them. One of the main goals of this text is to help you recognize pathophysiology based on signs, symptoms, and laboratory findings. Therefore, we also consider rare diseases, such as hereditary spherocytosis, that exemplify important physiological processes. We hope that you will gain both scientific knowledge about hematologic diseases, and a framework around which to organize information about the many other diseases that you will learn about.

Accompanying the text is a CD-ROM collection of images. Each slide relates to the text by a number, but may also be used for browsing as well.

Confusing Words and Concepts

The language of hematology has historical, multilingual, and multinational roots heavily infiltrated with abbreviations and jargon. Following are examples of the types of words you will encounter. These are similar-sounding but different words, and you should be alert to their meanings:

blood type A, A1, AB, etc., versus hemoglobin A_2, AS, etc.

reticulocyte versus reticulum cell

hemoglobin M versus blood type M versus M protein

megaloblast versus macrocyte

cryoglobulin versus cold agglutinin

aggregation versus agglutination

aplastic anemia versus aplastic crisis

intravascular hemolysis versus intravascular coagulation

myelocyte versus monocyte

steroid = corticosteroid = glucocorticoid, except when another steroid is specified

neutrophil = "seg" = "poly" = polymorphonuclear leukocyte = PMN

PART I
RED BLOOD CELLS

Introduction to Hematology

Archie MacKinney, Jr.

CHAPTER 1

OUTLINE

OBJECTIVE

- Explain the production and function of red cells, platelets, granulocytes, and lymphocytes to your patient.

OVERVIEW

Blood is beautiful. It is symbolic of life, courage, and sacrifice. Englishmen swear by it. The Romans loved to shed it in the arena. The ancient Hebrews made it sacred in their sacrifices. Its color fascinates flag-makers and artists. Students since Ehrlich have been delighted with the shapes and colors of red cells and leukocytes. The intellectual beauty of blood is apparent to the physiologist and the biochemist studying the orchestration of cells, gases, substrates, stimulators, and inhibitors. Here, we informally introduce four blood cells. Later chapters offer more complete discussions.

The Red Cell

The red cell is a masterpiece of design. Its thin flexible membrane, in the unusual shape of a biconcave disc, is nearly ideal for gas transport. The red cell is so pliable that it can pass through spaces half its diameter; yet its membrane is rugged enough to remain intact for 4 months and hundreds of miles. Like a good automobile tire, it is self-sealing. It carries no nucleus to impede gas exchange or add a metabolic burden. Only a few nonrenewable enzymes are used to maintain its membrane and respiratory pigment. It carries its respiratory pigment (hemoglobin) at concentrations near saturation. At the end of its 4-month life, the red cell is almost completely recycled.

The Neutrophil

If the red cell is benign and rather passive, the neutrophil is chemically explosive. It is an ameba-like phagocyte, loaded with a variety of potent enzymes. The first white cell on the scene of inflammation, it lives a short life of less than 24 hours after leaving the blood. After ingesting and digesting bacteria, the neutrophil self-destructs from the effects of its released enzymes and oxidants. A ready reserve of a cupful of neutrophils is kept in the bone marrow to fight large-scale infections.

The Lymphocyte

The lymphocyte is a reservoir of information. Its precursor has been selected to recognize self and not self. Lymphocytes are diverse, some long-lived, some short-lived, some B cells, some T cells, some helpers, some cytotoxic. The net result is robust cellular and humoral immunity.

The Platelet

The platelet is perhaps the strangest of all the blood cells. It is certainly the smallest, with a diameter that is one fourth that of the red cell. It is a cytoplasmic fragment of the largest hematopoietic cell, the megakaryocyte, containing a complex internal structure that includes structural filaments and specialized secretory granules. The platelet functions to plug holes in blood vessels. When a vessel wall is injured and its surface endothelium is disturbed, platelets adhere to the injury site and release chemical mediators that attract other platelets to form a gluey mass. This blood vessel "glue" is not tough enough to keep the blood from leaking out indefinitely, but the mass serves as an active site on which long fibrin strands form. Fibrin binds the platelets down, much as wire mesh holds the cork in a champagne bottle, until healing of the vessel wound is organized.

One may explain the complexity and functions of blood to patients in this way:

- Red cells carry oxygen.
- Neutrophils make bleach and fight infections.
- Lymphocytes are responsible for immunity.
- Platelets plug holes.
- The bone marrow is the factory in which these cells are made.

All of our subsequent discussion is laden with numbers. Hematology is a numerical science. Red cells, like beans, beg to be counted. And we have been able to sample them so easily and to count them with such accuracy that more detailed cellular knowledge has accumulated in hematology than in any other medical discipline. Hence, hematology is a good way to be introduced to the study of medicine.

The Bone Marrow

The adult bone marrow is the organ that produces red cells, white cells, and platelets. It is roughly the size of the liver (approximately 2 liters). Half of the marrow is fat; the other half is cells. Thus, there are about 1000 mL of hematopoietic cells (1×10^{12}), including 750 mL of granulocytes and their precursors, 250 mL of nucleated red cells, and 4×10^8 megakaryocytes. Monocytes, lymphocytes, and plasma cells are three minor cell types that make up the remaining marrow cells.

Peripheral Blood

The peripheral blood is the common conduit for cells made in the bone marrow. Red cells, granulocytes, and platelets are delivered into the circulation in similar numbers—1 to 2.5×10^{11} per day, or roughly 1 million of each cell type per second! However, their concentrations in the blood vary widely, reflecting their disappearance rates and their sites of action. Red cells function almost exclusively within the peripheral blood to transport gases (O_2, CO_2, CO, NO). Their numbers are high ($5 \times 10^6/\mu L$; 2.6×10^{13}/70-kg human!) and their circulation time long (120 days). In contrast, the neutrophils are 3 logs fewer ($5 \times 10^3/\mu L$), and their phagocytic work is done largely in the tissues, so that their intravascular transit time is very short ($t_{1/2} = 7$ hours). Platelets have intermediate numbers ($2 \times 10^5/\mu L$) and a 10-day circulation time.

The cells also have different flow patterns. Red cells move rapidly through the center of the vessel (axial flow), whereas platelets and white cells are pushed to the walls of the vessel. Half of the granulocytes and some platelets are rolling along the endothelium and are not available to the sampling needle. Consequently, the true number of granulocytes is twice as great as the number counted in a venous blood sample.

Counting Methods

Red cells are measured by three techniques:

- Counting individual cells (the red count)
- Measuring the amount of hemoglobin
- Estimating the fractional volume of blood occupied by red cells (the hematocrit)

TABLE 1-1. Normal Values of Red Cells in Adults*

	Hb (g/dL)	HCT mL/dL	RBC × 10⁻⁶per μL
Females	13.7 ± 2	41.0 ± 6	4.5 ± 0.7
Males	15.5 ± 2	46.0 ± 6	5.1 ± 0.7

Hb, hemoglobin; HCT, hematocrit; RBC, red blood cell.
*The differences between adult males and females are due to testosterone.

Counting of red cells, and also of white cells and platelets, can be performed manually using a calibrated microscope chamber by light scattering in a cuvette, or by electronic signal as cells pass through a calibrated orifice. The amount of hemoglobin is determined by lysing the red cells and measuring the free hemoglobin spectrophotometrically. The fractional volume of red cells, the hematocrit (HCT), is determined by centrifuging a sample of whole blood in a narrow tube and determining the percent of volume that is occupied by red cells. The reasons for using these three measurements will become clear in the next chapters. Values are given in Table 1-1.

The values of the red blood cell count, hemoglobin, and hematocrit are in part dependent on the plasma volume. We usually assume that the plasma volume is normal (about 40 mL/kg). If the plasma volume is reduced, as in hypertension and dehydration, these red cell numbers are falsely elevated. On the other hand, if the plasma volume is greatly increased, the red cell count, hemoglobin, and hematocrit will be falsely low. When both red cells and plasma are lost in acute bleeding, the hematocrit is normal, but the total blood volume is reduced. Under these varied conditions, measuring the total blood volume may be helpful.

Although red cells, white cells, and platelets are all counted as individual particles, white cells require a second procedure for quantification. They are sorted into different classes by counting 100 to 200 consecutive cells on a stained blood smear. This distribution into classes is called the **differential** and is reported in percent. The number of cells in each class per microliter of blood can be obtained by multiplying the percentages by the white blood cell count. Table 1-2 contains normal leukocyte values.

Counting Newly Made Cells

To study rates of production of cells, we should know how many new cells are delivered each day. New red cells, called **reticulocytes**, are easily identified by a special stain (new methylene blue) and are quantified as a percent of total red cells. New neutrophils and platelets cannot be accurately counted. Qualitatively, however, young neutrophils released under stress are band forms, and young platelets are greater than 2 μm in diameter on blood smears. Because of the

TABLE 1-2. Normal Adult Peripheral Blood White Cell Values

Cell Class	Mean/μL	Range/μL	Percent
Segmented neutrophils	3800	1600–6700	50
Lymphocytes	2600	1300–4200	35
Monocytes	410	110–810	6
Band neutrophils	370	50–1400	6
Eosinophils	200	0–575	3
Basophils	33	0–160	0.6
Total	7200	4400–11,500	100

difficulties in quantifying newly made neutrophils and platelets, delivery of these cells is less well understood.

Statistical versus Physiologic Ranges

Normal values for laboratory data are usually reported as the statistical mean plus or minus 2 standard deviations, but values above and below these limits are well tolerated. Thus, although the lower normal limit of hemoglobin is 12 g/dL, symptoms do not occur in otherwise healthy subjects until the hemoglobin reaches 10 g/dL. A less than normal range of hemoglobin or hematocrit value is called **anemia**. Hemoglobin below 10 g/dL, and especially below 7 g/dL is anemia that is often associated with weakness, easy fatigue, and shortness of breath. Similarly, low granulocyte counts do not predispose to infection until the absolute granulocyte count drops below 1000/μL. Platelet counts above 80,000/μL do not expose the patient to increased risk of bleeding; spontaneous bleeding is seen when the platelet count goes below 10,000/μL.

At the upper limits of the physiologic range, hematocrit values between 50% and 55% often produce no symptoms in otherwise healthy subjects, although cerebral blood flow is clearly decreased. At values above 55%, blood tends to stagnate and clot. Platelet counts above 1 million per microliter are commonly associated with clotting or, paradoxically, bleeding. Practically no symptoms are found with high leukocyte counts unless the cells are undifferentiated ("blastic"). White counts of blasts cells greater than 100,000/μL signal a medical emergency because of the risk of bleeding in the brain.

SUMMARY POINTS

Much of hematology is a numerical cell science, which incorporates much basic science in the evaluation and treatment of disease. There are three cells systems—white cells for infection and immunity, platelets for hemostasis and wound repair, and red cells for oxygen transport. The cells have wide physiologic ranges, a built-in safety feature. Chapter 2 discusses the origins of these cells.

Hematopoietic Stem Cells and Their Progeny

Archie MacKinney, Jr., Jonathan L. Finlay, Nasrollah T. Shahidi

OUTLINE

Totipotent and Pluripotent Stem Cells
Unipotent Stem Cells
Growth Factors
Control of Hematopoiesis
Stem Cell Transplantation

Differentiated Hematopoietic Cells
    Anatomy of Bone Marrow
    Ontogeny
    Sampling Methods
    Differentiated Cells of Marrow
Summary Points

OBJECTIVES

- Define stem cells. Give examples of totipotent, pluripotent stem cells and differentiated marrow cells.
- Name three growth factors used in medical practice.
- Cite examples of hematopoietic control mechanisms.
- Know how stem cells are used to treat disease.
- Know the differential of the normal bone marrow.

All differentiated hematopoietic cells (red cells, granulocytes, monocytes, lymphocytes, and platelets) are the progeny of a primitive stem cell. Roughly one marrow cell in 100,000 is a stem cell. Stem cells can be recovered from peripheral blood as well. Because stem cells resemble lymphocytes, they cannot be identified by morphology. Since the 1960s, tissue culture, marrow transplantations in animals, and cell surface markers have enabled characterization of these rare and undifferentiated cells. A series of International Workshops on Leukocyte Antigens has sorted through available monoclonal antibodies to classify cell surface proteins according to CD (cluster designation) numbers. Human stem cells have the unique characteristics of being CD34$^+$ CD38$^-$.

Stem cells are undifferentiated precursors that can sustain their own numbers as well as differentiate into functioning cells. The following is a hierarchy of potentialities:

- Totipotent stem cells can make all known cells of the blood and bone marrow except stromal cells.
- Unipotent stem cells can make one lineage.
- Pluripotent stem cells can make several cell lineages.
- Lymphoid stem cells makes both T cells and B cells and their myriad progeny.
- Myeloid stem cells can make granulocytes and monocytes, platelets, and red cells.

TOTIPOTENT AND PLURIPOTENT STEM CELLS

The bone marrow is a rapidly dividing tissue and has an enormous output: 1 to 2.5×10^{11} red cells, granulocytes, and platelets are produced daily by a 70-kg person. Under stress such as major blood loss, the hematopoietic system can increase its production of red cells up to five or six times. Continuous hematopoietic stem cell maturation is necessary to maintain the pools of mature cells. Stem cell self-replication, however, is also essential. Otherwise, the stem cell pool would become depleted. The basic characteristic of the primitive totipotent stem cell is that it can replicate itself and also differentiate into pluripotent stem cells.

Research suggests that the totipotent stem cell is normally in a dormant state and does not divide actively. The dormancy protects the stem cells from drugs that kill dividing cells and render it less susceptible to mutation. Thus, it is possible by chemotherapy for acute leukemia to kill all the visible cells in the bone marrow and yet to have bone marrow recover in 20 to 25 days from the virtually invisible stem cell pool.

Pluripotent stem cells have been identified in the mouse. When a mouse is exposed to a dose of ionizing radiation sufficient to destroy its hematopoietic cells and then receives a suspension of normal syngeneic bone marrow by intravenous injection, the animal will survive and its spleen will become a center of donor cell growth. After 7 to 8 days, visible nodules will be found on the spleen. Each nodule consists of a recognizable colony of hematopoietic cells and its precursors, with each of these colonies arising from a single cell. The donor cells taking root in the spleen are called spleen colony-forming units (CFU-S). The colonies that form may consist of cells of one lineage (i.e., erythroid, myeloid, or megakaryocytic), or they may consist of two or even three lineages. If these colonies are excised from one mouse's spleen and injected into another syngeneic irradiated mouse, similar colonies arise in the second mouse's spleen. Hence, the CFU-S include self-replicating and differentiating cells and fulfill both criteria for being uncommitted hematopoietic stem cells. Evidence for an even more primitive precursor, the totipotent CFU-LM (lymphoid-myeloid) comes from chromosome studies of mouse and human.

UNIPOTENT STEM CELLS

Committed, unipotent stem cells may be identified by their ability to form colonies of cells in a variety of in vitro systems. Human or mouse hematopoietic cells may be cultured on dishes in semisolid support media, using stimulatory factors favoring one or another of the hematopoietic cell lines (e.g., erythropoietin for erythroid colony growth or colony-stimulating factor (GM-CSF [granulocyte-macrophage colony-stimulating factor]) for myeloid colony growth). The cells in these colonies are derived from committed progenitor cells called CFU-C (colony-forming units–culture, because they were first found in tissue culture). They are unipotent stem cells in that all the cells within a colony are of a single type, except for CFU-GM, which can produce both neutrophils and monocytes.

Unipotent stem cells, not yet identifiable as erythroid or myeloid precursor cells, are already committed to one pathway. They proliferate and differentiate into morphologically distinct hematopoietic elements (e.g., erythroblasts, myeloblasts, and lymphoblasts) (Fig. 2-1).

Figure 2-1 shows a model of three stem cell compartments. The totipotent stem cell (CFU-LM) in the black box differentiates into CFU-GEMM (granulocytic-erythrocytic-monocytic-megakaryocytic) and CFU-L (lymphoid) stem cells in the dark gray pluripotent compartment. Unipotent stem cells are found in the light gray third compartment. The CFU-GM is unique because it produces both monocytic and granulocytic precursors. None of these three stem cell compartments is visible in the marrow. They are interpretations of bone marrow culture

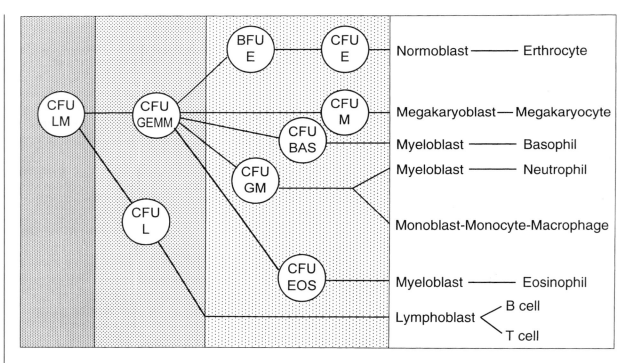

FIGURE 2-1.
Schematic flow of stem cells into differentiated compartments. CFU-LM, colony-forming unit–lymphoid-myeloid is the totipotent stem cell for lymphoid and myeloid cells. CFU-GEMM, CFU–granulocytic-erythrocytic-monocytic-megakaryocytic, is the stem cell for they myeloid series. BFU-E, burst-forming unit–erythroid, and CFU-E, CFU–erythroid, are successive erythroid stem cells. CFU-M, CFU-megakaryocyte, is the platelet stem cell. CFU-GM, CFU–granulocyte-macrocyte, is the stem cell of granulocytic and monocytic cells. CFU-BAS, CFU-basophil; CFU-EOS, CFU-eosinophil; CFU-GM, CFU–granulocyte-macrophage; CFU-L, CFU-lymphoid.

and animal studies. Only in the fourth compartment (white) do we find cells with enough differentiation to be recognized by ordinary microscopy. The importance of these compartments will become apparent when we study the malignancies of the bone marrow in later chapters.

The hematopoietic stem cell and progenitor cell pools are not limited to the bone marrow. Small numbers can be grown from the spleen and the peripheral blood. Lymphoid cells also can be grown from progenitor cells of the thymus and other lymphoid organs as well as from the bone marrow. The normal function of stem cells in extramedullary locations is not well understood, but they repopulate the bone marrow after local marrow areas have been injured by x-radiation.

GROWTH FACTORS

Colony stimulating factors (CSF) are so called because they were defined by bioassay in tissue cultures where colonies grew from single progenitors (CFU) that are stem cells. On the other hand, the lymphoid cells are usually grown in liquid media so that colonies are not formed and the term CSF would not be appropriate. The term **interleukin** (IL) is used for growth factors that stimulate lymphocytes. The term **cytokine** encompasses both CSFs and interleukins.

Cytokines are glycoproteins that are active at low concentrations. Cytokines usually interact with dimeric or trimeric transmembrane receptors that are linked to intracellular protein tyrosine kinases. The biology of these factors and receptors is complex. Some cytokines are synthesized by multiple tissues. A given cytokine affects the growth and differentiation of more than one cell type. Receptors share common subunits. The result is that cytokines have additive or synergistic effects and function as an orchestra rather than as solo players. Endocrine (stimulating cells at a distance), paracrine (stimulating at short range), and autocrine (self-stimulating) effects have been observed. In addition to stimulating growth of normal cells, cytokines may stimulate the growth of tumors, since some tumors have receptors for growth factors.

Erythropoietin, G-CSF (granulocyte colony-stimulating factor), and GM-CSF are already in clinical use, and a number of additional cytokines, including thrombopoietin, are in clinical trials. G-CSF and GM-CSF stimulate neutrophil production after chemotherapy for cancer. Some of the interleukins, such as IL-2, have been tested for their ability to direct the activities of lymphocytes and thus enhance immunity against cancer.

The genes for IL-4, IL-5, GM-CSF, IL-3, and M-CSF are on the long arm of chromosome 5, the deletion of which is associated with bone marrow failure (myelodysplasia). Some cytokines and their actions are listed in Table 2-1. The full list goes beyond IL-18. The human genome project will undoubtedly add new "players."

CONTROL OF HEMATOPOIESIS

In normal humans, blood cell production takes place exclusively in the bone marrow space. The nature of this microenvironment is incompletely understood. There appear to be fixed cellular niches in the bone marrow—presumably determined by bone marrow stromal cells, which include endothelial cells, adventitial cells, fibroblasts, and macrophages and also lymphocytes and fat cells. In long-term bone marrow tissue cultures, a layer of adherent stromal cells must be established before active proliferation of bone marrow stem cells occurs. Pluripotent stem cells adhere to the stroma and proliferate actively. BFU-E (burst-forming units erythroid) attachment is mediated by fibronectin, an extracellular adhesion protein. Unipotent stem cells appear to be nonadherent. Further evidence for a microenvironment is that the bone marrow fails to recover

TABLE 2-1. Some Growth Factors and Their Actions

Erythropoietin
Made by the kidney
Stimulates growth of colony-forming unit–erythroid and normoblasts

Thrombopoietin
Made by liver, kidney, spleen, and bone marrow
Regulates growth of megakaryocytes

Stem cell growth factor, C-kit ligand, steel factor, mast cell growth factor
Made by many cells
Synergizes with other factors to stimulate red cell, granulocyte, megakaryocyte, mast cell, and lymphocyte production

Granulocyte-macrophage colony stimulating factor (GM-CSF)
Made by a wide variety of cells, including leukemic myeloblasts (autocrine effect)
Stimulates granulocyte-macrophage, granulocyte, and macrophage colony formation and proliferation
Enhances adhesion, cytotoxic and phagocytic activity of neutrophils and monocytes

Granulocyte colony stimulating factor (G-CSF)
Made by a wide variety of cells
Stimulates formation of granulocyte colonies in vitro
Enhances activation of neutrophils
Acts to release marrow granulocytes and stem cells
Acts synergistically with interleukin-3 (IL-3) to stimulate megakaryocyte colonies, and with GM-CSF to stimulate granulocyte-macrophage colonies

Macrophage colony stimulating factor (M-CSF)
Made by a wide variety of cells
Stimulates growth of macrophage colonies in vitro
Supports macrophage survival in vitro and activates monocytes and macrophages
Increases replication of HIV in monocytes
Interacts with the receptor, which is the c-*fms* proto-oncogene product

IL-1, endogenous pyrogen, neutrophil-releasing factor
Made by monocytes
Induces synthesis of acute phase proteins by hepatocytes
Induces muscle proteolysis (recycling amino acids)
Causes fever (pyrogen)
Releases neutrophils from marrow stores
Causes decrease in serum iron
Increases bone resorption (osteoclast activating factor) and cartilage degradation
Stimulates proliferation of fibroblasts, osteoblasts, and other connective tissue cells
Induces IL-2 and IL-2 receptors
Decreases pituitary hormone production
Synergizes with IL-3, M-CSF, G-CSF, and GM-CSF to stimulate various stem cell classes

IL-2, T-cell growth factor
Made by T cells
Supports growth of T cells (autocrine)
Inhibits granulocyte-macrophage colony formation
Induces secretion of γ-interferon
Augments lymphocyte-activated killer activity

IL-3 (multi-CSF)
Made by T cells and stromal cells
Stimulates formation of granulocyte, macrophage, eosinophil, mast cell, natural killer cell (NK), and erythroid colonies
Synergizes with GM-CSF and M-CSF
Stimulates pulmonary alveolar macrophages to proliferate

TABLE 2-1. Some Growth Factors and Their Actions (Continued)

IL-4, B-cell stimulating factor-l (BSF-l)
Made by monocytes, T cells, etc
Induces resting B cells to proliferate in presence of anti IgM antibodies
Increases expression of class II MHC (major histocompatibility complex) molecules on
  resting B cells
Promotes secretion of IgG and IgE
Interacts with erythropoietin to stimulate erythroid colonies

IL-5, B-cell differentiating factor, eosinophil differentiating factor
Promotes differentiation of B cells
Stimulates eosinophil colony formation and differentiation

IL-6, BSF-2
Made by B, T cells
Induces differentiation of B cells and stimulates Ig secretion
Promotes growth of Epstein-Barr virus–infected B cells
Growth factor for myeloma cells (autocrine)
Stimulates growth of megakaryocytes

IL-7 to -18
Modulate B and T cells in various ways

---

after high-dose radiation (> 30 Gy), suggesting destruction of the stromal cells within the beam of radiation.

Control of hematopoiesis is further modulated by feedback inhibitors. In the presence of excessive concentrations of a CSF, macrophages or monocytes produce prostaglandins that may inhibit myelopoiesis. Lactoferrin secreted by granulocytes also blocks CSF production. T lymphocytes have been shown to be essential for normal erythroid colony growth. However, T-lymphocyte suppressor cells may inhibit erythropoiesis. For example, some patients with aplastic anemia appear to have immune suppression of hematopoiesis. Some cases of acquired red cell aplasia are associated with a T-cell tumor of the thymus called **thymoma**.

STEM CELL TRANSPLANTATION

An important frontier in medicine revolves around transplantation of hematopoietic stem cells. Stem cell transplantation is used mainly to reconstitute the patient's marrow after lethal chemotherapy and rarely to replace primary loss of stem cells. Stem cells can be harvested from the patient with Hodgkin's disease, for example. High-dose chemotherapy is given; and stem cells are given back intravenously as in a blood transfusion. In 6 weeks, the patient is possibly cured of the lymphoma, the marrow has been reestablished, and a nearly normal life resumes. This type of transplantation is called an **autologous** transplantation.

If the marrow has been damaged by previous treatment or contaminated with malignant cells, stem cell transplant from another individual (**allogeneic**) can be done. This requires the search for a donor matched for the major histocompatibility complex (MHC) on chromosome 6. The chance of a sibling being a match at both loci is 1:4. Because of marked linkage disequilibrium, the general population is likely also to contain individuals with the same two MHC haplotypes as a given patient. Thus, stem cell transplant registries have been created to identify matched unrelated donors for patients who do not have sibling match. Allogeneic stem cell transplantations work both because of the intensive therapy undergone before transplantation and the graft-versus-tumor effect of the transplanted immune system. A patient with acute leukemia, for example, is treated with chemotherapy to kill all visible leukemia cells. After the remission is induced, a sibling-matched stem cell transplantation is done. The patient is treated with otherwise lethal chemotherapy and radiation therapy to remove the last traces of malignancy. Life is preserved by the donated stem cells. The major complication is caused by the transplanted immune system attacking the host and causing graft-versus-host disease (GVHD). Allogeneic bone marrow transplant recipients, therefore, must be carefully followed up for years.

Some of the diseases that we will discuss arise from abnormal stem cells. These include the malignancies of the marrow such as the acute leukemias, chronic myelogenous leukemia, and polycythemia vera; myelodysplastic states such as refractory anemia; and nonmalignant disorders such as paroxysmal nocturnal hemoglobinuria and aplastic anemia.

DIFFERENTIATED HEMATOPOIETIC CELLS

Anatomy of Bone Marrow

The bone marrow is a complex space separated into incomplete compartments by bony trabeculae. The bone marrow cells grow in these compartments outside the blood vessels, supported by fat and reticular cells. Mature red cells, granulocytes, and platelets enter the veins through the cytoplasm of endothelial cells, which form the walls of thin venous sinusoids. Their precursors are excluded from the circulation because of specific adhesion to cells and extracellular matrix of the bone marrow stroma.

Ontogeny

In the embryo, blood cell production begins in primitive mesenchyme and the yolk sac. The liver and, to a lesser extent, the spleen take over this function after the tenth week of gestation. After the fourth fetal month, production of blood cells begins in the bone marrow. At birth, active marrow has receded from the liver and spleen but fills most of the marrow cavity. By adulthood, however, the growth of the bone cavity has exceeded the growth of hematopoietic tissue, so that the active red marrow is confined to the flat bones (skull, pelvis, and ribs), the vertebrae, and the proximal ends of the femurs and humeri. A malignancy of the marrow like multiple myeloma can therefore destroy bone in all of these sites. Red marrow can expand into the fatty, yellow medullary spaces of the round bones (femur, humerus) when the long-term demand for cells increases. The liver and spleen can also resume hematopoiesis in some pathologic states.

Sampling Methods

The bone marrow is sampled by two techniques: aspiration and biopsy. The dense particles of hematopoietic cells, fat, and endothelial cells can be aspirated through a needle and smeared on slides or coverslips. The smear gives excellent cell detail. Biopsy entails cutting out a core of bone marrow, including some trabecular bone, with a large-bore cutting needle. The biopsy shows the marrow architecture and adherent cells that cannot be aspirated, such as cancer and fibrous tissue. Both needle aspirate and needle biopsy are widely used, and usually both are obtained in the same procedure entering the ilium through the posterior crest.

Differentiated Cells of Marrow

More than 50% of marrow cells are granulocytes and their precursors. Their proportions make an easily remembered series of 4s: 1% myeloblasts, 4% promyelocytes, 12% myelocytes, 16% metamyelocytes, and 20% bands and segmented neutrophils {#1–6}.

Nucleated red cells make up about 25% of marrow cells: 4% are pronormoblasts, and 18% are normoblasts. The granulocyte-to-erythrocyte ratio (G/E) is the sum of the granulocyte precursors divided by the sum of the normoblast precursors: 53%/22%, 2.3/1 (range, 2/1–3/1) {#12–15}. Lymphocytes make up 10% to 20% of marrow cells {#10}, and plasma cells represent less than 3%. Monocytes account for less than 1% {#9}. Megakaryocytes are not measured as a percentage because of their scarcity, but two to five per low-power field is a normal estimate.

The granulocyte-to-erythrocyte (G/E) ratio is one of the important indices of total granulocyte and red cell production. An increase in the G/E ratio suggests hyperplasia of the granulocytes when the marrow is normally cellular or hypercellular. When the marrow is hypocellular, an increased G/E ratio suggests a decrease in red cell production.

The hallmark of a normal marrow is cellular diversity. At first glance, the normal marrow should contain about 35% easily recognizable metamyelocytes, segmented neutrophils, and bands. If the marrow is populated by cells with round nuclei rather than those of differentiated granulocytes, the following possibilities should be considered:

- Erythroid cells, plasma cells or lymphocytes {#91} are increased.
- Neutrophils are decreased {#101}.
- Cancer cells replace normal marrow cells{#98}.
- Blasts of the myeloid or lymphoid series predominate {#100}.

Marrow examination is also useful for the recognition of the following:
- Megaloblastosis (immature-appearing red cell nuclei with mature cytoplasm) {#21}
- Myelofibrosis (marrow replacement by fibrous tissue) {#91}
- Pathologic inclusions in macrophages (histoplasmosis {#74}, Gaucher's disease {#75}, Neimann-Pick's disease)
- Aplasia of one or more blood elements (#87} *or*
- Megakaryocyte numbers (immune thrombocytopenic purpura) {#49}

In addition to the routine polychrome stains, the bone marrow specimen can be stained for iron with Prussian blue by a simple, inexpensive process {#20}. The absence of stainable iron is important for the diagnosis of iron deficiency, one of the most common causes of anemia in humans.

SUMMARY POINTS

Stem cells are essential to life. The orchestration of growth factors and environmental niches necessary to maintain the stem cells and their progeny is one of the most interesting and important areas of modern biology. Stem cell transplantation offers the best chance for cure of a number of malignancies. Study of the bone marrow is important for diagnosis of many blood diseases.

CHAPTER 3

Erythropoiesis and the Analysis of Anemia

Robert D. Woodson

OUTLINE

OBJECTIVES

- Define G/E ratio.
- Calculate the reticulocyte index.
- Define the shift cell and its significance.
- Explain the physiology of acute versus chronic anemia.
- Understand the morphologic classification of anemia.
- Understand the kinetic classification of anemia.

Anemia is a common medical problem, and its pathophysiology is well understood. This chapter introduces red cell differentiation and maturation, control of red cell production, and methods of classifying anemia. Later chapters take up the membrane, enzymes, and hemoglobins in more detail.

RED CELL DIFFERENTIATION AND MATURATION

Red cell production (erythropoiesis) depends on stem cell differentiation into two successive erythropoietin-responsive cells. Under erythropoietin stimulation, these cells in culture form burst-forming units (BFU-E) and then the more mature colony forming units (CFU-E), as diagrammed in the stem cell chapter (see Fig. 2-1). In the normal marrow, these hematopoietic stem cells develop into the earliest morphologically recognizable erythroid progenitor, the **pronormoblast**.

Approximately 8 days elapse from the pronormoblast stage to the release of a mature red cell into the circulation (the normoblast). Five days are spent in division and 3 days in reticulocyte maturation. During its growth period, the normoblast divides three to four times at about 24-hour intervals. The normoblast synthesizes hemoglobin and changes color on staining from deep blue (RNA) to pink (hemoglobin) and decreases in size (Fig. 3-1). The nucleus then undergoes involution and is extruded, engulfed, and digested by an adjacent macrophage. The developing normoblast proceeds through four phases based on nuclear and cytoplasmic changes.

- The **pronormoblast** {#12} has a generous amount of royal blue cytoplasm with no recognizable hemoglobin and has a diameter of 20 to 24 μm.
- The **basophilic normoblast** is smaller {#13}, 16 to 18 μm in diameter, with blue cytoplasm and a conspicuous Golgi apparatus.
- The **polychromatophilic normoblast** {#14} has blue-gray cytoplasm, reflecting the mixture of RNA and hemoglobin, and a checkerboard-appearing nucleus (12 to 15 μm in diameter).
- The **orthochromatic normoblast** {#15} has pink-gray cytoplasm and a pyknotic nucleus. Hemoglobin synthesis is nearly complete. Three or four repeated divisions have reduced the normoblast volume from 900 to 90 femtoliters (fL) and its diameter from 20 to 8 μm.

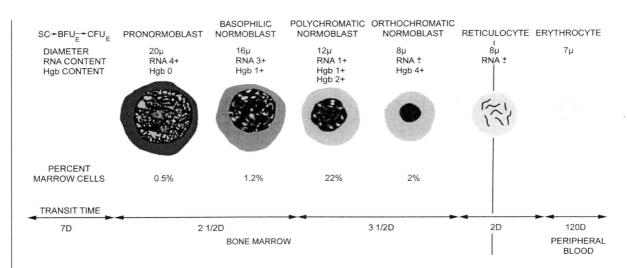

FIGURE 3-1.

Maturation sequence of the red cell. Note changes in number, size, hemoglobin (Hgb) and RNA content, and time in marrow and blood compartments. SC, serum creatine, BFU$_E$, burst-forming units-erythroid; CFU$_E$, colony-forming units-erythroid

The conspicuous event occurring during normoblast maturation is hemoglobin synthesis, which involves synthesis of both heme and globin. Heme synthesis begins with the condensation of succinate and glycine to yield δ-aminolevulinic acid, which is catalyzed by δ-aminolevulinic acid synthetase in the mitochondria. This enzyme appears to be regulated by erythropoietin and requires pyridoxal phosphate (vitamin B_6) as a cofactor. Figure 3-2 shows the synthesis of porphobilinogen from δ-aminolevulinic acid. Four molecules of porphobilinogen condense to form the tetrapyrrolic ring compound uroporphyrinogen, which is then converted to coproporphrinogen. These steps, beginning with the condensation of δ-aminolevulinic acid, occur in the cytosol. The final steps occur in the mitochondria, where coproporphyrinogen is converted to protoporphyrin and iron is inserted to yield heme (Fig. 3-3).

Meanwhile, α and β globins are synthesized on ribosomes. Heme and globin synthesis are closely linked. When globin synthesis is deficient, heme synthesis is correspondingly reduced, and vice versa. Assembly of the hemoglobin tetramer from two α chains and two β chains, each bearing heme groups, occurs then.

When the orthochromatic normoblast extrudes its nucleus, it is called a **reticulocyte**. Reticulum is a collection of RNA-rich mitochondria and ribosomes that appears as nodular blue strands when stained by supravital dyes such as new methylene blue {#31}. Reticulocytes require about 4 days to mature into red cells—about 3 days of this period is normally spent in the marrow and 1 day in the peripheral blood. Inasmuch as approximately 1% of the circulating red cells are replaced daily (the red cell life span is 120 days) and since the newly released erythrocyte is identifiable as a reticulocyte for about 24 hours, about 1% of circulating red cells are normally reticulocytes.

Almost 25% of hemoglobin is synthesized during the reticulocyte stage. Hemoglobin synthesis stops when the hemoglobin has reached the astonishing concentration of 340 g per liter of red cells. During this time the RNA (reticulum) is degraded. Morphologically, the reticulocyte changes from a large, irregular spherical cell with redundant membrane to the familiar biconcave disc form.

Young reticulocytes in the marrow display abundant RNA. They have bluish cytoplasm (polychromatophilia) {#17} when stained with ordinary Wright's or Giemsa stains. The more mature reticulocytes normally present in peripheral blood are indistinguishable from mature red cells with Wright's or Giemsa stains. Hence, larger bluish red cells in the peripheral blood signal early release from the marrow and suggest increased erythropoietin activity or a breakdown in the marrow barrier. When seen in the peripheral blood smear, these cells are called **polychromatophilic macrocytes** or "shift cells."

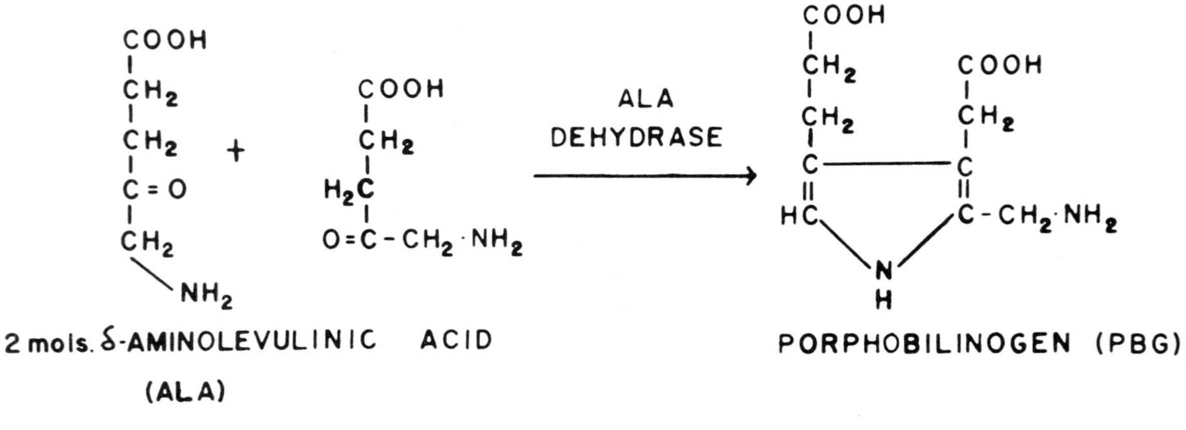

FIGURE 3-2.
Synthesis of porphobilinogen from δ-aminolevulinic acid.

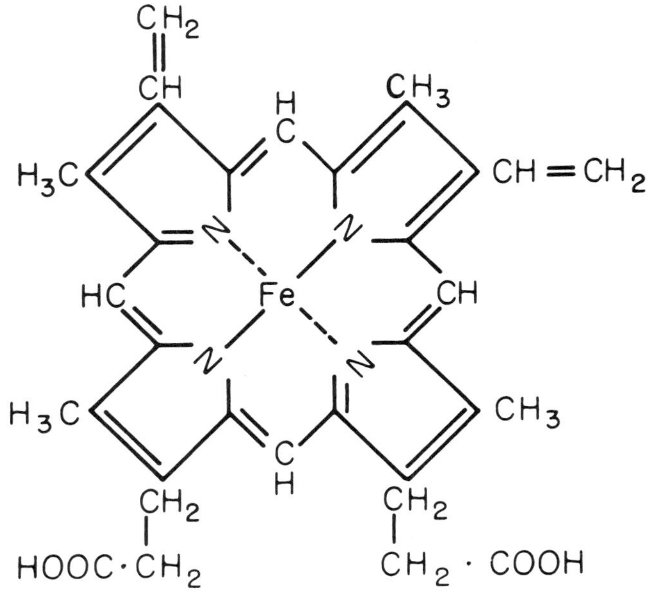

FIGURE 3-3.
Heme (ferroprotoporphyrin 9), ready for binding to an α- or β-chain.

During normal erythropoiesis, approximately 10% of the red cell precursors are destroyed in the marrow. This destruction was discovered by the appearance of tracer molecules in hemoglobin breakdown products shortly after their incorporation into developing red cells (**Fig. 3-4**). Exaggerated intramarrow cell death occurs in vitamin B_{12} or folic acid deficiency, thalassemias, and other marrow disorders.

ERYTHROPOIETIN

Red cell production is regulated by erythropoietin. Erythropoietin is normally present in blood and excreted in urine in small amounts. The level of erythropoietin varies inversely with the hematocrit (Fig. 3-5). When the hematocrit is below 20%, the levels increase by a factor of 100 to 1000. When subjects are hypertransfused or develop autonomous (erythropoietin-independent) production of red cells, erythropoietin falls to low levels. Erythropoietin levels are believed to be modulated by an oxygen sensor that monitors microvascular or tissue Po_2. Kidney peritubular cells are the probable source of erythropoietin. Erythropoietin increases in response to a lowered Po_2 in the renal microvasculature. This includes anemia, acute blood loss, and conditions that shift the oxygen dissociation curve to the left (decreased oxygen release). It is now recognized that extrarenal sources of erythropoietin exist. Thus, months after total nephrectomy, erythropoietin again is found in serum, and the hematocrit gradually rises to the high 20s. Extrarenal erythropoietin probably comes from the liver, which is also a source of this hormone in the fetus.

High erythropoietin levels act on the marrow in several ways. Its predominant action is to increase differentiation of pronormoblasts from stem cells, leading to increased output of red cells. Erythropoietin also accelerates the maturation of normoblasts, shortening the intermitotic interval and increasing the rate of hemoglobin synthesis. Finally, increased erythropoietin promotes the release of reticulocytes at an earlier stage of development. Hence, the presence of large

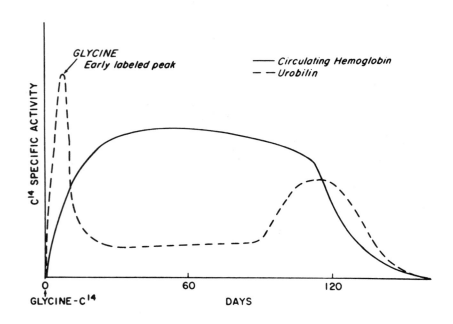

FIGURE 3-4.
Incorporation of glycine-2-14 C in red cells, measuring activity in circulating red cells and fecal urobilin. The early labeled peak indicates physiologic loss of red cells within the marrow. The late labeled peak coincides with the death of the cohort of red cells at 120 days. (From Williams WJ, et al. *Hematology*, 2nd ed. New York: McGraw-Hill, p. 238, by permission.)

young reticulocytes (polychromatophilic macrocytes or shift cells) in peripheral blood is a useful sign of increased erythropoietin.

RED CELL LIFE SPAN AND DEATH

Normal human red cells circulate for about 120 days, after which they are destroyed by a macrophage in the spleen or, if the spleen is absent, in the liver. Erythrocyte death is related to aging processes. These processes include a decrease in activity of enzymes, a decline in adenosine triphosphate (ATP) level, an increase in cell density and mean corpuscular hemoglobin concentration (MCHC), and a decrease in deformability as the cell becomes spherocytic. Immunoglobulin accumulation on aging erythrocytes also may play a role in phagocytosis by macrophages. Hemoglobin catabolism is discussed at length in Chapter 6.

ERYTHROKINETICS

Normally, production of new red cells and removal of old cells are exactly balanced so that the hematocrit is stable. Changes in hematocrit, if changes in plasma volume are excluded, are due to a change in the rate of production, destruction, or blood loss.

The Granulocyte-to-Erythrocyte Ratio

The granulocyte-to erythrocyte ratio (G/E ratio) is the ratio of granulocytic precursors to nucleated red blood cells in an aspirate of bone marrow. Since it is a ratio, it is useful only when marrow granulocyte production is normal. In the

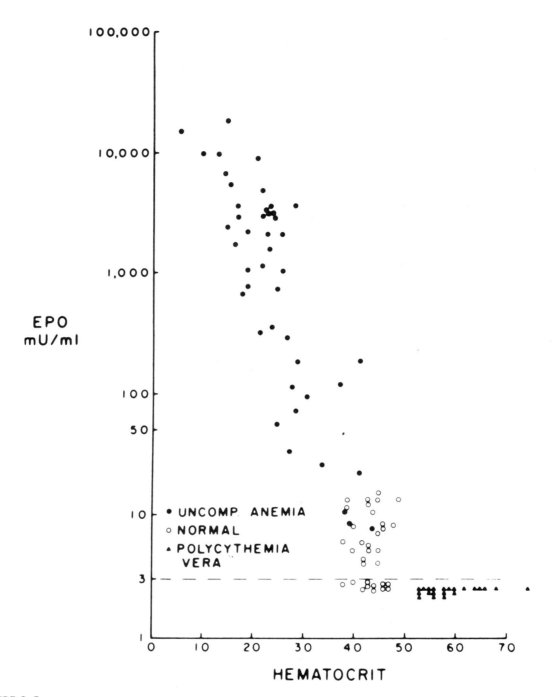

FIGURE 3-5.

The relation between hematocrit and plasma erythropoietin titers. Patients with anemia not complicated by kidney disease or inflammation, normal subjects, and patients with polycythemia vera are indicated. EPO, erythropoietin. (From Erslev AJ, et al. Plasma erythropoietin in health and disease. *Ann Clin Lab Sci* 10:250.)

normal state, the G/E ratio is about 3:1 {#84}. The ratio provides an estimate of erythroid marrow activity. For example, when an increase in erythroid activity is sufficient to double or triple output of erythrocytes from the marrow, this ratio decreases to about 3:2 and 1:1, respectively. Conversely, when erythrocyte output falls by 50%, the ratio changes to 6:1.

The Reticulocyte Index

The reticulocyte index is the most useful everyday measure of effective marrow production. The release of one reticulocyte signals effective production of one red cell by the marrow. In contrast, the G/E ratio and plasma iron turnover represent total red cell production. The clinical laboratory reports express reticulocytes as a percentage of circulating red cells, and two corrections are applied to derive the actual reticulocyte output. First, the reticulocyte percentage is multiplied by the number of erythrocytes per microliter to obtain the absolute retic count. This value in normal people is about $50,000/\mu L$ ($1.0\% \times 5 \times 10^6$ erythrocytes/μL). A second correction accounts for changes in the maturation time of reticulocytes in peripheral blood. When erythropoietin stimulation is increased, reticulocytes are released from the marrow prematurely. This increases the time a reticulocyte spends in the blood and inflates the absolute number of reticulocytes, as illustrated in Figure 3-6. Accordingly, the second correction is applied only when immature reticulocytes (polychromatophilic macrocytes, or shift cells) are observed in peripheral blood.

When the hematocrit is 25%, reticulocytes are released about 24 hours earlier than normally (see Fig. 3-6), and it is necessary to divide the absolute reticulocyte count by two. The resulting value is called the "corrected absolute reticulocyte count." At hematocrits of 35% and 15%, the absolute reticulocyte count should be divided by 1.5 and 2.5, respectively. The corrected absolute reticulocyte count provides an accurate indication of red cell production. For example, a value of $150,000/\mu L$ suggests that the marrow is producing cells at three times the normal rate; a value of $25,000/\mu L$ suggests that it is producing erythrocytes at half the normal rate.

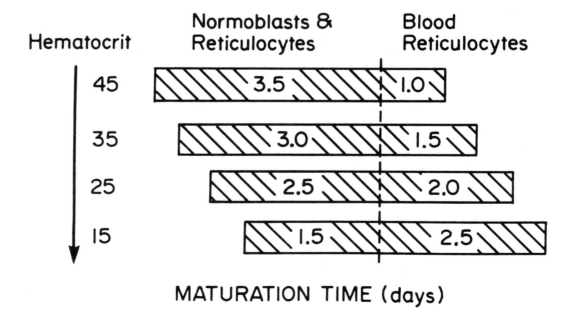

FIGURE 3-6.
The time normoblasts and reticulocytes spend in the marrow and blood at different hematocrits. The horizontal dashed line indicates the marrow barrier. As the hematocrit decreases, there is progressively shorter marrow time and longer blood maturation time. (From Bothwell TH, et al. *Iron Metabolism in Man*, 2nd ed, Oxford: Blackwell, p. 238.)

The ratio of the doubly corrected reticulocyte count to 50,000 is termed the **reticulocyte index**. The formula is as follows:

$$RI = \frac{reticulocytes}{100} \times RBC\ count \times \frac{1}{50,000} \times \frac{1}{maturation\ time}.$$

PATHOPHYSIOLOGY OF ANEMIA

In normal subjects, the concentration of hemoglobin, the volume of red blood cells per unit volume of blood (hematocrit), and the number of red cells per unit volume of blood are closely regulated. Actual values, which differ with age and sex, are given in Table 3-1. A decrease below these levels is **anemia**; an increase is **erythrocytosis**.

Note the elevated values in the newborn with high indices, and physiologic anemia in the 1- to 2-year-old with low indices. The differences between adult men and women are due to testosterone.

A slow decline in hematocrit to 30% usually produces no symptoms in normal sedentary subjects. However, the capacity for aerobic activity such as competitive athletics or heavy work is sharply limited by even mild anemia. When the hematocrit falls below 30%, weakness, fatigue, and breathlessness are common. Hematocrits below 25% are poorly tolerated, especially in the elderly, and transfusions may be required. Anemia may critically limit oxygen delivery to organs whose blood supply have been compromised by vascular disease. For example, patients may have chest pain (angina) or pain in the legs (claudication) when their hematocrit falls below 30%, but not when the hematocrit is higher.

Acute blood loss does not immediately change the measurements of red cells. Instead, symptoms and signs are related to the amount of blood lost. Tachycardia and drop in blood pressure occur when the amount is more than 20% of the blood volume (1 liter in a 70-kg adult). If more than 30% of the blood volume is acutely lost, air hunger, cold clammy skin, thready pulse and other signs of shock appear. If more than 50% of blood volume is lost, death occurs unless the blood volume is replaced immediately.

Normal Response of Marrow to Anemia

The marrow acts to reverse anemia. Acute anemia causes a drop in oxygen transport to the kidney and a logarithmic rise in erythropoietin. This, in turn, leads to appearance of extra reticulocytes in the blood within 12 hours. This influx of new

TABLE 3-1. Normal Values for Red Corpuscles at Selected Ages

Age	RBCs $\times 10^{-6}$ (per μL)	Hb (g/dL)	HCT (mL/dL)	MCV (fL)	MCH (pg)	MCHC (g/dL)
1 day	5.1	19.5	54.0	106	38	36
→60 days	4.7	14.0	42.0	90	30	33
6–12 mo	4.6	11.8	35.5	77	26	33
1–2 yr	4.5	11.4	35.0	78	25	32
3–10 yr	4.6	12.6	37.0	80	27	34
Adults						
Women	4.5 ± 0.7	13.7 ± 2	41.0 ± 6	87 ± 05	30 ± 2	34 ± 2
Men	5.1 ± 0.7	15.5 ± 2	46.0 ± 6	87 ± 05	30 ± 2	34 ± 2

Hb, hemoglobin; HCT, hematocrit; MCH, mean corpuscular hemoglobin; MCHC, mean corpuscular hemoglobin concentration; MCV, mean corpuscular volume; RBCs, red blood cells.

cells does not raise the hematocrit significantly, but it does show that the erythropoietin level is responding. The rise in erythropoietin also causes an increase in the rate of differentiation of erythroid cells from their committed precursors.

One or 2 days after the abrupt onset of anemia from bleeding or hemolysis, the number of early erythroid forms (pronormoblasts and basophilic normoblasts) increases in the marrow, followed over the next couple of days by normoblasts in later stages of development {#97}. By 5 to 7 days, the reticulocyte index increases; after 7 to 10 days, the marrow response is complete, and a new plateau of production is established. If the erythropoietic stress is severe, however, erythroid marrow expansion may go on for months. The degree of response is proportional to the severity of the anemia. This is shown in Figure 3-7, in which output of red cells by the marrow is expressed in multiples of basal red cell production. **Table 3-2** shows similar changes in G/E ratio and reticulocyte index. These normal responses of the marrow to anemia require an adequate supply of iron, vitamin B_{12}, and folic acid. If the nutritional supply is marginal, the response will be blunted.

When the marrow expands, it encroaches on marrow fat. If the expansion is marked and long-lasting, the erythroid marrow expands into bones that do not normally contain active marrow. If marked and persistent expansion occurs

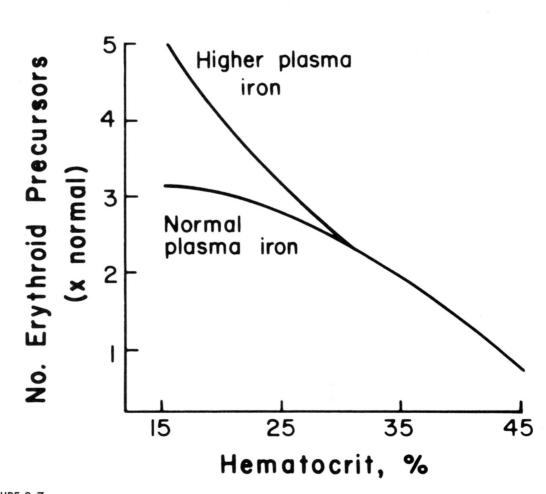

FIGURE 3-7.

The response of normal erythroid marrow to anemia. The response depends on adequate iron availability. The higher levels of response (five or more times normal) are not observed unless serum iron is higher than normal, as in hemolysis.

during childhood, bone structure is altered to accommodate the increased mass of marrow. This is discussed in later chapters.

Analysis of Anemia

Anemia may be analyzed by the size and shape of the red cells (morphology) or by their rates of production (kinetic analysis).

Morphologic Analysis

RED CELL INDICES

The erythrocyte can be characterized by ratios of three measurements; the hemoglobin, the hematocrit, and the red cell count.

- Mean corpuscular volume (MCV) is the hematocrit (volume) divided by erythrocyte count. This value is useful in the primary classification of anemia.
- Mean corpuscular hemoglobin (MCH) is the hemoglobin concentration divided by erythrocyte count. This value is useful in assessing hemoglobin synthesis.
- Mean corpuscular hemoglobin concentration (MCHC) is the hemoglobin concentration divided by hematocrit.

Normal values for indices are given in Table 3-1. The derivation of the indices is given in Appendix II.

Anemias may be classified by indices. When all the red cells are large (macrocytic; MCV > 100 fL), defects in DNA synthesis are most likely. When red cells are small (MCV < 80), poor hemoglobin production is the basic problem. The next two chapters develop a differential diagnosis of conditions that can cause microcytic and macrocytic anemias; the macrocytic anemias are discussed further in Chapter 4 and the microcytic anemias in Chapter 5.

A second part of morphologic analysis of anemia is to study the red cell smear for shape changes not suggested by the indices. The blood smear may show any of 10 or more abnormal shapes (e.g., sickle cells, spherocytes, broken cells, targets). **Anisocytosis** is the term for many different sizes of red cell. When red cells of many different shapes are seen, the term **poikilocytosis** is used. In addition, there may be abnormalities of platelets or white cells that give important clues to the cause of anemia.

Kinetic Classification

Anemias may also be classified by the gross rate of production of marrow cells (G/E ratio) and the effective release of red cells to the circulation (reticulocyte count). This classification has four parts: decreased production, decreased delivery, increased destruction, and blood loss.

TABLE 3-2. Appropriate Response to Anemia

HCT (%)	G/E Ratio	Reticulocyte Index*
45	3:1	1
35	3:2	2
25	1:1	3
15	1:1–1:2	3–5

*Expressed in multiples of normal values, which are assigned a value of 1. The indicated production levels are achieved only after the anemia has been present for 7 to 10 days.

DECREASED PRODUCTION (HYPOPROLIFERATIVE ANEMIA)

In hypoproliferative anemia, the rate of production of erythrocytes by marrow is lower than expected for the degree of anemia. In industrial terms, the car dealers are calling for 50,000 pickup trucks, but the assembly line is delivering only 8000. Aplastic anemia is a particularly serious form of hypoproliferative anemia in which red cell production totally fails. Other kinds of hypoproliferative anemia are discussed in Chapter 5.

DECREASED DELIVERY (INEFFECTIVE ERYTHROPOIESIS)

In ineffective erythropoiesis, developing erythrocytes are destroyed within the marrow or immediately after they are released to the circulation. In industrial terms, the factory is running a full assembly line, but few trucks are coming off the ramp because they are rejected by the inspectors. There is a major disparity between high rates of total production (e.g., G:E ratio 1:1) and low rates of output (reticulocyte index < 2%) (Table 3-3; see also Table 3-2). The most common examples in this category are folic acid and B_{12} deficiency anemias (see Chapter 4) and the thalassemias (see Chapter 7).

INCREASED DESTRUCTION (HEMOLYTIC ANEMIA)

Hemolytic anemia means that the red cells die after perhaps 10 to 30 days in circulation instead of the normal life span of 120 days. In industrial terms, the assembly line is going night and day because the trucks last only 1 year instead of 10. The erythroid marrow compensates by accelerated production beyond what is expected for the degree of anemia (Tables 3-2 and 3-3). If the rate of hemolysis exceeds the marrow production capacity, anemia develops. A dramatic example of hemolytic anemia is a drug-mediated process in which an autoantibody attacks the red cells and causes rapid, acute illness.

BLOOD LOSS ANEMIA

Blood loss anemia is due to external or internal bleeding. When blood loss is acute, the blood counts do not accurately reflect the loss of red cells for 24 to 72 hours, the time required to reexpand the blood volume by body water and plasma proteins (Fig. 3-8). Seven to 10 days are required for the bone marrow to reach the level of production demanded by the anemia (Tables 3-2 and 3-3).

In practice, we take three steps in the investigation of anemia after the history and physical examination are completed. (1) The red cells are sized by an electronic particle counter, and the MCV (mean corpuscular volume) is determined. On the basis of the MCV, anemias are classified as macrocytic, microcytic, or normocytic. **Macrocytic anemias** are associated with defects in cell division such as vitamin B_{12} or folic acid deficiency. Microcytic anemias are associated with

---

TABLE 3-3.   Kinetic Analysis of Anemia

	Reticulocyte Index	Marrow G/E ratio
Normal	1	3/1
Bleeding, acute	1	3/1
Hemolysis	3–6	<1/1
Ineffective hematopoiesis	<2	1/1
Hypoproliferation	<2	>3/1

Modified from Hillman RS, Finch CA. Red Cell Manual. Philadelphia: FA Davis, 1985.

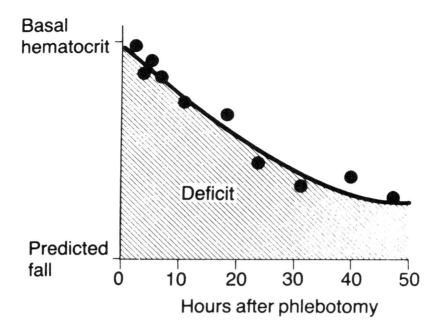

FIGURE 3-8.

After a sudden loss of whole blood, the fall in hematocrit is a gradual process, which depends on the rate of mobilization of albumin and water from extravascular sites. Full expansion of the blood volume and the lowest hematocrit value may not be reached for 48 to 72 hours. (From Williams WJ, et al. *Hematology*, 3rd ed. New York: McGraw-Hill, p. 668.)

defects in hemoglobin synthesis, such as iron deficiency or thalassemia. (2) The blood smear is examined for abnormalities in red cells and in other cells as well. (3) We use kinetic analysis when the other methods are not productive, estimating red cell growth by the reticulocyte count and the total cell production by the bone marrow G/E ratio.

SUMMARY POINTS

The biochemistry of the red cell is understood in detail. As the cell matures, one can visualize the formation of hemoglobin and the fading of RNA in the bone marrow. The nucleus becomes pyknotic and is extruded, and the cell is delivered to circulate for 4 months. Thus, a relatively small volume of marrow cells, perhaps 300 mL, expands into 2200 mL of circulating cells—about 2 trillion. Anemia represents a failure of this elegant system. It may be caused by decreased production, decreased delivery, increased destruction, or blood loss. Anemia may be analyzed by examining the size and shape of the erythrocytes in the blood or by examining kinetic parameters.

CASE DEVELOPMENT PROBLEM: CHAPTERS 1, 2, AND 3

Some cyclists in the Tour de France illegally injected themselves with erythropoietin (EPO) to increase production of red cells. It is well known from studies of racehorses that increased hematocrit (HCT), to a point, improves performance. The team doctors suggest target HCT at the upper limits of normal in males (50% to 52%). Unfortunately, some cyclists with HCT > 50% have experienced strokes at night or acute myocardial infarction during the race. These thrombi are probably due to a combination of factors: physiologic bradycardia of trained athletes (pulse rate < 30/min), dehydration and hemoconcentration during the race, and shifts in blood flow from brain, gut, and kidney in favor of muscle and bone during severe exercise. With no sensitive test to detect EPO "doping," the racing commission has banned cyclists with HCT > 50%. The racers might therefore attempt to drink a lot of fluid before being tested so that the plasma volume would increase and the hematocrit would be falsely decreased.

1. (a) What is hemoconcentration? (b) What is hemodilution?
2. How long before the race must the cyclist start EPO?
3. How can the race commission apply the HCT < 50% rule fairly?
4. Would nutritional supplements in addition to EPO aid in erythropoiesis?

CASE DEVELOPMENT ANSWERS

1. (a) Hemoconcentration is lowering of the plasma volume caused by loss of water and plasma components from the intravascular space. Sweating and hyperventilation or repeated vomiting can result in large losses of fluid and electrolytes. This increases the concentration of red cells (HCT). (b) On the other hand, if the cyclists drink a large amount of fluid before being tested, the plasma volume will increase and the HCT will be falsely decreased (hemodilution).
2. At least 2 weeks and preferably longer. To increase the red cells mass, the bone marrow must become hyperplastic. Once the red cells are made, they have a long life span, so the EPO does not have to be taken continuously.
3. Monitor the weight as well as the HCT. If the cyclist is overhydrated, the weight will increase, and the HCT will decrease.
4. Red cell production requires iron, folic acid, and vitamin B_{12}. These athletes have difficulty eating 5000 to 7000 kcal needed to bicycle the daily 80- to 150-mile stages. Their nutritionists should make sure the diet contains enough folic acid.

Vitamin B_{12} (Cobalamin*) and Folic Acid (Folate)

Robert F. Schilling

CHAPTER 4

OUTLINE

OBJECTIVES

- Compare and contrast macrocytosis and megaloblastosis and describe morphology of various cells.
- List five mechanisms of vitamin deficiency.
- Trace the metabolism of vitamin B_{12} and folic acid from food sources through adsorption pathways and storage sites to enzyme activities.
- Define pernicious anemia. Explain the hazard of overlooking the diagnosis of B_{12} deficiency.
- Describe diagnostic tests for B_{12} and folic acid deficiency.

* Vitamin B_{12} and cobalamin are used as synonyms.

A key event in a rapidly dividing tissue such as the bone marrow is the synthesis of new DNA. Any process that inhibits DNA synthesis blocks production of all replicating cell lines. In the bone marrow, a block in DNA synthesis results in a nucleus that is immature for the degree of maturation in the cytoplasm. Red cell precursors with this abnormality are called *megaloblasts* rather than normoblasts. Megaloblastosis is most commonly due to the shortage of folic acid or vitamin B_{12}. These vitamin deficiencies lead to a shortage of thymidine, which in turn leads to retarded DNA synthesis and megaloblastic anemia. Megaloblastic anemia results in large red cells called *macrocytes*.

DEFINITIONS

Macrocytic anemia is a subset of anemia in which the nonnucleated erythrocytes are larger than 100 femtoliters (fL), although some laboratories may consider 95 fL as the upper limit of normal. This condition is found in association with illnesses such as liver disease, alcoholism, hypothyroidism, and several forms of marrow damage as well as in B_{12} and folic acid deficiency. Macrocytes are red cells released before they have divided enough times to be normal-sized. There are two probable mechanisms for decreased divisions: early release forced by demand for new red cells, and retarded DNA synthesis. For example, because reticulocytes are considerably larger than mature red cells (some young ones may be 150 fL), hemolytic anemia with a high reticulocyte count may be macrocytic on that basis alone. In megaloblastic anemia, the red cells are macrocytic, presumably because retarded DNA synthesis has reduced the number of cell divisions that normally occurs as the cytoplasm matures.

Megaloblastic anemia is a specific subset of the general class of macrocytic anemias. Megaloblastosis is the visible change in nucleated cells that results from a lag in nuclear maturation relative to cytoplasmic maturation. It is the morphologic counterpart of reduced DNA:RNA and thymine:uracil ratios noted in biochemical assays of megaloblastic marrows.

Folic acid deficiency is probably the most common cause of megaloblastic anemia in the general population, but cobalamin deficiency may be a more common cause in parts of the world where intake of animal protein, the dietary source of vitamin B_{12}, is low. Megaloblastic anemia due to vitamin deficiency is a manifestation of advanced deficiency. In a referral hospital with a large proportion of cancer patients, however, the most common cause of megaloblastic change is cancer chemotherapy. Megaloblastosis is seen commonly after chemotherapy with methotrexate. Marked macrocytosis and hypersegmentation of neutrophils occur in patients treated with hydroxyurea. Table 4-1 gives other examples.

TABLE 4-1. Drugs Associated With Megaloblastosis

Associated Megaloblastosis	Drug Examples
Common	Dihydrofolate reductase inhibitors: methotrexate
	Purine analogues: 6-mercaptopurine
	Pyrimidine analogues: 5-fluorouracil (5-FU), zidovudine (AZT)
	Ribonucleotide reductase inhibitors: hydroxyurea
Uncommon	Anticonvulsants: diphenylhydantoin
	Drugs that interfere with B_{12} absorption: phenformin, neomycin
	Heavy metals: arsenic poisoning
	Oxidants: nitrous oxide

Megaloblastosis is best seen in the erythroid cell. Instead of having a small, compact nucleus, orthochromatic megaloblasts have a large nucleus with finely dispersed chromatin, much younger than expected for the degree of hemoglobinization of the cytoplasm {#21–23}. A second feature is the presence of giant bands in the bone marrow. A third feature is hypersegmentation of the neutrophils in the peripheral blood. In normal people, most neutrophils have two, three, or four lobes, and less than 5% have five lobes. Neutrophils with six or more lobes are seen in megaloblastosis {#24}. The peripheral blood expressions of megaloblastosis (macrocytosis and neutrophil hypersegmentation) may occur with minimal anemia. Hypersegmentation of neutrophils should lead to a search for the cause—most likely B_{12} or folate deficiency or some drug known to cause megaloblastosis.

DEFICIENCY OF FOLATE OR VITAMIN B_{12}

Vitamin deficiency is almost invariably the result of one or more of the following five processes:

- *Inadequate intake* of folic acid is common among alcoholics and institutionalized patients. Strict vegetarians ingest very little vitamin B_{12} and should take a vitamin pill containing B_{12}. Other highly restricted diets lacking in meat and fresh vegetables may produce folic acid deficiency.
- *Malabsorption* of vitamin B_{12} may be due to a lack of intrinsic factor. Drugs may prevent removal of glutamic acid residues on folic acid in food and thereby impair its absorption.
- *Increased utilization or loss* occurs in pregnancy and hemolysis, thus increasing the need for folate. These are extremely rare causes of vitamin B_{12} deficiency.
- *Drug inhibition* of the physiologic function of the vitamin can occur when certain drugs are taken. For example, methotrexate is a folic acid antagonist. Nitrous oxide inactivates some of the cobalamin and may be hazardous in subjects with marginal stores.
- *Genetic defects* of transcobalamin II are rare congenital disorders of B_{12} metabolism.

VITAMIN B_{12}: THE RED VITAMIN

History

The concept of ill health due to inadequate intake of food is as old as mankind, but the concept of diseases due to specific deficiencies was slow to gain recognition in the medical world. Two centuries ago, a Scottish naval surgeon, James Lind, proved that fresh lemons and limes cured and prevented scurvy among sailors, but the next clear proof of a specific disease due to a specific nutritional deficiency was not recognized until the early 20th century, when thiamine deficiency was shown to cause beriberi among rice-eating peoples of Southeast Asia. Pernicious anemia was well described morphologically and clinically for at least half a century before it was shown to be caused by a nutritional deficiency. However, the distinguished American physician, Austin Flint, wrote in 1860 that the disorder was probably due to a failure to assimilate some necessary nutrient from the diet. Dr. Flint also proposed to accept the credit for his idea as soon as someone could do the work necessary to prove its validity! Unfortunately, he did not live long enough to see the proof offered by Minot and Murphy in 1926.

During and immediately after World War I, George Whipple and Frieda Robscheit-Robbins studied the anemia induced in dogs when blood was removed each day. Their work was intended to determine the most efficacious diet for the regeneration of blood, and they found, of course, that refeeding the blood to the dog was most efficacious. The next most effective diet was one that was high in liver. George Minot, an investigative physician in Boston, knew of the work of Whipple and Robscheit-Robbins and was of the opinion that pernicious anemia might be a special kind of nutritional deficiency. Minot's view was contrary to the current dogma, since patients with pernicious anemia usually did not appear undernourished and in fact were sometimes moderately obese. But when Minot and Murphy fed a half-pound of lightly cooked liver (!) each day to patients with pernicious anemia, the patients showed a remarkable hematologic improvement. Minot and Murphy's reward for their documented and confirmed observation was international acclaim and a Nobel Prize. Thus, it had been established as early as 1926 that some substance in liver was curative for patients with pernicious anemia. An injectable liver extract was prepared soon afterward. The injection of liver extract every 2 to 4 weeks prevented death and neurologic disease and corrected anemia in patients with pernicious anemia.

For several decades before the therapeutic triumph of Minot and Murphy, it was known that patients with pernicious anemia had severe atrophy of the gastric mucosa. Also, their gastric juices were known to be scanty and lacking in acid and peptic activity. William Castle postulated that the gastric pathology might be playing a causal role in pernicious anemia, and he proved this with brilliantly conceived and controlled therapeutic trials. Feeding about 0.25 kg of hamburger to a patient daily for 10 days failed to improve the reticulocyte count or anemia. During the next 10 days, however, he fed the patient the same quantity of hamburger with normal human gastric juice, and generated an impressive reticulocyte response, increase in hemoglobin, and sense of well-being. We now know that the function of gastric "intrinsic factor," a phrase coined by Castle, is to bind dietary B_{12} and facilitate its absorption in the ileum.

The identification of the anti–pernicious anemia principle in liver had to wait until 1948. In that year, scientists at American and British pharmaceutical firms simultaneously and independently reported the isolation and crystallization of vitamin B_{12}. Each of these groups had demonstrated that the purified vitamin was extremely effective in the treatment of pernicious anemia. The first reports showed that, on one occasion, the injection of as little as 10 micrograms (μg) of vitamin B_{12} led to a significant hematologic improvement. Vitamin B_{12} was thus the most potent vitamin known at that time.

It was soon demonstrated that the red vitamin contained cobalt bound into a tetrapyrrole ring, somewhat analogous to the iron in heme. A second Nobel prize related to vitamin B_{12} was awarded to Dorothy Hodgkin for her x-ray crystallographic studies demonstrating the exact structure of the vitamin (molecular weight 1350), as diagrammed in Figure 4-1. Commercial vitamin B_{12} is derived from microbial synthesis, an efficient and inexpensive process compared with chemical synthesis; a quantity sufficient to treat a pernicious anemia patient for a whole year costs no more than a couple of dollars.

Physiology

The typical daily Western diet contains 5 to 30 μg of vitamin B_{12} in animal, bird, and fish products, of which the liver and kidney are especially rich sources. Muscle contains 0.5 to 2.0 μg of vitamin B_{12} per 100 g. Vitamin B_{12} in food is not absorbed as well as aqueous B_{12}. It is probable that peptic digestion contributes to the freeing of B_{12} from binding proteins in food.

Two to five micrograms of vitamin B_{12} are absorbed daily. Some of the B_{12} first complexes with *R binders* in the stomach. In the duodenum, B_{12} is released from the R binders by pancreatic digestion and binds to *intrinsic factor*. R binders are related to transcobalamins I and III, which are B_{12}-binding proteins found in serum. They are called R binders because their electrophoretic mobility is more

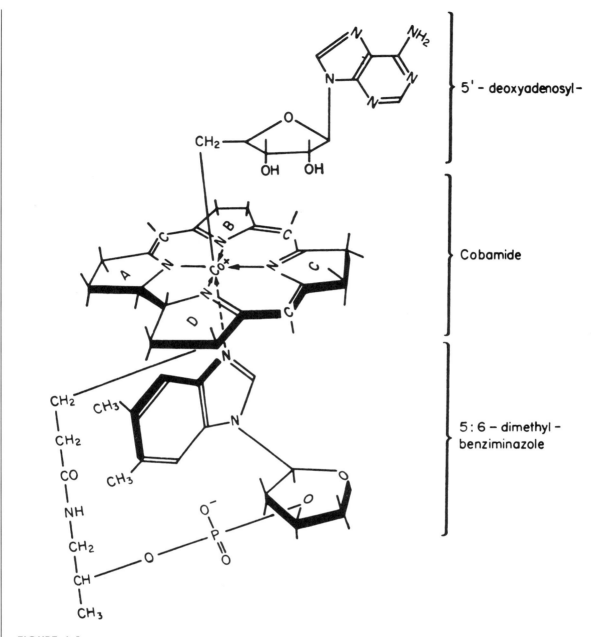

5' - deoxyadenosyl-

Cobamide

5:6 - dimethyl - benziminazole

FIGURE 4-1.

Structural formula of deoxyadenosyl cobalamin. Cyanocobalamin has a CN group ligated to the cobalt in a place of deoxyadenosyl, and methylcobalamin would have a methyl group at that locus.

rapid than that of transcobalamin II. The function of this intervening R binder reaction is unknown, but speculation is that R binders help dispose of inactive cobalamin analogues.

Intrinsic factor (IF) is a labile glycoprotein secreted by gastric parietal cells. Although vitamin B_{12} is very stable, it requires intrinsic factor for absorption. When complexed with B_{12}, intrinsic factor is protected from degradation by enzymes in the small intestine. It is of interest that colonic bacteria synthesize B_{12}, but that this B_{12} is not absorbed. The IF-B_{12} complex is adsorbed to brush border receptors in the ileum, and the vitamin enters the circulation via the ileal cells. In the absence of intrinsic factor, only 1 to 2% of B_{12} is absorbed, but with intrinsic factor 60% to 90% of a 1-μg test dose of aqueous B_{12} will be absorbed. From the ileum, B_{12} is carried by *transcobalamin II* to the liver, in which some of the vitamin is stored. However, most of the serum B_{12} is bound to transcobalamin I, a protein whose function is unknown.

The human body ordinarily contains 2000 to 5000 μg of vitamin B_{12}. Approximately 0.1% to 0.2% of the body store is lost daily, so the biologic half-life of the vitamin is in approximately 1 $^1/_2$ years, and clinical deficiency becomes apparent only after several years of grossly inadequate absorption. Megaloblastic anemia and neurologic disease due to vitamin B_{12} deficiency probably occur after body stores of the vitamin have decreased to less than 20% of normal.

Biochemistry

Cyanocobalamin, a stable form of vitamin, was the first cobalt-containing organic compound shown to have a biologic role. Students of animal husbandry knew that cobalt was an essential nutrient for sheep. After isolation, crystallization, and partial characterization of cyanocobalamin from liver in 1948, the role of cobalt in the maintenance of life of all animals and many bacteria began to emerge. Plants do not require or synthesize vitamin B_{12}. Some bacteria require an external source of vitamin B_{12}, others synthesize their own, and some bacteria neither require nor synthesize cobalamin.

Commercial pharmaceutical vitamin B_{12} is extracted from the culture broth of *Streptomyces* or other microbes. During purification, the cyano group is added to produce the stable cyanocobalamin molecule. The addition of radioactive cobalt during fermentation yields radioactive B_{12}, a useful diagnostic reagent for studying intestinal absorption of B_{12} and a standard reagent in radioligand assays of vitamin B_{12} concentration in serum, etc. The cobalt–cyano ligand can be broken readily in the body, and a methyl or 5′-deoxyadenosyl group attached. These latter two forms of vitamin B_{12} are thought to be the most important for biologic activity in mammals, but cyanocobalamin and hydroxocobalamin also have been identified in humans. It is obvious that many chemical variants must exist for a molecule as large and complex as vitamin B_{12}. Feces and rumen fluids contain numerous analogues of vitamin B_{12}. Some of these have been shown to lack biologic activity in humans while retaining vitamin B_{12} activity in some microorganisms. In a few instances, analogues have been demonstrated to act as antivitamins. The existence and role of inactive vitamin B_{12} analogues in humans have yet to be convincingly demonstrated. Human feces contains numerous analogues.

The mechanism by which B_{12} deficiency leads to relative failure of DNA synthesis is not understood in humans because no B_{12}-dependent ribonucleotide reductase has been described in mammalian cells. In mammals, only two reactions clearly requiring vitamin B_{12} have been identified: The reversible conversion of methylmalonyl CoA to succinyl CoA is dependent on adenosylcobalamin (Fig. 4-2). Deficiency of methylmalonyl CoA synthetase is thought by some investigators to be the cause of the neurologic disease in B_{12} deficiency.

The methylation of homocysteine to form methionine requires enzyme-bound methylcobalamin and 5-methyltetrahydrofolate [5-CH_3 H_4 PTE GLU_5] as a methyl donor (Fig. 4-3). Methionine provides a methyl group for modification of myelin basic protein; a deficiency of methionine is believed by some to decrease synthesis of myelin, leading to demyelination of the posterior and lateral columns of the spinal cord. However, since homocysteine accumulation in serum is regularly seen in folate deficiency as well as in B_{12} deficiency (see Fig. 4-3), the failure of this enzyme reaction does not explain the extreme rarity of neurologic disease in folate deficiency and the frequency of neurologic disease in cobalamin deficiency.

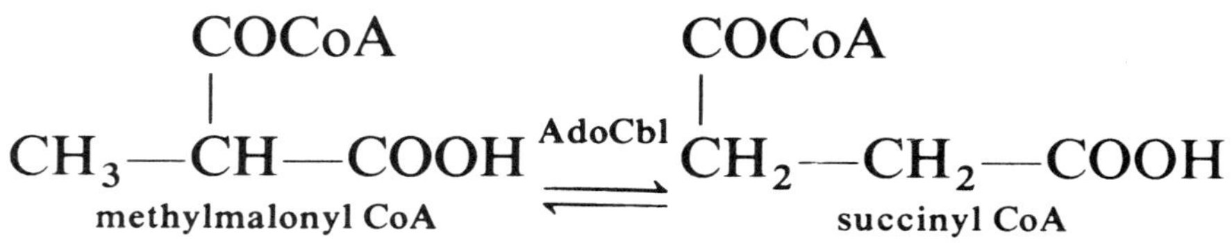

$$\underset{\text{methylmalonyl CoA}}{\overset{\displaystyle\overset{\text{COCoA}}{\underset{|}{}}}{CH_3{-}CH{-}COOH}} \xrightarrow[]{\text{AdoCbl}} \underset{\text{succinyl CoA}}{\overset{\displaystyle\overset{\text{COCoA}}{\underset{|}{}}}{CH_2{-}CH_2{-}COOH}}$$

FIGURE 4-2.

Conversion of methylmalonyl CoA to succinyl CoA by adenosylcobalamin.

The enzyme-bound cobalamin serves as a methyltransferase. The interdependence of vitamin B_{12} and folate in this methyl transfer is shown schematically in Figure 4-3, which indicates that the methyl group of methylcobalamin is from methyltetrahydrofolate (abbreviated in Fig. 4-3 as 5 - CH_3 H_4 Pte Glu_5. There is evidence that the sera of vitamin B_{12}-deficient patients contain higher than expected levels of methyltetrahydrofolate. This "trapping" of folate in the serum as methyltetrahydrofolate is thought to result in an intracellular deficit of a tetrahydrofolate needed as a cofactor for thymidylate synthetase, which is essential for DNA synthesis. It is believed that the active forms of intracellular folate are polyglutamates and that the enzyme that adds glutamic acid residues to folate cannot use methyltetrahydrofolate as a substrate. Tissue levels of folate polyglutamates are low in B_{12} deficiency, whereas plasma levels of methyltetrahydrofolate are elevated. Thus, it appears that B_{12} deficiency leads to a functional folate deficiency in dividing cells. Formyltetrahydrofolic acid can correct

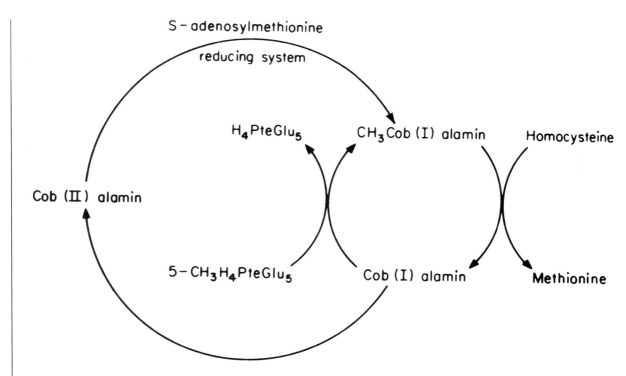

FIGURE 4-3.

Linkage of folate and cobalamin in the methylation of homocysteine to form methionine.

B_{12} deficiency in vitro. If intracellular folate deficiency is the shared biochemical defect in B_{12} and folate deficiency, the morphologic identity of the megaloblastic abnormalities in these two conditions is understandable.

New and elegant methods of quantifying serum or urine homocysteine and methylmalonate (MMA) have shown inverse correlations between concentrations of these intermediates and B_{12} supplies. Note (as indicated in Fig. 4-3) that homocysteine accumulates in the plasma when either vitamin is lacking, but MMA accumulates as a result of B_{12} deficiency, not folate deficiency. Measurement of MMA is likely to become a useful test in the evaluation of unexplained peripheral neuropathy, especially in patients who have no hematologic clues of megaloblastosis.

Mechanisms of Vitamin B_{12} Deficiency

The most common cause of B_{12} deficiency in the Western world is an acquired loss of intrinsic factor, also known as "pernicious anemia." In humans, intrinsic factor is secreted only by gastric parietal cells. Parietal cells may be lost by autoimmune destruction of the gastric mucosa, by physical or chemical injury, or by surgical removal. Autoimmune destruction is common. Loss of parietal cells causes eventual B_{12} deficiency as well as achlorhydria (pH of gastric juice greater than 6.5 after pharmacologic stimulation), and achylia gastrica (no gastric juice). The release of B_{12} from the food we eat is partially dependent on proteolysis by pepsin in the stomach. Patients with injured stomachs that lack intrinsic factor also have defects in peptic proteolysis.

The risk of vitamin B_{12} deficiency from inadequate intake is greatest in strict vegetarians who eat neither eggs nor milk products. In fact, the human is a nearly obligate partial carnivore, if such a phrase describes an organism that eats something from each of the meat, fish, and egg food groups. There are few true vegetarians in the United States, so dietary insufficiency is rarely a cause of megaloblastic anemia or neonatal B_{12} deficiency. Strict vegetarians should be advised to take vitamin pills containing vitamin B_{12} and folate.

Because B_{12} is avidly taken up and biochemically altered by many microorganisms, one might expect some patients with intestinal disease accompanied by massive bacterial overgrowth to suffer from B_{12} malabsorption and deficiency. This is the case in several anatomic and physiologic disorders of the gut, especially large diverticula of the small intestine or a surgically created blind loop ("blind loop syndrome"). Anaerobic organisms such as bacteroides avidly bind vitamin B_{12}, even when it is coupled to intrinsic factor, rendering the vitamin unavailable for absorption. Patients with hypogammaglobulinemia may also have excessive numbers of bacteria in the gut. Fish tapeworm infestation is common in Finland, and B_{12} deficiency often follows because the worm is a successful competitor for B_{12}.

The pancreas also plays a role in B_{12} absorption: patients with extensive chronic pancreatitis or with cystic fibrosis often fail to absorb B_{12} when given an oral test dose. The malabsorption is corrected by the simultaneous oral administration of pancreatic extract or trypsin. Clinical B_{12} deficiency, however, is very rare in those patients.

At the ileum, B_{12} is transferred from its intrinsic factor complex into the circulation and cells of the body. Patients who have lost their ileal function through surgical removal or bypass or because of extensive inflammatory destruction of the mucosa, as in regional ileitis (Crohn's disease) may become deficient because of a failure to absorb vitamin B_{12}. Thus, structural injury to the gastrointestinal tract (destruction of the gastric mucosa, injury to the pancreas, blind loop or giant diverticula of the small intestine, or destruction of the ileum) leads to B_{12} deficiency more commonly than dietary nutritional deficiency or genetic metabolic derangement.

A genetic deficiency of transcobalamin I does not lead to vitamin B_{12} deficiency, whereas lack of transcobalamin II is associated with severe megaloblastic anemia early in life.

Nitrous oxide ("laughing gas") is a widely used anesthetic. The use of nitrous oxide for anesthesia in unrecognized subclinical B_{12} deficiency has led to severe neuropathy. Recreational use of nitrous oxide has led to macrocytosis and neuropathy indistinguishable from B_{12} deficiency. Nitrous oxide reduces the activity of methionine synthetase, probably by inactivating the B_{12} coenzyme portion of the molecule. Nitrous oxide also destroys methyl cobalamin. This appears to be a new mechanism for developing megaloblastic anemia. It responds to treatment with vitamin B_{12} as expected.

Serology

About 90% of sera from patients with pernicious anemia contain autoantibodies to gastric parietal cells, but these antibodies have low specificity. Anti-parietal cell antibodies are relatively common in patients with myxedema, diabetes, gastritis, and several other conditions. Autoantibodies to intrinsic factor are present in only about 60% to 70% of sera from patients with pernicious anemia, but they have high specificity. (The problem of specificity versus sensitivity is ubiquitous in laboratory tests and x-ray interpretation and even in physical examination.) The presence of intrinsic factor antibodies is almost diagnostic of "pernicious anemia," but not of vitamin B_{12} deficiency. A formal definition of pernicious anemia is *autoimmune or idiopathic gastric atrophy sufficient to cause vitamin B_{12} mal*absorption due to lack of intrinsic factor. Because of the long biologic half-life of this vitamin, it is possible to diagnose pernicious anemia in a person who is not yet anemic and not deficient in vitamin B_{12}. Further, antibodies to parietal cells and to intrinsic factor are present even after the patient's B_{12} deficiency has been treated. Similarly, achlorhydria, achylia, and gastric atrophy are not corrected by the administration of vitamin B_{12}, because they are the cause, not the result of vitamin deficiency. The failure to absorb vitamin B_{12} is permanent in patients with pernicious anemia, and the condition can therefore be diagnosed by testing a patient's ability to absorb B_{12}, even after anemia and neurologic disease have been corrected by vitamin B_{12} injections.

Pernicious Anemia

"Pernicious" anemia is a misnomer because the disease is simple to treat with an injection of vitamin B_{12}. Vitamin B_{12} deficiency is a disease of the second half of life, the incidence being roughly one new case per year per 4000 people over 40 years of age. There also is a hereditary form of lack of functional intrinsic factor, known as "juvenile pernicious anemia." This rare condition is inherited as a recessive trait, resulting in nonfunctional intrinsic factor.

In addition to the usual physical findings of anemia, the pernicious anemia patient may complain of a sore tongue, which is often smooth, red, and glistening because of lack of papillae. The tongue symptoms and appearance improve promptly after the correction of the vitamin B_{12} deficiency. Patients may complain of paresthesias and difficulty walking in the dark and may appear neurotic. Neurologic examination often reveals absence of vibratory sensation and proprioception. In advanced stages, the neurologic aspects of vitamin B_{12} deficiency may cause spastic paralysis of lower extremities, loss of sphincter control, and dementia—a severe derangement of thought processes sometimes called "megaloblastic madness."

Vitamin B_{12} deficiency leads to demyelination of lateral and dorsal spinal cord tracts (Fig. 4-4). Persons with mild to moderate neurologic deficits can be expected

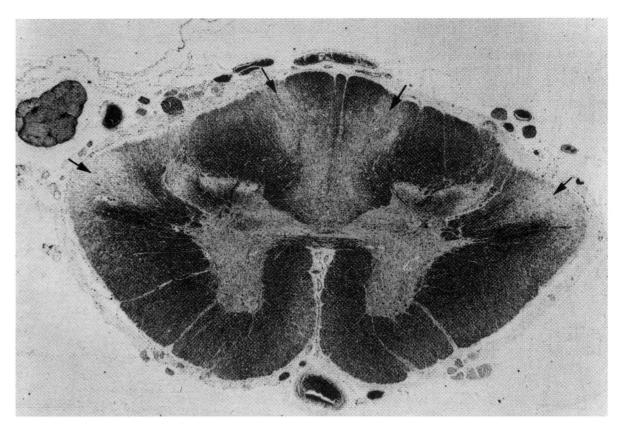

FIGURE 4-4.
Degeneration of the posterior and lateral columns of the spinal cord in vitamin B12 deficiency. The arrows point to areas of demyelination and loss of nerve fibers. (From Kass LS. *Pernicious Anemia*. Philadelphia: WB Saunders.)

to make a complete recovery after B_{12} therapy, although the time required to recover full function may be as much as 12 to 16 months. Recovery from advanced neurologic damage (inability to walk; incontinence) is unlikely to be complete. Neurologic disease in a patient with megaloblastic anemia is highly suggestive of B_{12} deficiency rather than folate deficiency. It is not necessary to have significant anemia or neurologic disease to make the diagnosis of megaloblastic disease due to B_{12} deficiency. In some patients, the neurologic disease is prominent with little or no anemia, whereas others have prominent anemia with normal neurologic examinations. In patients with megaloblastic anemia, the absence of posterolateral column disease should not be interpreted as evidence of folic acid deficiency. If a patient with B_{12} deficiency is treated with folate, neurologic disease may progress to irreversible crippling without evident anemia.

Cell Production

Since vitamin B_{12} and folate are essential to DNA synthesis, one would expect all multiplying cells to be affected with analogous biochemical and morphologic defects. Megaloblastosis is most easily recognized in erythroid and myeloid cells. Pancytopenia (decreased red cell, platelet, and granulocyte production) may occur in those with severe deficiency. Macrocytosis and dissociation of maturation in nucleus and cytoplasm leave as is have also been described in cells from other rapidly growing tissues such as skin, tongue, testis, bronchus, stomach, and cervix. The fetus and newborn also have special need for B_{12}. There are cases of infants who became B_{12}-deficient while nursing from mothers who were strict vegetarians or who had gastric bypass for obesity. It is prudent to give B_{12} supplements to such mothers.

The kinetic classification of megaloblastic anemia is ineffective erythropoiesis, and markedly elevated serum lactic dehydrogenase is seen in some florid cases. Red cell destruction is mainly in the marrow rather than in the blood (see Chapter 3). Circulating red cells also have a modestly shortened life span. The erythroid marrow is hypercellular with a 1:1 G/E ratio, and the total marrow mass is greatly increased. Plasma iron turnover is increased by a factor of 4 to 10. The serum bilirubin and serum iron may be increased as expected in red cell destruction, but the absolute reticulocyte count is decreased because few new cells are released.

Methods and Principles of Vitamin B_{12} Absorption Tests

The most common cause of B_{12} deficiency is malabsorption, not dietary deficiency. There are several different mechanisms of B_{12} malabsorption, and a radioactive B_{12} absorption study is a common diagnostic procedure to sort them (Table 4-2).

Because of the chemical stability of B_{12}, it is safe to assume that radioactivity administered as vitamin B_{12} represents intact vitamin if detected in stool, blood, urine, liver, or the body as a whole. Measurement of any of the latter samples has been shown to estimate vitamin B_{12} absorption from an oral dose of 0.5 to 2.0 μg of B_{12}. The radioactivity in the total stool collected for the 7 days after a test dose represents unabsorbed B_{12}, and the difference between radioactivity in the test dose and that in the stool represents the absorbed B_{12}. With a whole body counter, the radioactivity at 1 to 3 hours after oral ingestion is 100%; that remaining in the body after 7 days also represents absorbed B_{12}. Radioactivity in serum or plasma at 10 hours after oral ingestion represents absorbed B_{12}. The two latter techniques are not widely used because of technical difficulties.

The test that is most widely applied for the study of B_{12} absorption is the urine radioactivity test (Schilling test). Radioactivity appearing in the urine after an oral dose of radioactive B_{12} represents absorbed vitamin. Because absorbed B_{12} is normally bound to plasma transcobalamins, no radioactive vitamin is filtered at

TABLE 4-2. Results of Vitamin B_{12} Absorption Tests

Condition	B_{12} and water	B_{12} and Intrinsic Factor	B_{12} after 7–10 Days of Antibiotics	B_{12} and Pancreatic Extract	Food B_{12}*
Normal	N	N	N	N	N
Lack of pepsin	N	N	N	N	Low
Lack of intrinsic factor (e.g., pernicious anemia)	Low	N	Low	Low	Low
Blind loop syndrome (bacterial overgrowth)	Low	Low	N	Low	?Low
Lack of pancreatic secretions	Low	Low	Low	N	?Low
Lack of or bypass of ileum†	Low	Low	Low	Low	Low

N, normal absorption; Low, less than normal absorption.
Radioactive vitamin B_{12} is administered orally, and absorption is estimated by one of the methods described in the text.
*Radioactive B_{12} incorporated into egg or chicken serum.
†There are rare patients in whom the mechanism of vitamin B_{12} malabsorption is unexplained. For example, we do not know the cause of vitamin B_{12} malabsorption in children with congenital selective B_{12} malabsorption (the Imerslund-Gräsbeck syndrome), since they have normal intrinsic factor and pancreatic functions and do not have recognized ileal disease or bacterial overgrowth.

the glomerulus (molecular weight of B_{12} is 1350). However, if a large quantity (1000 μg) of nonradioactive vitamin B_{12} is injected 2 hours after the oral dose, the transcobalamins will be saturated, much of the absorbed radioactive B_{12} will be unbound, and about one third of the absorbed radioactive vitamin will appear in urine in the next 24 hours. The molecular size of B_{12} is such that unbound vitamin passes the glomerular filter efficiently. Urine radioactivity in this test has been shown to correlate closely with B_{12} absorption determined by stool or whole body counting. Performance of this test also corrects B_{12} deficiency; hence, serum for vitamin B_{12} assay must be drawn before this test. It is obvious that severe renal impairment (creatinine >2 mg/dL) will yield a spuriously low urine radioactivity. It is prudent to know the blood urea nitrogen (BUN) or creatinine before performing these tests. A complete 24-hour collection of urine is essential. Correction of the failure to absorb B_{12} by the simultaneous administration of intrinsic factor is good evidence for pernicious anemia or total gastrectomy.

Methods and Principles of Assaying Serum for B_{12} or Folate

There are two general methods of assay:

1. Use of microorganisms that require the vitamin for growth. *Lactobacillus leishmanii*, *Euglena gracilis*, and *Escherichia coli*] are most commonly used for estimation of vitamin B_{12} concentration.
2. Competitive binding inhibition (one subset of this is termed radioligand assay).

It is important to understand the general principles of a competitive binding inhibition assay because a subset of this class of procedures, the radioimmunoassay, is widely used in diagnostic and research laboratories in many fields of medicine in addition to hematology. Reduced to the simplest steps, this procedure requires a protein that possesses specific binding sites for the compound to be assayed (e.g., vitamin B_{12}) and a radioactive form of the same compound. For example, to a tube containing a protein with binding capacity for 100 pg of vitamin B_{12}, add a serum containing an unknown amount of vitamin B_{12} and 100 pg of radioactive vitamin B_{12}. Separate the free vitamin from the protein bound by absorbing on charcoal or by dialysis, or by gel filtration. The vitamin in the unknown serum will reduce the protein binding of radioactive vitamin, and the reduction of binding is quantitatively related to the amount of vitamin in the unknown serum.

Low serum B_{12} concentration may exist for years without the development of clinical disease. However, it is advisable to look at a blood smear and do simple neurologic tests in such patients so that this treatable cause of dementia and neuropathy is not overlooked. Measurements of serum homocysteine and MMA are useful in defining metabolic evidence of cobalamin deficiency. Bear in mind that as tests for clinically significant cobalamin deficiency, these measurements appear to have excellent sensitivity but less than desirable specificity. Too many subjects have elevated serum levels of these metabolites while showing no other evidence of cobalamin deficiency.

FOLIC ACID

History

Within a few years after the demonstration of the remarkable efficacy of liver in the treatment of pernicious anemia, researchers realized that not all megaloblastic anemia was due to a deficiency of the factor present in injectable liver extract.

In the 1930s, Lucy Wills, a young physician from London, went to Bombay to study megaloblastic anemia, which was common in late pregnancy in India. She demonstrated in a convincing manner that injections of purified liver extract (so wonderfully efficacious in pernicious anemia in London) did not benefit the megaloblastic anemia of pregnancy in Bombay. She did find that eating generous amounts of "marmite" (a yeast extract) led to impressive hematologic and subjective improvement. From this observation came the term "Wills factor" to identify that beneficial nutrient in yeast. In 1946, folic acid was identified and synthesized by scientists at Lederle Laboratories studying growth factors for certain bacteria. It soon became apparent that Wills factor was folic acid.

Metabolism and Biochemistry

Pteroylmonoglutamic folic acid is a small molecule (molecular weight 440) that is absorbed in the small intestine, especially in the jejunum (Fig. 4-5). Both passive diffusion and active transport have been demonstrated. Yeast is the richest non-medicinal source of folate, but many vegetables, dairy products, and seafoods are excellent dietary sources. Food folate found in spinach, beans, broccoli, and other green leafy vegetables is in the polyglutamate form. An intestinal brush border conjugase cleaves all but the last glutamate and thus enhances absorption. Since the daily food intake of folate is 200 to 400 μg and the daily nutritional requirement is about 50 μg, we infer that some food folate is not available to the host or that some of the excess absorbed folate is excreted in the urine. The vitamin is stored in the liver and other cells. The biologic half-life of folic acid is less than 1 month. Increased loss of folate occurs in patients dialyzed for chronic renal failure.

Although polyglutamate forms of folate in the diet probably are deconjugated to the monoglutamate form before absorption, once in the cells of the body, polyglutamate forms are resynthesized. Folate coenzymes transfer single carbon units in various oxidation states, such as methyl and formyl and formate, in a large variety of essential processes. For example, the methylation of deoxyuridine monophosphate to deoxythymidine monophosphate is catalyzed by thymidylate synthetase in a reaction linked to dihydrofolate reductase. The presence of these enzymes has been demonstrated in mammalian bone marrow. Other reactions requiring folic acid coenzymes are serine conversion to glycine, histidine catabolism, methionine synthesis from homocysteine, and purine synthesis.

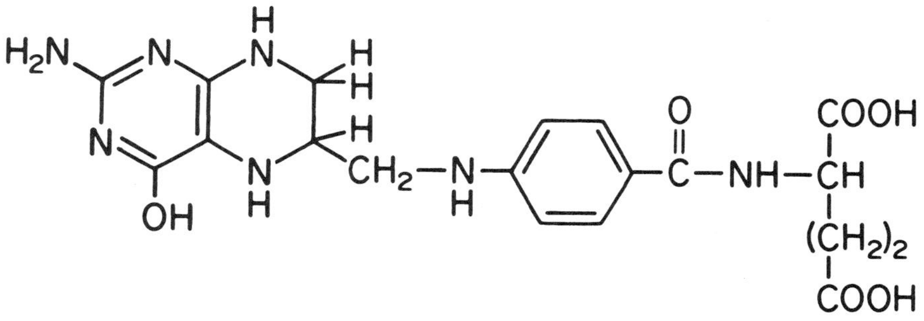

FIGURE 4-5.
Chemical structure of folic acid (pteroylglutamic acid.).

Mechanisms of Deficiency

Diet and Malabsorption

Diets composed exclusively of tea and toast or brandy and beer rapidly lead to folate deficiency. Food folate can be lost because it is easily oxidized when vegetables are cooked in boiling water. One physician investigator intentionally induced folic acid deficiency in himself in 3 months merely by thoroughly boiling his food and discarding the water. Other causes of folic acid deficiency are more complex. Serious decrements in folate absorption occur in sprue, probably due to defective active transport or lack of the deconjugase.

Pregnancy

Increased metabolic requirement and accelerated turnover of folate explain the folic acid deficiencies in pregnancy, chronic hemolytic anemia, and myeloproliferative disorder such as myelofibrosis. The incidence of folic acid deficiency in pregnancy varies from 2% to 50% in different reported series, and subclinical folate deficiency in the mother has been implicated in neural tube defects (spina bifida) in the fetus. Powerful evidence exists that extra folate given *very early* in pregnancy reduces the number of babies born with spina bifida. Folate is now being added to cereal grains so that all who eat bread and cereal will derive added folate. Some experts are concerned that this public health policy decision may result in neurologic disease in some people with undetected cobalamin deficiency. It is wise to remember that neuropathy due to cobalamin deficiency is very treatable, and therefore serum cobalamin levels should be checked in most older patients with newly developed neurologic disease.

Alcoholism and Drugs

Folic acid deficiency in alcoholics is probably the result of several factors: decreased intake, decreased absorption, possibly an antagonistic effect of ethanol at the intracellular enzyme level, and probably decreased storage in an injured (cirrhotic) liver. Megaloblastic anemia in alcoholics is almost always caused by folic acid deficiency.

Some drugs, when taken over an extended period of time, have been associated with an increased incidence of folate deficiency and megaloblastic anemia. Phenytoin, an anticonvulsant taken daily by thousands of people in the Western world, is statistically associated with a lower serum folate level, mild to moderate macrocytosis, and, rarely, frank megaloblastic anemia. It is not clear whether the tendency to folate deficiency is due to inhibition of the folate deconjugase or to diminished absorption of the monoglutamate. Treatment of such megaloblastic anemia with modest doses of oral folate is effective. However, some evidence indicates that rapid correction of the folate deficiency increases the likelihood of seizures in such patients. The use of oral contraceptives has been associated with megaloblastosis in a few women, but is so rare that it may be fortuitous.

Serum Folate

The diagnosis of folate deficiency is suggested by a low serum folate level, especially when combined with the hematologic findings. Low serum folate levels are common in elderly people and the seriously ill, regardless of age. The normal serum concentration is 4 to 10 ng/mL (9 to 23 nmol/L). Low serum folate increases the likelihood of the patient becoming clinically folate-deficient if not supplemented. The evidence that measurement of red cell folate is a useful clinical procedure is not convincing, and its use as a routine diagnostic test should be discouraged until further research establishes its usefulness.

Ramifications of Marginal Folate Status

It has been 35 years since severe arteriosclerosis was first recognized in a child who died of congenital homocysteinuria, a condition manifesting extreme hyper-homocysteinemia. In the last 15 years moderate/mild elevation of plasma homo-cysteine has proved to be a significant independent risk factor for stroke, myocardial infarct, and peripheral vascular disease. Such elevations are not rare in persons with serum B_{12} and folate and pyridoxine in the range of normal. Supplemental folate, and to a lesser extent B_{12}, and pyridoxine will lower the homocysteine level in such patients. It is likely that supplemental folate (as fortified cereal grain or as a vitamin pill) will be shown to reduce the incidence of stroke and myocardial infarct in the general population. The indirect evidence for this is convincing.

SUMMARY POINTS

Both B_{12} and folic acid contribute to donation of single carbons in interlocking metabolic pathways, and anemia due to deficiency of one is identical morpho-logically with deficiency of the other. Folate has a short half-life in the body and must be replenished frequently. Vitamin B_{12} deficiency can lead to irreversible neurologic damage. The diagnosis of each is medically important. Convenient ways of cataloging B_{12} deficiency are to associate it with structural defects and injury to the gut (stomach, ileum, worms, blinds loops, and jejunal diverticula) and of folate deficiency are to associate it to metabolic problems such as malabsorption, poor diet, increased demand, and competing drugs.

SUGGESTED READINGS

Chanarin I. *The Megaloblastic Anemias*, 3rd ed. Oxford: Blackwell Scientific Publications, 1990.
Jandl JH. *Blood: A Textbook of Hematology, 2nd ed.* Boston: Little, Brown, 1996.

CASE DEVELOPMENT PROBLEM: CHAPTER 4

History: A 60-year-old carpenter presented with a complaint of progressive weak-ness of 6 months' duration. The year before he had had a normal physical exam and normal blood counts.

Physical examination: Extreme pallor of skin and mucous membranes and redness of the tongue with atrophy of marginal filiform papillae were noted.

Laboratory data: 1.0 million RBC/μL (1.0×10^{12}/L); HCT 12% (.12 L/L); Hb 4.2 g/dL (42 g/L); 3000 WBC/μL (3.0×10^9/L); 90,000 platelets/μL (90×10^9/L); reticulocyte count 2% (2×10^{10}/L). The marrow was hypercellular with G/E ratio of 1:1.

1. Calculate the mean corpuscular volume (MCV); indicate the normal ranges.
2. Calculate the reticulocyte index.
3. Describe this anemia morphologically and kinetically.
4. This anemia is most likely due to a deficiency of _____ or _____ .
5. Predict the appearance of the peripheral smear.
6. Predict the appearance of the marrow.
7. How do you reconcile a hypercellular marrow with a G/E ratio of 1:1 with a reticulocyte index of less than 0.2?

$$\frac{20,000}{50,000 \times 2.5}$$

What is the kinetic classification now?

8. Can you distinguish between folic acid and vitamin B_{12} deficiency on the basis of the peripheral smear and bone marrow?
9. What further history would help you distinguish between folic acid deficiency and vitamin B_{12} deficiency?
10. What tests should be ordered? List the pathophysiologic processes that may lead to a deficiency of folic acid or a deficiency of vitamin B_{12}.
11. Describe the pathophysiology of this anemia in detail. Include theories of the cause; the reason for the lack of absorption; the pathophysiology of the anemia, granulocytopenia, and thrombocytopenia; and the pathophysiology of the neurologic deficit.

CASE DEVELOPMENT ANSWERS

1. MCV = HCT/RBC = 120 fL (normal 87 ± 5).
2. $\dfrac{.02 \times 1.0 \times 10^{12}/1}{5 \times 10^{10}/1} \times \dfrac{1}{2.5} = .15$

   (The 2.5 in the denominator is the allowance for the maturation time of reticulocytes in severe anemia.)
3. Macrocytic; lack of production.
4. Folic acid; B_{12}.
5. Marked anisocytosis and poikilocytosis, oval macrocytes, occasional nucleated red cells, which may be megaloblastic; Howell-Jolly bodies; hypersegmented neutrophils; thrombocytopenia.
6. Marked hypercellularity with G/E of 1:1, megaloblastic maturation of red cell series, giant bands and metamyelocytes.
7. The kinetic abnormality in folic acid or B_{12} deficiency is ineffective erythropoiesis. Although there is a great deal of marrow activity, the cells produced are so defective that they are destroyed within the marrow cavity and are not released into the peripheral blood.
8. No.
9. Investigate the patient's diet, surgeries, and neurologic symptoms.
10. The house staff ordered a serum folic acid and B_{12} level. Results of these tests would not be available for a week. Therefore, a Schilling test was performed. The serum B_{12} level was 100 pg/mL; serum folic acid was 9 ng/mL. In Part 1 of the urine radioactivity test (Schilling test), 1% of the orally administered radioactivity appeared in the 24-hour urine collection. In Part 2 (with intrinsic factor), 12% was in the 24-hour urine.

CHAPTER 5

Iron Metabolism and Hypoproliferative Anemias

Robert D. Woodson, Archie A. MacKinney, Jr.

OUTLINE

OBJECTIVES

- Describe the path of iron from food intake to incorporation into the red cell.
- Know the cause of iron deficiency and its significance in different groups—men, pre - and post - menopausal women, babies.
- Understand anemia of iron deficiency in context of other hypoproliferative anemias.
- Understand syndromes of iron overload (hemochromatosis).
- Understand iron poisoning.

IRON METABOLISM

Iron is an essential element in oxygen transfer and electron transport. Iron deficiency is one of the most common problems in medicine, with 25% affected in many populations. In most cases, blood loss, not poor nutrition, is the cause.

Food Iron Availability

The average American diet contains 7 mg of iron per 1000 calories. The person who consumes 2400 calories ingests about 14 mg of iron and absorbs about 10% of this amount.

Roughly 5% of dietary iron is present as **heme** iron, which is derived from hemoglobin and myoglobin. Although comparatively small in amount, it accounts for 25% to 33% of the iron normally absorbed, the fraction increasing further in iron deficiency. The heme molecule, with its iron atom, is absorbed intact. The iron is liberated in the intestinal mucosal cell, probably by heme oxygenase, which cleaves the porphyrin ring. Absorption of heme iron is not affected by the many factors that affect nonheme iron absorption.

Nonheme iron in food is in various chemical forms, from which it is liberated in ionic form during digestion. Availability of iron for absorption is affected by the mix of foods present, some of which enhance, while others inhibit, absorption. Enhancers of nonheme iron absorption include heme iron (meat, poultry, and fish), ascorbic acid, and some sugars. Naturally occurring inhibitors include carbonates (soft drinks), tannate (tea), oxalate (spinach, rhubarb), phosphates, polyphenols and phytates (vegetables and egg yolk phosphoprotein). Many of these are anions that make iron insoluble. For example, when tea or coffee is drunk with a meal, absorption of nonheme iron falls by 50% to 75%. EDTA (ethylenediaminetetra-acetic acid), a cation chelator in soft drinks and prepared foods, is a powerful antagonist of absorption. Clay, which is sometimes ingested by people from the rural South, sharply curtails iron absorption. When medicinal iron is taken with a meal, its fractional absorption approaches that of nonheme iron derived from the diet. If antacids are given with the iron, the iron is poorly absorbed. Ferric salts are poorly absorbed, probably because of low solubility at the alkaline pH of the duodenum.

Influence of Dose

The amount of iron absorbed is in part determined by the amount ingested. When ferrous sulfate is administered, the percent absorbed decreases as the dose rises, but the absolute amount absorbed increases. This is true of excessive doses, which may produce gastrointestinal bleeding and shock or death.

Gastrointestinal Tract

Release of iron during digestion makes iron available for absorption. Hydrochloric acid promotes absorption of the nonheme component of dietary iron. Thus, persons with achlorhydria absorb nonheme iron less than normal. Biliary and pancreatic factors probably have no effect beyond their role in digestion.

The duodenum and upper jejunum comprise the major sites of iron absorption. At least two proteins are important in this process, the divalent cation transporter of the brush border (also known as Nramp2) and the HFE protein. The amount of iron absorbed is determined primarily by the body's need for iron, although the exact mechanism is still under investigation. In general, mucosal cells of the intestinal crypts are believed to "sense" the body's iron level. As they migrate to the villi, they carry this information along, where they absorb iron in accord with this set point. However, the ability of the mucosal system to limit iron absorption is finite, and large amounts of ferrous iron are absorbed if ingested. This is important because the body lacks any method for excreting iron. In addition to body iron status per se, mucosal absorption appears to be independently increased by the rate of erythropoiesis and by hypoxia.

Iron Distribution

Iron is distributed in normal adults as shown in Table 5-1. The largest quantity is present in the form of hemoglobin iron. One milliliter of packed cells contains 1.2 mg iron. The second largest fraction is in stores. Iron is present in a large number of metalloenzymes, most notably the cytochromes and flavins. The amount of storage iron is about 1000 mg in males, but is lower in females, ranging from 200 to 400 mg. Most storage iron is present as ferritin, with the remainder (20% to 30%) as hemosiderin.

Iron Balance

In the normal steady state, iron absorption and loss are balanced. Iron in men and nonmenstruating women is lost through desquamating cells of skin (including hair and nails), kidney, and intestine, and a small amount through intestinal blood loss (0.5 to 1 mL/day). Total iron losses average about 1 mg per day in an adult male.

Iron balance is appreciably affected by growth, menstruation, pregnancy, and lactation. During a baby's first year of life, the iron required by the rapidly expanding red cell mass and muscle may exhaust the iron stores, whereas the diet may not yet provide sufficient iron (Fig. 5-1). This is more likely in premature infants, who begin extrauterine life with less iron. The probability of iron deficiency in babies also depends on child feeding practices. A milk diet provides relatively little iron (0.1 to 0.2 mg/dL); however, human milk has twice the iron available than does cow's or goat's milk (unless fortified with iron). Young children are iron-deficient in many parts of the world. Surveys in the United States show that 9% of children 12 to 36 months are iron-deficient, and 3% having iron deficiency anemia. These rates are significantly higher among the poor and among minorities.

During the reproductive years, the average menstrual blood loss is 30 mL per month, but some women lose as much as 500 mL. Since 1 mL of packed cells contains 1.2 mg iron, the average menstrual loss is about 14 mg iron (30 mL blood × 40 mL red cells/mL blood × 1.2 mg/100 mL packed cells). Thus, the average menstruating woman requires an additional 0.5 mg per day (14 mg/

TABLE 5-1.   Distribution of Iron in Healthy Adults

Functional compounds	
Hemoglobin	2230 mg
Myoglobin	140 mg
Tissue enzymes	8 mg
Transport	
Transferrin	4 mg
Stores (ferritin, hemosiderin)	
Males	1000–1400 mg
Females	200–400 mg

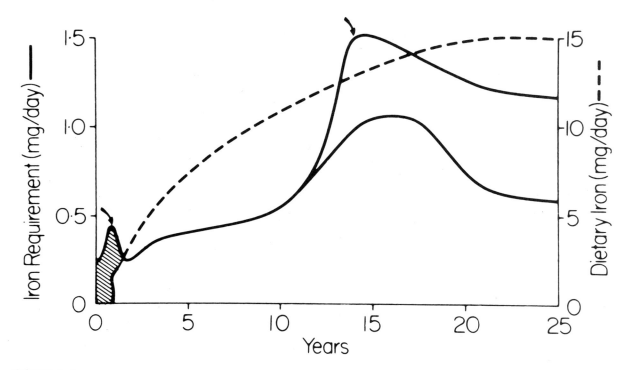

FIGURE 5-1.

Iron requirement. The daily iron requirement at different ages is indicated by the black line. At age 12, the line divides into the requirements for females (*upper solid line*) and males (*lower solid line*). The dashed line indicates the available iron in the normal Western diet. The shaded area during the first year of life indicates the period of negative iron balance when the infant outgrows his or her iron supply. The arrow also shows the other critical period when losses are likely to exceed supplies. (From Bothwell TH, et al: *Iron Metabolism in Man.* Oxford: Blackwell, 1979:15.)

28 days), but this requirement may reach 2.5 mg per day in those with heavy menses. Since normal absorption is 1.0 to 1.5 mg per day and since maximal dietary absorption is essentially capped at 3 to 3.5 mg per day even with an optimal diet and the stimulus of iron deficiency, iron balance is obviously tenuous in women and negative iron balance is common. Surveys of menstruating US women show that about 10% lack iron stores and 3% to 5% have suboptimal hemoglobin values because of iron deficiency. In Third World countries, much higher percentages of women lack iron stores and are anemic.

TABLE 5-2.   Iron Needs in Pregnancy

Expanded red cell mass	480 mg
Formation of fetus and placenta	400 mg
Average blood loss (without episiotomy) at delivery	85 mg
Total	965 mg
Expanded red cell mass returned after parturition	480 mg
Total	485 mg

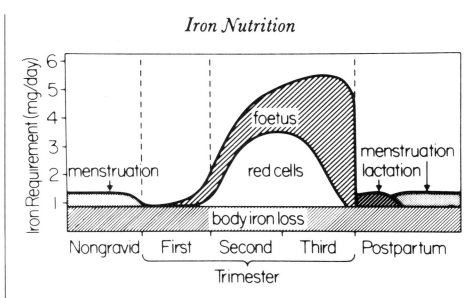

Iron Nutrition

FIGURE 5-2.
Daily iron requirements during pregnancy. The requirements for expanding the red cell mass, fetal needs, and lactation are laid on the basal daily iron loss and menstruation. (From Bothwell TH, et al. *Iron Metabolism in Man*. Oxford: Blackwell, 1979:21.)

The tendency toward negative iron balance in women is compounded by pregnancy and lactation (Table 5-2; Fig. 5-2). Although menses cease during pregnancy, the increase in maternal red cell mass (about 400 mL red cells, 480 mg iron), the fetal and placental requirements for iron (350 to 400 mg), and the blood loss attending delivery (averaging 200 mL, 85 mg iron) amount to about 1000 mg of iron beyond basal requirements. The iron of the expanded red blood cell mass is returned to the body at the end of gestation, making the net loss about 500 mg. Therefore, each pregnancy uses approximately 500 mg of iron beyond the normal daily requirements.

Lactation requires an additional 0.5 to 1.0 iron mg per day. Since these demands exceed iron stores in virtually all women with even the first pregnancy, it is accepted practice to monitor blood counts and provide iron supplements during pregnancy and lactation and for some months thereafter. Data on iron deficiency during pregnancy are not available for the general population; however, the iron deficiency anemia among low-income pregnant women is 9%, 14%, and 27% during the first, second, and third trimesters, respectively. Fortunately, the low iron stores of the mother do not prevent the fetus from capturing its necessary iron except in extremely severe iron deficiency.

Ferrokinetics

Once iron enters the circulation, it remains in a closed loop, as shown in Figure 5-3. The major features of this pathway are transport through plasma, uptake by red cell precursors in marrow, release of this iron from marrow in red cells, entrapment of senescent red cells by macrophages with salvage of iron from heme, and return of iron from macrophages to plasma. There is also a pool of storage iron in the macrophages that partially exchanges with the iron being processed from effete red cells. Finally, cells need a method to control uptake and disposition of iron. We will examine each of these aspects in turn.

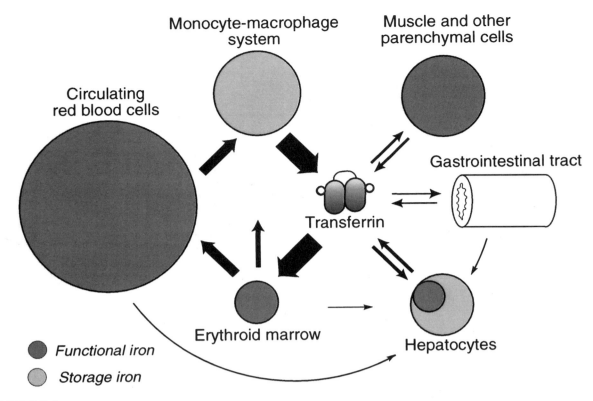

FIGURE 5-3.

Pathways of internal iron exchange. The four thickest arrows show the major pathways of iron movement with the areas of circles denoting the relative amount of iron in each pool. The vertical arrow represents the normally small amount of iron movement from developing normoblasts directly to macrophages; this comprises both transport of excess cytoplasmic iron and transfer of all iron from those few normoblasts that are normally destroyed. When ineffective erythropoiesis is present (*vertical line*), this normoblast-to-macrophage pathway becomes the dominant iron pathway. (From Brittenham GM. RBC Function and disorders of iron metabolism. In Scientific American Medicine, Editors: David C. Dale, MD, FACP, and Daniel D. Federman, MD, MACP 1997.)

Plasma Transport

Ferric ions are carried in plasma by **transferrin**, a glycoprotein with a molecular weight of 76,000, which is synthesized in hepatocytes and macrophages. Each molecule contains two iron-binding sites. This iron-transferrin complex is responsible for the normally salmon-pink color of normal plasma. Transferrin has a very high association constant for iron ($K_a \sim 10^{24}$), which means that there is an average of about one free ferric ion in the entire circulating blood volume! This is noteworthy because ionic iron is extremely toxic. About one third of the transferrin sites are ordinarily occupied by iron. The average serum iron (SI; the clinical measure of iron bound to transferrin in serum) concentration is about 100 μg/dL. The total iron-binding capacity, iron bound to transferrin plus the apotransferrin iron binding capacity) is normally about 300 μg/dL.

Iron Uptake by Erythroid Cells

Iron is transported primarily to developing normoblasts and reticulocytes in the bone marrow, which have a voracious iron requirement, but also to all other cells. Transferrin attaches to **transferrin receptors**, on the cell membrane (Fig. 5-4). After binding, the transferrin-transferrin receptor complexes cluster together, and an invagination of the cell membrane forms, leading to an endosome. A proton pump lowers the endosomal pH to ~5.5, which allows the Fe^{+3} to dissociate. The Fe^{+3} is reduced to Fe^{+2} and diffuses across the endosomal membrane to the cytosol, where it is either directly inserted into a waiting proto-porphyrin molecule to form heme or is complexed by another protein, ferritin, until needed for heme synthesis. The endosome then rejoins the cell membrane. The transferrin receptor remains in the cell membrane, and the transferrin is recycled to the plasma (see Fig. 5-4). Over the several days of life as a normoblast and reticulocyte, each cell takes up about 1 billion iron ions by this process. Occasional normoblasts display aggregates of iron (hemosiderin) visible by light microscopy when stained with Prussian blue. Such normoblasts are called **sider-oblasts**. Once hemoglobin synthesis is complete, the larger iron particles are removed by macrophages. The red cell, with nearly all of its iron contained in hemoglobin, then circulates in the blood for 120 days.

Intracellular Iron Regulation

The method used by erythroid and other cells to maintain appropriate iron homeostasis is of considerable biologic interest. A moment's reflection suggests that a cell's relative need for transferrin receptors and for ferritin molecules is reciprocal: when cellular iron is low, more transferrin receptor is needed for the cell to sequester extracellular iron; when it is high, more ferritin is required to store unneeded iron. The appropriate balance is maintained through the action of

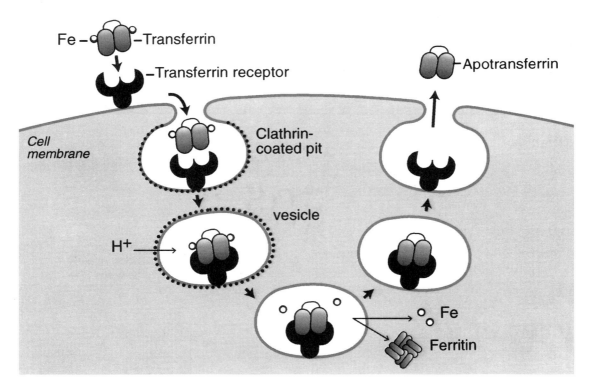

FIGURE 5-4.

Iron delivery from transferrin to normoblasts and other cells. Transferrin molecules with two iron molecules have a higher affinity for the transferrin receptor and are thus the more likely iron donor. Following transferrin binding, invagination and endosome formation occur, after which the iron is released and taken up by waiting heme or ferritin molecules (see text for details). Apotransferrin molecules are then released to the plasma, and the transferrin receptor molecules reassume their location on the cell membrane. (From Brittenham GM. RBC function and disorders of iron metabolism. In: David C. Dale, MD, FACP, Daniel D. Federman, MD, MACP, eds. *Scientific American Medicine*, 1997.)

cytoplasmic iron regulatory proteins (IRP1, IRP2). When cellular iron concentration is low, iron-binding by these cytosolic IRPs results in a change in IRP configuration such that the IRP attaches tightly to the iron-responsive element (IRE) of the messenger RNAs (mRNAs) for both transferrin receptor and ferritin (Fig. 5-5). This IRE, located in the untranslated portion of the message, has a highly specific stem-loop configuration (Fig. 5-6).

Attachment of the IRP to this IRE *suppresses* translation of ferritin mRNA but *stabilizes* tranferrin receptor mRNA against attack by housekeeping endonucleases. The result is fewer ferritin molecules synthesized but more transferrin

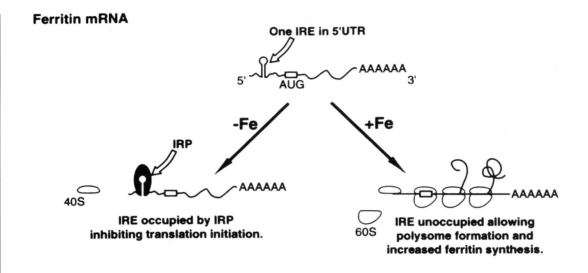

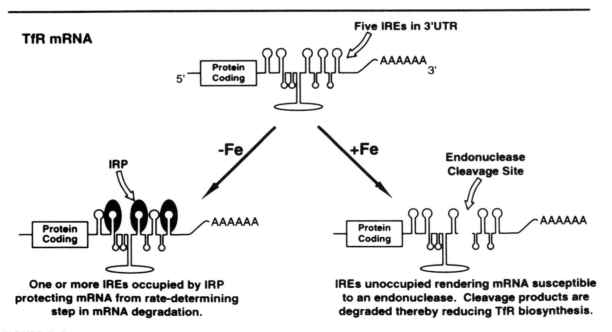

FIGURE 5-5.

Model of interaction between iron regulatory proteins (IRPs) and iron regulatory elements (IREs) of mRNA for ferritin and transferrin receptor (see text). (From Harford JB, Rouault TA. RNA structure and function in cellular iron homeostasis. In: Simons RW, Grunberg-Manago M, eds. *RNA Structure and Function.* Cold Spring Harbor, NY: Cold Spring Harbor Laboratory Press, 1998:575–602.)

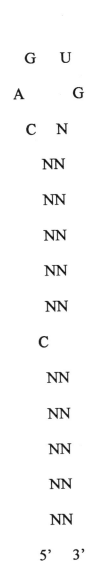

```
        G   U

      A       G

        C   N

          NN

          NN

          NN

          NN

          NN

        C

          NN

          NN

          NN

          NN

          NN

        5'  3'
```

FIGURE 5-6.
Stem-loop configuration of the iron regulatory element of mRNA.

receptors produced. The opposite occurs when cellular iron is high. This elegant system thus functions to maintain iron homeostasis in the appropriate range. The same IRP/IRE system also modulates translation of the mRNA for δ-aminole-vulinic acid synthase (see Chapter 3), a key enzyme in heme synthesis whose production also requires coordination with iron availability, and the membrane divalent cation transport protein (see Nramp2). In fact, cloning this 22 or so base-pair IRE into other genes causes their protein products to be similarly modulated by the ambient iron level. This system thus illustrates a fundamental mechanism through which physiologic coordination of distinct intracellular systems is achieved at the translational level.

Removal of Senescent Red Cells and Iron Recycling

The next step in the iron cycle occurs at the end of red cell life. After circulation of the erythrocyte for 120 days, senescent red cells are trapped in macrophages. The cell is lysed, hemoglobin is degraded, and iron is released from the heme ring (Fig. 5-3).

Delivery of Iron to Plasma

Iron is then released by the macrophage to serum transferrin at an appropriate rate by the macrophage. This has been studied in experiments in which heat-killed red cells containing radioactive iron are injected into experimental animals. Such nonviable red cells are removed from the circulation within a few minutes. After about half an hour, the time required for catabolism of cells and contained hemoglobin, iron release to plasma transferrin begins. About half of the radioactive iron is released relatively rapidly ($t_{1/2}$ = 34 minutes), whereas the remainder equilibrates with iron stored in the macrophages and is released gradually ($t_{1/2}$ = 7 days). This released iron then circulates back to the marrow, completing the circuit. As discussed in the following text, the serum iron level—and thus red cell production—is limited by the rate of iron release from the macrophage.

Summary of Ferrokinetics

Under normal conditions (equal erythrocyte production and destruction rates, stable hematocrit), the various components of this iron cycle also are in equilibrium. Thus, the quantity of iron removed by normoblasts and reticulocytes from transferrin per unit time (minus a small amount lost from "normal" intramarrow erythrocyte destruction) equals the quantity of iron delivered to the circulation in the form of mature red cells. This in turn is equal to the amount of iron returning per unit time from senescent red cells to macrophages, which finally is equal to that released per unit time from macrophages to transferrin. As one might expect, the amount of iron delivered to normoblasts per unit time has a precise relation to the amount of hemoglobin produced per unit time; determination of this step of ferrokinetics can be used to obtain a highly accurate measurement of red cell production by marrow.

Iron Storage

Iron is stored in two forms: ferritin and hemosiderin. **Ferritin** comprises a polyhedral protein shell (molecular weight 440,000) containing up to 4500 ferric salt molecules. The iron-ferritin crystal yields a characteristic pattern on electron microscopy, facilitating identification of iron storage sites. This unique appearance has led to its widespread use as a marker in electron microscopy, since ferritin can be conjugated to other proteins.

Ferritin conserves iron and protects cell constituents from this highly reactive ion. Apoferritin synthesis is stimulated within 10 minutes by entry of iron into cells. The half-life of the protein is 2 to 3 days. Ferritin is found in almost all tissues. Ferritin also circulates in plasma in nanogram quantities. Plasma ferritin is mainly derived from macrophages, and the plasma ferritin level normally serves a good index of body iron stores. Ferritin is elevated in relation to stores, however, in inflammation and liver disease.

Hemosiderin is the term applied to the form of storage iron visible by light microscopy. Predominantly found in macrophages in the bone marrow, liver, and spleen, hemosiderin is seen in unstained tissue sections as refractile yellow particles and as deep blue particles when stained with Prussian blue. It is probably formed by aggregation of partially denatured and deproteinized ferritin. Hemosiderin can also be seen in normoblasts and rarely in red cells.

THE HYPOPROLIFERATIVE ANEMIAS

The hallmark of hypoproliferation is *lower than expected* marrow erythroid cellularity and red cell production for the degree of anemia. Although production parameters (reticulocyte index and G/E ratio) may be normal or even increased compared with levels seen in normal subjects, they are, nevertheless, *lower than expected* for the degree of anemia. Such assessment of erythroid production must be made after anemia (in the case of anemia of sudden onset) has been present for 7 to 10 days, because production parameters will necessarily be in the hypoproliferative range until the marrow has had time to respond.

The hypoproliferative anemias are due to three basic mechanisms: an insufficient supply of iron for hemoglobin synthesis, relatively low erythropoietin levels for the degree of anemia, and marrow damage.

Insufficient Iron Supply

Iron Deficiency Anemia

Iron deficiency is one of the hypoproliferative anemias: the G/E ratio remains in the normal range, and the reticulocyte index does not increase as expected. This indicates that formation of normoblasts, as well as production of hemoglobin, is decreased by iron deficiency. In fact, a therapeutic application of this concept is that disorders of excessive red cell production can be controlled by deliberate induction of iron deficiency.

Iron deficiency is defined as the absence of stainable iron (hemosiderin) in macrophages. *The mechanism of iron deficiency is almost always blood loss.* Exceptions to this rule are (1) the 18-month-old child whose rapid growth exceeds dietary iron availability and (2) the patient who absorbs iron poorly because the stomach or duodenum has been altered by disease or surgery.

In contrast to younger women, in whom iron deficiency is usually a consequence of menstrual losses or pregnancy, iron deficiency in adult men and postmenopausal women is nearly always due to gastrointestinal blood loss. Lesions that commonly lead to blood loss include esophageal hiatus hernia and esophagitis, ulcers of the stomach and duodenum, inflammatory bowel disease, hemorrhoids, and carcinoma of the colon and stomach. Aspirin may also cause blood loss and iron deficiency by increasing normal gastrointestinal blood loss (0.5 mL/day) to 5 mL per day. Gastrointestinal parasites are a major cause of blood loss in many parts of the world. The serious nature of many of these disorders makes accurate correct determination of the cause of iron deficiency a necessity.

Iron deficiency begins with negative iron balance (Table 5-3, Fig. 5-7). Only when stores have been completely exhausted do further iron losses produce the typical laboratory signs of iron deficiency. At this point, the macrophage is unable to release sufficient iron to sustain the plasma iron level. Transferrin receptor increases and ferritin decreases through the action of cellular IRPs. Plasma transferrin rises. These changes in serum iron and iron binding capacity are shown graphically in Figure 5-8. The drop in serum iron limits hemoglobin synthesis, and anemia—initially normocytic and normochromic—results. As iron deficiency becomes more severe, red cells become smaller (reduced mean corpuscular volume [MCV]), the concentration of hemoglobin in individual red cells falls (mean corpuscular hemoglobin [MCH]), and the hemoglobin content per unit cell volume (MCHC) is reduced. Such cells are recognizable in peripheral blood smears as hypochromic microcytes; when iron deficiency is severe, a minority of cells are extremely small or misshhapen (poikilocytosis).

Iron deficiency affects body organ function in many ways, some overt, some subtle. Work capacity, exercise tolerance, and productivity decline in direct proportion to the decrease in hemogobin (Figs. 5-9 and 5-10). This is of considerable

TABLE 5-3. Stages in Development of Iron Deficiency or Inflammation[*]

State	Iron Stores	Hb (g/dL)	MCV (fL)	MCH (pg)	Fe (µg/dL)	TIBC (µg/dL)	Fe Saturation (%)	Ferritin (µg/L)	Transferrin Receptor	RBC Morphology	Polychromatophilic Macrocytes
Iron deficiency											
Normal	N	15	90	30	100	300	33	100	N	N	A
Iron depletion	D	15	90	30	100	300	33	22	N	N	A
Borderline deficiency	A	15	90	30	50	300	17	10	I	N	A
Mild iron deficiency	A	13	80	27	35	350	10	8	I	N	P
Severe iron deficiency	A	7	65	23	23	450	5	6	I	Microcytosis, hypochromia, poikilocytosis	P
Inflammation											
Normal	N	15	90	30	100	300	33	100	N	N	A
Acute inflammation (hours to days)	N	15	90	30	50	280	15	300	N	N	A
Persistent inflammation (wk)	I	9	65	23	20	220	15	300	D?	Microcytosis, hypochromia	A or Inf

A, absent; D, decreased; Inf, infrequent; I, increased; N, normal; P, present. Fe, iron; Hb, hemoglobin; MCH, mean corpuscular hemoglobin; MCHC, mean corpuscular hemoglobin concentration; MCV, mean corpuscular volume; RBC, red blood cell; TIBC, total iron-binding capacity.
*Although shown here as the simple concentrations, the serum transferrin/log ferritin ratio is the most sensitive indicator of early iron deficiency.

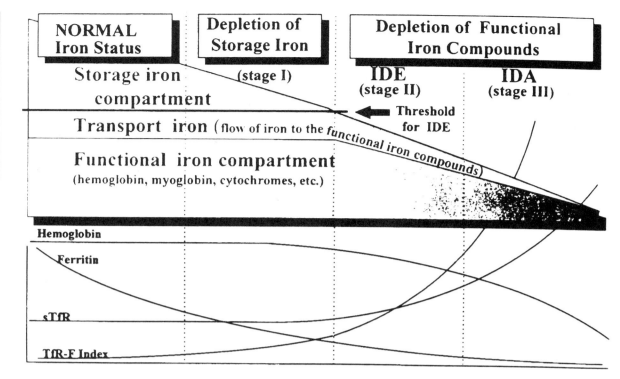

FIGURE 5-7.

Changes in iron parameters in normals' iron depletion and progressive iron deficiency. IDE, iron-deficient erythropoiesis; IDA, iron-deficient anemias, sTfR, serum transferrin receptor. TfT-F index is the ratio sTfR to log ferritin, a sensitive index of early iron depletion. From Suominen P, et al. Serum transferrin receptor and transferrin receptor-ferritin index identify healthy subjects with subclinical iron deficits. *Blood* 1998;92:2934.

economic importance in developing countries, where iron deficiency is common and physical labor very important. Since iron is present in many enzymes (e.g., cytochromes, cytochrome oxidase, xanthine oxidase, catalase, succinate dehydrogenase, peroxidases), it is not surprising that iron deficiency affects tissues other than erythrocytes. Nearly half of the enzymes of the Krebs cycle contain iron or require it as a cofactor.

Severe iron deficiency is associated with cheilosis (fissures at the angles of the mouth), atrophy of lingual epithelium, and brittle fingernails and toenails, which are flat or concave (spoon nails). Experimental evidence in animals indicates that severe iron deficiency impairs skeletal muscle function during exercise. This effect is in addition to the anemia per se and appears to result from depletion of the iron-containing mitochondrial enzyme, α-glycerophosphate dehydrogenase. Catecholamine and triiodothyronine (T_3) metabolism are also perturbed by iron deficiency. Of very great importance is the fact that iron deficiency produces abnormalities in brain metabolism. An important body of evidence now shows delayed sensory development, motor function, and language skills in young children with iron deficiency. These deficits do improve slowly with correction of iron deficiency, but children do not reach normal levels for some years. Other studies indicate an effect of iron on cognition in teen-age girls who are iron-deficient but not anemic; iron supplementation produces significant improvement on psychometric tests in the iron versus placebo-treated subjects. Frank iron deficiency is known to interfere with ability to withstand serious infection. Finally, iron deficiency sometimes creates a desire to eat substances such as ice, clay, or starch, a disorder called **pica**. This odd perversion may result in young children chewing on painted surfaces with lead poisoning as outcome.

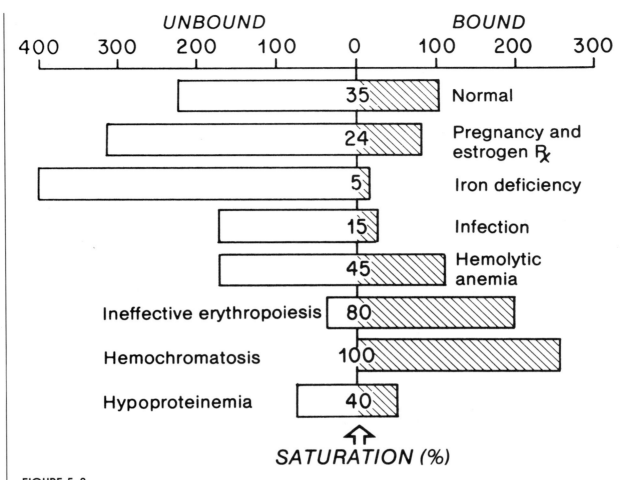

FIGURE 5-8.
Transferrin-bound iron and unsaturated iron-binding capacity in various disease states. Total iron-binding capacity is the sum of the two sides of the bar diagram. The number on the bar diagram refers to the % saturation.

Iron deficiency is readily treated by oral ferrous salts (sulfate, fumarate, succinate, or gluconate) or by polysaccharide iron complex. As above, iron absorption is enhanced as a result of iron deficiency. Ordinarily, improvement in hemoglobin concentration begins within 2 to 3 weeks. Iron dextran can be given parenterally, but this treatment has risks and is usually unnecessary. In terms of the population as a whole, the multiple consequences of iron deficiency have prompted a new public policy in the United States of fortifying grains with iron to increase dietary iron intake.

Anemia of Inflammation

Inflammation that lasts for weeks regularly leads to anemia. Usually, the hematocrit ranges from 25% to 32%. Although iron deficiency is the most common cause of anemia worldwide, anemia of inflammation is the second most common cause and the most common type of anemia in hospitalized persons. Inflammation may be due to infection, such as pneumonia, to a collagen vascular disease such as rheumatoid arthritis, or to a malignant tumor, even when symptoms of inflammation are not apparent.

Anemia of inflammation (sometimes known by the misnomer "anemia of chronic disease") is due to several mechanisms: reduced release of iron to transferrin by macrophages (Fig. 5-8) and lower erythropoietin than appropriate for the

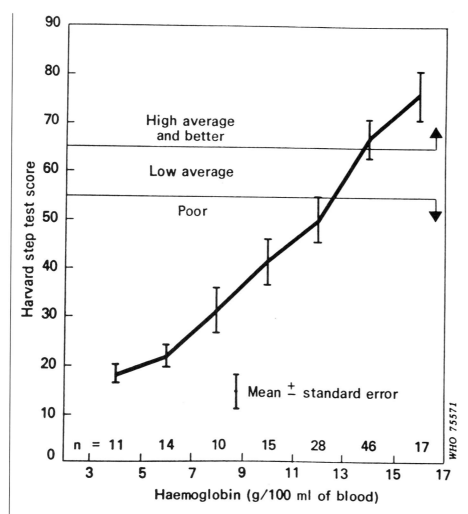

FIGURE 5-9.

Exercise capacity in subjects with iron deficiency anemia. (From Viteri FE, Torún B. Anemia and physical work capacity. *Clin Haematol* 1974;3:609.)

degree of anemia. These in turn appear to be due to inflammatory cytokines, particularly interleukin 1 (IL-1), tumor necrosis factor, and γ-interferon. Within a few hours of the onset of acute inflammation, a sharp decrease occurs in the early component of iron release from macrophages to transferrin (Fig. 5-11), as described above. Both serum iron and total iron-binding capacity decrease (Fig. 5-12), but the decrease in the former is proportionately greater (Fig. 5-8). The drop in iron saturation decreases iron supply to normoblasts, and marrow erythroid cellularity decreases. This situation is confirmed by ferrokinetic measurements, which show low values for the degree of anemia. Microcytic, hypochromic red cells, as seen in iron deficiency, may be observed after inflammation has been present for a few weeks. This drop in serum iron also has a major payoff: it deprives bacteria and parasites, the most common causes of inflammation, of an essential factor for growth, tilting the balance in favor of the host. This protection is apparently a matter of degree, since absolute iron deficiency can also impair resistance to some infections (see earlier under Iron Deficiency Anemia).

The second pathophysiologic explanation for the anemia of inflammation is that erythropoietin is lower than expected (Fig. 5-13). As a consequence of the relatively low erythropoietin, polychromatophilic macrocytes (shift cells) are often scant or absent. There is also evidence of diminished erythropoietic

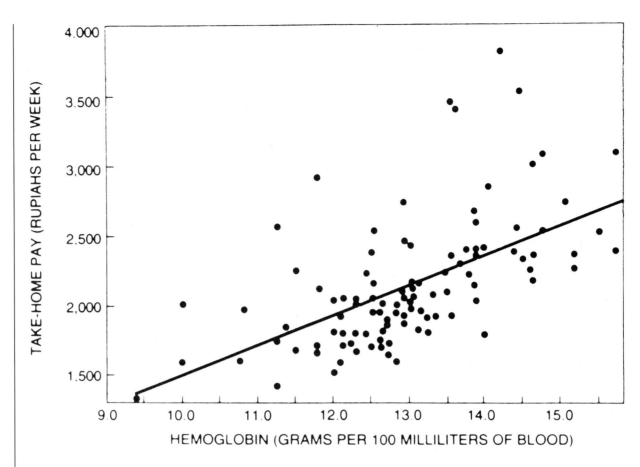

PRODUCTIVITY of Indonesian rubber tappers varies with hemoglobin levels. The diagonal line marks the association between income and hemoglobin.

FIGURE 5-10.

Take home pay as a function of hemoglobin concentration in Indonesian rubber workers. (From Scrimshaw NS. Iron deficency. *Sci Am* 1991;265:46–52.)

response to erythropoietin in vitro. A third potential mechanism is that the increased cytokines may directly suppress erythropoiesis in vivo as they do in marrow cultures.

Table 5-3 shows the changes observed in relatively mild and moderate anemia of inflammation. The similarity of changes to those of iron deficiency is a reflection of related pathophysiologic mechanisms. The anemia of inflammation can often be differentiated from iron deficiency anemia by a low total iron-binding capacity, elevated serum ferritin, and the paucity or absence of shift cells. When these tests are inconclusive or when both conditions might be present, the correct diagnosis or diagnoses can be facilitated by measuring circulating transferrin receptor (high in iron deficiency, normal in inflammation) or by checking for stainable iron in marrow macrophages. Anemia of inflammation is not corrected by iron therapy but by treatment of the underlying abnormality.

Low Erythropoietin Anemias

Chronic Renal Failure

Anemia usually appears when the creatinine clearance falls from the normal adult level of about 100 mL per minute to about 25 mL per minute, indicating a 75%

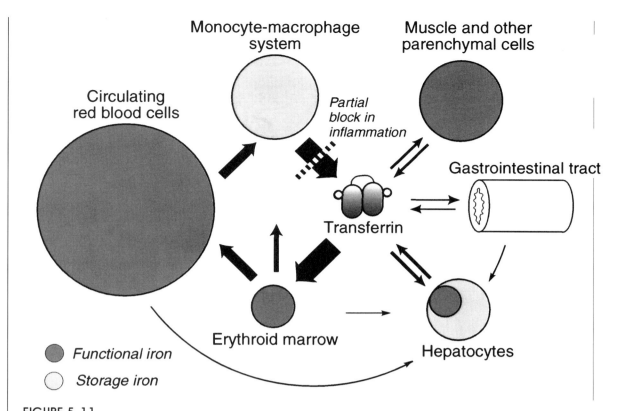

FIGURE 5-11.
Partial block in iron release (*dotted line*) from macrophages to transferrin when inflammation is present. (Modified from Brittenham GM. RBC function and disorders of iron metabolism. In David C. Dale, MD, FACP, and Daniel D. Federman, MD, MACP, eds. *Scientific American Medicine*, 1997.)

loss of renal function. The severity of anemia correlates roughly with the degree of renal failure and is largely due to destruction of the renal erythropoietin-producing mechanism (Fig. 5-14). Other factors may contribute to the anemia, such as mild shortening of the red cell life span, blood loss in hemodialyzing equipment, right shift of the oxygen dissociation curve (see Decreases Hemoglobin Oxygen Affinity) and inflammation. Red cell indices usually are normal. Burr cells may be observed (see Appendix I). Young reticulocytes usually are not observed in the circulation, despite the severity of the anemia, because erythropoietin levels are depressed.

Injections of recombinant erythropoietin dramatically improve anemia in patients with chronic renal failure. This treatment both eliminates the need for transfusions and improves the quality of life for chronic renal failure patients.

Endocrine Deficiencies

Several hormones beside erythropoietin influence erythroid marrow activity. At puberty, hemoglobin in males increases by an average of 2 g/dL as a result of the increase in testosterone. When testosterone levels fall (old age or castration), male and female hemoglobin values tend to coincide.

Mild to moderate anemia often is observed in hypothyroidism and panhypopituitarism. The exact mechanism of the anemia is not known. Limited studies show that erythropoietin tends to be lower than expected for the degree of anemia, and young reticulocytes are not present in circulating blood. Red cells

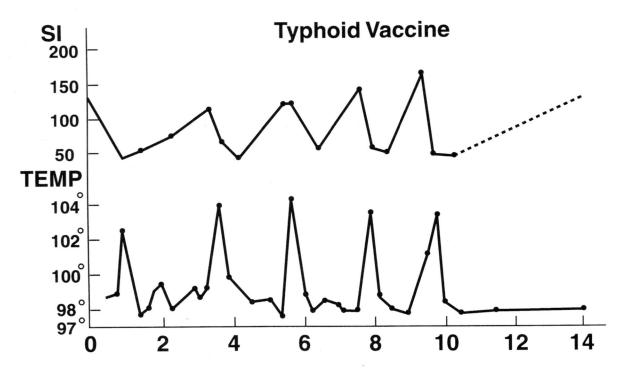

FIGURE 5-12.
The effect of induced fever by Typhoid vaccine on plasma iron in a human subject. With each temperature elevation, the plasma iron drops sharply and returns to normal shortly after cessation of fever. SI, serum iron. (From Cartwright GE, Wintrobe MM. The anemia of infection XVII. *Adv Intern Med* 1952;5:165.)

are usually normal in size and appearance. The abnormalities are reversed by treatment with the deficient hormones.

Protein/Calorie Malnutrition

Malnutrition regularly causes anemia. The exact mechanism is unknown, but the assumption is that red cell production participates in the atrophy that many tissues undergo. Erythropoietin levels are low for the degree of anemia. Limited data suggest that red cell production is otherwise normal, since blood loss in such patients results in reticulocytosis and a rise in hemoglobin to the level prevailing before blood loss.

Decreased Hemoglobin Oxygen Affinity

A rare but physiologically instructive cause of anemia is a rightward shift of the oxygen dissociation curve due a hemoglobin mutation or to an increased level of erythrocyte 2,3-bisphosphoglycerate. This is the opposite of erythrocytosis caused by a leftward shift of the oxygen dissociation curve (see Chapter 8). In this instance, the amount of oxygen released from blood with a right-shifted oxygen dissociation curve for a given drop in PO_2 is greater than normal. As a result, the kidney generates less erythropoietin so as to maintain hemoglobin below normal, thus maintaining its own oxygen tension in the normal range.

Mild right shifts of the oxygen dissociation curve also are observed in children. This is due to higher levels of 2,3-bisphosphoglyceric acid in red cells

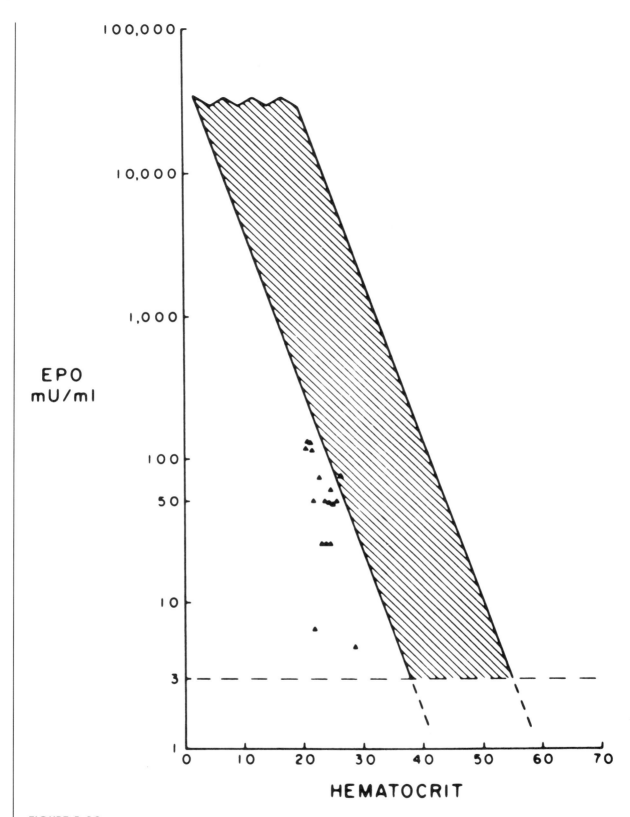

FIGURE 5-13.
Relation between hematocrit and plasma erythropoietin in inflammation. The cross-hatched area shows the normal range of values. (From Erslev AJ, et al. Plasma erythropoietin in health and disease. *Ann Clin Lab Sci* 1980;10:250.)

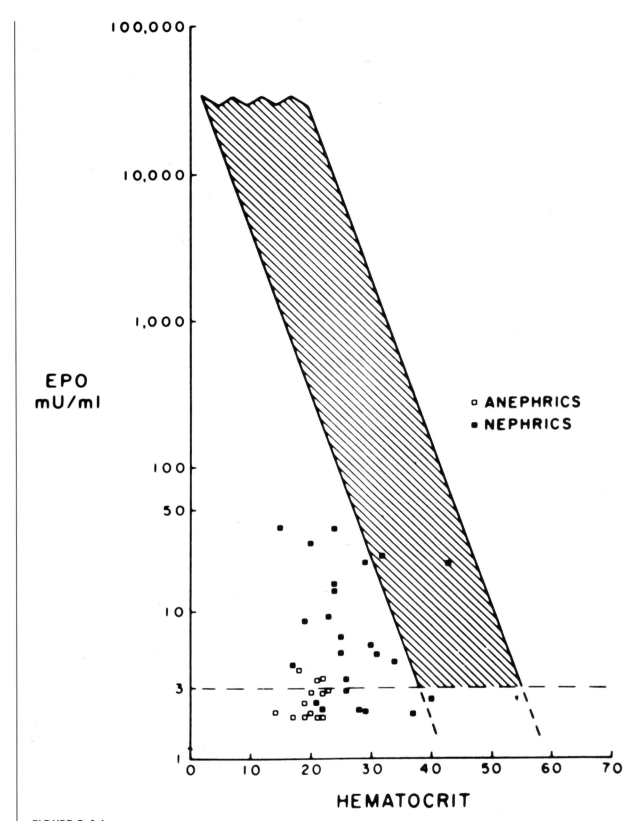

FIGURE 5-14.
Relation between hematocrit and plasma erythropoietin in patients with chronic renal failure, with and without kidneys. The cross-hatched area shows the normal range of values. (From Erslev, AJ, et al. Plasma erythropoietin in health and disease. *Ann Clin Lab Sci* 1980;10:250.)

(see Chapter 6), which in turn is a consequence of higher serum phosphate levels. This right shift is one reason why the hematocrit is lower in children than in adults.

Anemias Due to Marrow Damage

Aplastic Anemia

Aplastic anemia is a heterogeneous group of conditions in which the marrow is severely hypocellular. By definition, the red cell series plus one or more additional cell lines, that is, granulocytes and/or megakaryocytes, is involved. The diagnosis of aplastic anemia is made from the combination of low hematocrit, white cell count or platelet count, and markedly reduced cellularity on bone marrow examination. As in other hypoproliferative anemias, the reticulocyte index is low for the degree of anemia. The serum iron is elevated because of the marked decrease or absence of erythroid precursors to take up iron from transferrin (Fig. 5-8).

Pure Red Cell Aplasia

Pure red cell aplasia is a disorder in which there is complete or very nearly complete absence of erythrocyte precursors from the marrow. Reticulocytes are virtually absent. Other cell lines in the marrow and peripheral blood are normal. As with aplastic anemia, there are multiple causes of pure red cell aplasia. An acute transient form of red cell aplasia is caused by a parvovirus and is important in patients with hemolytic anemia. (see Chapter 6). A congenital form of pure red cell aplasia, known as Blackfan-Diamond syndrome, occurs in young children and can often be treated effectively by corticosteroids. Adult forms of the disease are usually due to immune disorders. Some adult cases are associated with a thymoma, and many of these patients are helped by thymectomy. IgG antibodies directed against normoblasts have been found in other patients, who often are helped by treatment with immune suppressants; T cells with activity against erythroid precursors have also been identified.

Myelophthisic Anemia

Myelophthisis (phthisis = wasting) refers to a group of conditions in which the marrow is replaced by foreign cells. The classic example is myelofibrosis in which the marrow spaces are replaced by fibroblasts. Another example is metastasis to the marrow by malignant cells, as in small cell carcinoma of the lung. In Gaucher's disease, abnormal macrophages may crowd out other marrow elements.

Severity of anemia, thrombocytopenia, and leukopenia depend on the degree of marrow injury. The anemia is normochromic and normocytic. Red cells often are abnormal in appearance, with "tear drop" forms. Immature granulocytes, megakaryocyte fragments, and nucleated erythrocytes regularly appear in the peripheral blood, presumably as a result of structural disorganization of the marrow or extramedullary hematopoiesis or both.

IRON OVERLOAD

The body does not excrete excess iron. When the total amount of storage iron reaches 15 to 20 g, evidence of toxicity can usually be identified. **Hereditary hemochromatosis** is a common and important genetic disease of iron storage. The disease is usually inherited as an autosomal recessive. The mutant gene, termed HFE, is strikingly homologous with the human leukocyte antigen (HLA) histocompatibility genes and closely linked to them on chromosome 6. Approximately 10% to 12% of whites are heterozygotes but phenotypically normal; 2 to 3 per 1000 are homozygous. This mutation is uncommon to nonexistent in nonwhites. In homozygotes, accumulation of iron from the normal diet reaches 15 to 50 g by age 50. It is estimated that a mere doubling of daily iron absorption is sufficient to cause this disease. Note that serum iron rises and transferrin saturation approaches 100% in early decades of life, often before much iron has been stored (Fig. 5-8); ferritin also rises to high levels but generally reaches abnormal levels at a later point in time. Women are relatively spared, a fact undoubtedly due to losses from menstruation and pregnancy.

The abnormality is due a single base substitution (G845A), yielding the mutant HFE protein cys282tyr. The normal HFE protein plays a major role in regulating intestinal iron absorption and in iron kinetics in the macrophage. This protein is normally expressed on the surface of cells, where it is found in a complex with β_2-microglobulin and with the transferrin receptor. When the mutation is present, the protein folds improperly, does not associate with β_2-microglobulin, and remains in the endoplasmic reticulum. Since knock-out of either the HFE gene or the β_2-microglobulin gene in mice causes increased iron absorption closely mimicking the human disease, the HFE–β_2-microglobulin– transferrin receptor complex clearly is needed for normal iron uptake regulation. Exactly how this abnormality dysregulates iron absorption in the duodenum is still unclear.

Homozygotes present with organ failure due to the excessive iron. It is assumed that, when iron stores exceed the sequestration capacity of the protective proteins, iron exists in a "free" state and causes tissue damage, presumably through its ability to catalyze redox reactions with free radical generation. The most commonly affected organs are the liver (cirrhosis, carcinoma); heart (cardiomyopathy, congestive heart failure); endocrine glands (especially diabetes mellitus, but also adrenal, gonadal, pituitary, and other endocrinologic disorders); and synovia (arthropathy). These manifestations are totally preventable by early detection and preventive treatment. The former must be done by routine screening of white and mixed populations (transferrin saturation, ferritin) followed by testing the proband and appropriate relatives for the mutant HFE gene. Such screening should be done in late adolescence or early adulthood and repeated a couple of decades later (including after menopause in women).

Treatment before tissue damage occurs is straightforward: weekly phlebotomies of 500 cc until iron deficiency appears, then phlebotomies frequently enough to maintain ferritin in the normal range (usually several times per year). Iron removal by aggressive phlebotomy is also important once tissue damage has occurred, because it increases life expectancy and often brings about improvement of organ function (Fig. 5-15). Because moderate vitamin C often increases iron toxicity in all iron overload states, intake of this vitamin should be carefully monitored.

Iron overload occurs in a number of other settings. One type is found in Africans and African Americans. The cause is not known, but there is indirect evidence for a genetic basis. Increased iron absorption and overload also occur in patients who have anemia due to ineffective erythropoiesis. This commonly occurs in persons with the inherited disease thalassemia and in some persons with the acquired disorder myelodysplastic syndrome (Chapter 12). Iron overload from increased absorption in these disorders is often compounded by transfusions needed to treat the anemia. Finally, iron overload occurs when sufficient blood transfusions have been given for anemia due to marrow disease (i.e., anemia not due to blood loss). Evidence of organ toxicity is identifiable when about 100 units of blood have been given. In all of these conditions, the organ damage is similar to that seen in hereditary hemochromatosis. Iron can be removed by regular phlebotomy in patients with the African/African American variety of iron overload and in some patients with mild anemia due to ineffective erythropoiesis. In those in whom this is impossible, daily injection of a chelator

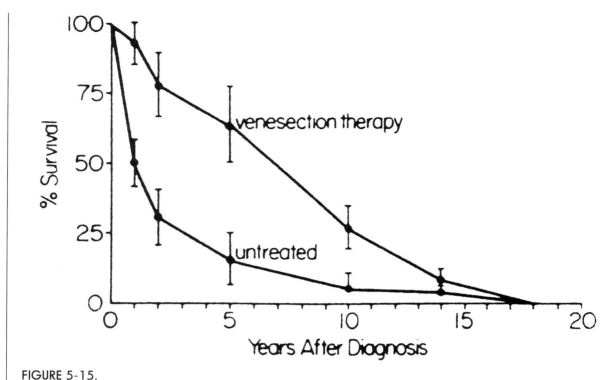

FIGURE 5-15.

Life-table survival curves after diagnosis in treated and untreated groups of patients with idiopathic hemochromatosis. The vertical lines at each time interval represent ± 1 SE (From Bothwell TH, et al. *Iron Metabolism in Man*. Oxford: Blackwell, 1979:154.)

of iron, deferoxamine is necessary to induce urinary and gastrointestinal iron loss and to minimize organ damage. The latter treatment is of great importance in those with thalassemia major, because untreated patients otherwise die in their teens or 20s from iron-induced heart or liver failure.

Acute iron poisoning is a preventable cause of death in young children. The potentially toxic dose is about 20 mg of iron per kilogram of body weight. Iron tablets may resemble candy (M&M's), and as few as three adult tablets, together containing less than 300 mg of iron, would exceed this level in a child of 12 kg. With major toxicity the gastrointestinal mucosa undergoes necrosis leading to nausea, vomiting, and bloody diarrhea. Shock and coma follow, in part due to loss of body fluids into the gut, but also due to the toxic effect of ferrous ions on the circulation. Emergency removal of iron from the gastrointestinal tract and administration of the chelator desferrioxamine have improved the survival of these gravely sick children.

SUMMARY POINTS

Iron is essential to life, but paradoxically cannot be free in the body because of its toxicity. Elegant methods are used by the body to conserve iron and to shield it with transport and storage proteins. Iron deficiency is a worldwide problem, which is easily recognized and treated. It is common in young children and in women in the child-bearing years as a result of result of an imbalance between supply and demand. In older women and men, iron deficiency is commonly a result of gastrointestinal losses, of which cancer is the greatest concern. Early treatment of hemochromatosis prevents all complications.

A simple numeric mnemonic for iron uses orders of magnitude (1, 10, 100, 1000):

1 mL of RBC contains ~1 mg of iron.

1 mg of iron is absorbed daily (10% of ~10 mg of dietary iron).

Serum iron is 100 μg/dL; serum ferritin is 100 μg/L.

Storage iron is 1000 mg in men.

SUGGESTED READINGS

Baer AN, Dessypris EN, Krantz SB. The pathogenesis of anemia in rheumatoid arthritis. *Semin Arthritis Rheum* 1990;19:1209.

Baumann Kurer S, Seifert B, Michel B, et al. Prediction of iron deficiency in chronic inflammatory rheumatic disease anaemia. *Br J Haematol* 1995;91:820–826.

Bothwell TH, Charlton RW, Cook JD, Finch CA: *Iron Metabolism in Man*. Oxford: Blackwell, 1979.

Bruner AB, Joffe A, Duggan AK, et al. Randomised study of cognitive effects of iron supplementation in non-anaemic iron-deficient adolescent girls. *Lancet* 1996;348:992–996.

Eschbach JW, Egrie JC, Downing MR, et al. Correction of the anemia of end-stage renal disease with recombinant human erythropoietin. *N Engl J Med* 1987;73:316.

Harford JB, Rouault TA. RNA structure and function in cellular iron homeostasis. In: Simons RW, Grunberg-Manago M, eds. *RNA Structure and Function*. Cold Spring Harbor, NY: Cold Spring Harbor Laboratory Press, 1998:575–602.

Lozoff B, Brittenham GM. Behavioral alterations in iron deficiency. *Hematol/Oncol Clin North Am* 1987;1:449–464.

Scrimshaw NS. Iron deficiency. *Sci Am October* 1991, 46–52.

Soemantri AG, Pollitt E, Kim I. Iron deficiency anemia and educational achievement. *Am J Clin Nutr* 1985;42:1221–1228.

Suominen, P, Punnonen K, Rajamaki A, Irjala K. Serum transferrin receptor and transferrin receptor-ferritin index identify healthy subjects with subclinical iron deficits. *Blood* 1998;92:2934–2939.

U.S. Department of Health and Human Services, Centers for Disease Control and Prevention (CDC). Recommendations to prevent and control iron deficiency in the United States. *MMWR Morb Mortal Wkly Rep* 1998; No. RR-3:47.

CASE DEVELOPMENT PROBLEMS: CHAPTER 5

Problem I

History: A 43-year-old accountant presented with a chief complaint of breathlessness and fatigue. He reported daily bright red blood with bowel movements for 20 years.

Physical examination: a pale man in no distress. BP: 130/80; pulse 80. The examination results were negative except for "spoon nails" and large, bleeding hemorrhoids.

Laboratory data: Hemoglobin 4.7 g/dL; hematocrit 15.9%; RBC count $3.26 \times 10^6/\mu$L; WBC count 7800/μL; platelet count 407,000/μL; reticulocyte count 3.0%.

1. Calculate the erythrocyte indices and compare them with the normal ranges.
2. Predict the appearance of the peripheral smear.

3. Calculate the reticulocyte index, assuming this patient's normal red cell count is $5.0 \times 10^6/\mu L$.
4. How would you characterize the anemia morphologically? Kinetically?
5. What is the most likely diagnosis?

Iron studies revealed a serum iron of 10 $\mu g/dL$, an iron-binding capacity of 495 $\mu g/dL$, and a ferritin of 13 $\mu g/L$. A bone marrow aspirate showed a normally cellular marrow with a G/E ratio of 2:1 and small red cell precursors with ragged bluish cytoplasm. Iron stain showed no stainable iron in the macrophages and no siderocytes.

6. What is your final diagnosis?
7. (a) What are normal iron stores in an adult? (b) How much iron is contained in 1 mL of blood? (c) Should one look for other sources of blood loss?

This patient was begun on ferrous sulfate 300 mg three times daily by mouth. Hemorrhoidectomy was also performed.

8. Describe the expected patient response to oral iron.
9. Listed below in random order are the steps in the development of iron deficiency anemia. Rearrange the steps in proper order:
   - Decrease in tissue (enzyme) iron
   - Normochromic, normocytic anemia
   - Increase in serum transferrin receptor
   - Negative iron balance
   - Decrease in iron stores
   - Fall in plasma iron concentration and rise in iron-binding capacity, increase in serum transferrin receptor
   - Hypochromic microcytic red cells

Problem II

History: A 35-year-old executive secretary with a past history of duodenal ulcer disease and one previous episode of upper gastrointestinal bleeding was hospitalized by her physician after 12 hours of hematemesis (vomiting blood). Otherwise, she had been in good health.

Physical examination: Supine BP 110/70, pulse 110, respiration 18; temperature 37° C; sitting BP 80/40, pulse 135. She is a well-developed, well-nourished female complaining of epigastric pain and nausea. Examination of the head, neck, chest, and heart resulted in negative findings. Abdomen: tenderness in the epigastrium; hyperactive bowel sounds. There was no hepatosplenomegaly. Rectal exam was negative except for black guaiac-positive (test for hemoglobin) stool.

Laboratory data: Hematocrit 39%; smear of peripheral blood: normocytic, normochromic red cells with occasional polychromatophilic macrocytes (shift cells); urinalysis negative.

1. (a) What do you infer from the pulse and blood pressure? (b) What difference do you note between this patient and the man in problem I?
2. Explain why the hematocrit was not decreased.
3. (a) What do the shift cells on the smear indicate? (b) How soon after a bleeding episode should shift cells appear?

The patient was given 1000 mL of normal saline intravenously. Her blood pressure and pulse promptly improved. Her blood was typed, and 3 units of packed red blood cells were transfused. She was given a H$_2$-blocker. She did not continue to bleed.

4. Why was this patient given a blood transfusion?

On the third hospital day, the patient's condition was stable, and the following data were obtained: Upper gastrointestinal endoscopy: 1 cm duodenal ulcer, with significant gastric outflow obstruction. A test for *Helicobacter pylori* was performed. Hemoglobin 9 g/dL; hematocrit 28%; RBC count $3.1 \times 10^6/\mu L$; WBC count 6500/μL; normal differential; platelet count 400,000/μL;

smear: normocytic, normochromic with moderate numbers of polychromatophilic macrocytes; reticulocyte count 4.8%; stool guaiac 2+.

5. Calculate the reticulocyte index (RI) and the erythrocyte index.
6. (a) How would you classify this patient's anemia in kinetic terms? (b) In morphologic terms?
7. Why is the RI low for the severity of the anemia 3 days after the bleeding episode?
8. What should the bone marrow show 3 to 4 days after acute hemorrhage of this severity?

Since there was extensive scarring with significant gastric outflow obstruction, the patient was advised to have subtotal gastrectomy. To avoid further transfusion, the surgeon elected to delay the operation until hematocrit had risen to about 35%. Since *H. pylori* was positive, treatment with appropriate antibiotics was begun, and the H_2-blocker was replaced with a hydrogen pump inhibitor.

9. If after several weeks the hematocrit fails to rise as expected, what causes of persistent anemia would you consider?
10. What lab tests would help you distinguish between or among them?

CASE DEVELOPMENT ANSWERS

Problem I

1. Mean corpuscular volume (MCV) = 49 fL (normal 82 to 92 fL); mean corpuscular hemoglobin (MCH) = 14 pg (normal 26 to 34 pg); mean corpuscular hemoglobin concentration (MCHC) = 29% (normal 32% to 36%).
2. Severely microcytic, hypochromic red cells, frequent shift cells, occasional misshapen cells, platelets increased.
3. RI = .03 × 3,260,000 × 1/2 × 1/50,000 = 0.98.
4. Hypochromic, microcytic. Hypoproliferative.
5. Iron deficiency anemia.
6. Iron deficiency anemia.
7. (a) Approximately 1000 mg in males and 0 to 300 mg in females. (b) 0.5 mg iron/mL whole blood. (c) Although hemorrhoidal bleeding of this duration is an adequate explanation of advanced iron deficiency, men over 40 should be screened for other gastrointestinal lesions. Endoscopic studies of the esophagus, stomach, duodenum, and colon were normal. In chronic blood loss, the blood volume is normal and the patient is not in acute danger. The anemia is better corrected slowly.
8. Expected is a modest rise in reticulocytes after 7 days of treatment with oral iron. In this patient, the hematocrit reached 34% on the 21st day of treatment and 44% on the 64th day. The platelet count declined to 240,000/μL over the same time period.
9. The correct sequence is:
   • Negative iron balance
   • Decrease in iron stores
   • Fall in serum iron concentration, rise in iron-binding capacity, increase in serum transferrin receptor
   • Decrease in marrow sideroblasts
   • Normochromic, normocytic anemia
   • Hypochromic microcytic anemia
   • Decrease in tissue (enzyme) iron

Problem II

1. (a) Tachycardia and postural hypotension of this magnitude mean that effective blood volume is significantly below normal. This may be caused by poor pump (severe heart failure), autonomic insufficiency, some drugs, or decreased blood volume. A decrease in blood volume sufficient to cause symptoms is most likely due to major acute blood loss (>15% of the total blood volume). (b) This situation differs from that of the previous patient, who had chronic blood loss but normal blood volume.

2. During hemorrhage, patients lose equal amounts of red cells and plasma, so the hematocrit does not change immediately. The hematocrit falls when the blood volume is restored by mobilization of extravascular fluid. This reequilibration requires about 48 hours to reach completion.

3. (a) The appearance of shift cells on the peripheral smear is an indication of increased erythropoietin acting on the marrow. It indicates renal hypoxia due to low blood volume or anemia. (b) Shift cells begin to appear approximately 12 hours after significant bleeding.

4. The patient's blood volume was severely decreased and should be replenished in the interest of safety.

5. $RI = \dfrac{\% \text{ reticulocytes}}{100} \times RBC \text{ count} \times \dfrac{1}{\text{maturation time}} \times \dfrac{1}{50{,}000}$.

   $= .048 \times 3{,}100{,}000 \times 1/2 \times 1/50{,}000 = 1.5$

   MCV = 90; MCH = 29; MCHC = 32; RI = reticulocyte index.

6. (a) When the reticulocyte index is low, the kinetic classification would have to be hypoproliferative anemia, ineffective erythropoiesis, or effective erythropoiesis with insufficient time passed for the expected marrow response. (b) Because the indices are normal, the morphologic classification is normocytic, normochromic.

7. A healthy person with adequate iron stores and hematocrit that dropped to 28% should be able to increase marrow production and reticulocyte production index to two to three times normal. However, this requires 7 to 10 days after onset of anemia. Three days after hemorrhage, one would not expect to see full-scale marrow activity.

8. The marrow should show some erythroid hyperplasia with a G/E ratio of 2:1 to 1:1 by 3 to 4 days posthemorrhage. This discrepancy between marrow response and RI reflects the time necessary for normoblast maturation and delivery of erythrocytes to the circulation.

9. If the hematocrit fails to respond, one would think of continuing hemorrhage or a new inflammatory process. Depleted iron stores would also prevent an adequate marrow response.

10. Repeating stool guaiacs, reticulocyte count, and serum ferritin would help distinguish among continuing hemorrhage, iron deficiency, and inflammation.

CHAPTER 6

The Red Cell Membrane and Hemolysis

Elizabeth B. Silverman

OUTLINE

OBJECTIVES

- Describe the red cell membrane and list its functions.
- Discuss the three basic mechanisms of hemolysis.
- Describe the complications of hemolysis.
- Discuss the diagnosis of hemolysis.
- Describe the heredity, pathophysiology, and clinical features of hereditary spherocytosis.
- Identify the major causes of the traumatic hemolytic anemias, and describe the peripheral blood findings.
- Discuss the pathophysiology of paroxysmal nocturnal hemoglobinuria.

> *Comparative hematology suggests that without the red cell membrane, the activity of man could hardly have exceeded the torpid pace of the lugworm.*
>
> Samuel E. Lux
> *Seminars in Hematology* 1979;16:21

THE RED CELL MEMBRANE

Many invertebrates have no red cells. Their respiratory pigments are dissolved in the plasma. In vertebrates, hemoglobin is confined within a membrane, resulting in the 400% increase in oxygen carrying capacity needed to satisfy the demands of mammalian metabolism.

"Packaging" of hemoglobin not only makes high hemoglobin concentration possible, but protects hemoglobin from oxidation and enables red cell 2,3-diphosphoglyceric acid (DPG) to modify hemoglobin affinity for oxygen. Having a red cell membrane, however, carries the risk of breaking the membrane and lysing the red cell, that is, **hemolysis**. This is the first of three chapters that cover the major types of abnormalities that can lead to hemolysis: membranes, hemoglobins, and enzymes.

The red cell membrane is made up of equal quantities of lipids and proteins (Fig. 6-1).

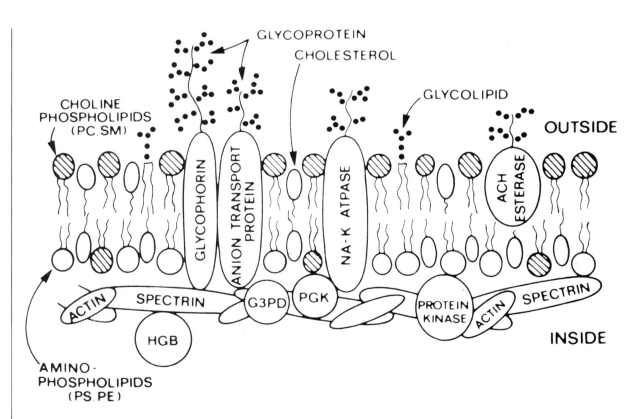

FIGURE 6-1.

A schematic cross-section of the red cell membrane. Glycophorin A, a glycoprotein with a large number of sialic acid residues, confers a negative charge on the red cell membrane. (From Beck WS. *Hematology*, 2nd ed. Cambridge: MIT Press, p. 270.)

Lipids

The lipids are organized in an asymmetric bilayer, with the choline phospholipids (phosphatidylcholine, sphingomyelin) concentrated in the outer half of the bilayer and the aminophospholipids (phosphatidylserine, phosphatidylethanolamine) in the inner half. Cholesterol and glycolipids are interspersed among the phospholipids. The membrane cholesterol and phospholipids are partially exchangeable with plasma lipids. Consequently, the membrane is susceptible to size and shape change based on plasma lipids as well as osmotic and chemical factors. The lipid bilayer is in a fluid state permitting flexibility of the red cell membrane.

Membrane Proteins

The major membrane proteins have been characterized and divided into two groups: the integral proteins and the structural proteins.

Integral Proteins

The integral proteins traverse the lipid bilayer or are attached to it by a glycolipid anchor. These include:

- Receptor and antigen-bearing proteins such as glycophorin A
- Transport proteins such as sodium-potassium adenosine triphosphatase (ATPase) and calcium ATPase
- The anion transport protein, which facilitates chloride and bicarbonate movement
- "Channel" proteins, which facilitate diffusion of glucose into the cell
- Glycolipid anchored proteins, such as decay accelerating factor, which protect the red cell from lysis by complement

Structural (Cytoskeletal) Proteins

The structural proteins are confined to the inner surface of the membrane and consist primarily of spectrin, actin, and ankyrin, as well as some enzymes. The spectrin-actin network supports the lipid bilayer and stabilizes the positions of the membrane-spanning proteins. This network thus assumes a dominant role in maintaining membrane shape and flexibility.

Accessory Membrane Functions

To maintain its osmotic equilibrium, the red cell must actively pump out sodium and water. Extrusion of Na^+ and inward transport of K^+ are accomplished by the membrane enzyme Na^+-K^+ ATPase. Intracellular potassium is maintained at very high concentrations, requiring active transport of K^+ into the cells. The erythrocyte also maintains a very low intracellular concentration of calcium by actively extruding calcium via the membrane Ca^{2+}-Mg^{2+} ATP-dependent calcium pump. This pump is activated by the calcium-binding protein, calmodulin.

HEMOLYSIS: GENERAL CONCEPTS

The normal human red cell emerges from the marrow and circulates in the peripheral blood for approximately 120 days (100 to 130 days). At the end of its life span, it is removed from the circulation by the macrophages of the liver and spleen. *Hemolysis is defined as an erythrocyte survival time less than 100 days.*

Mechanisms of Hemolysis

There are three basic pathophysiologic mechanisms of hemolysis:

- Loss of red cell deformability
- Phagocytosis by macrophages
- Disruption of membrane integrity

When red cells are removed prematurely from the circulation by macrophages of the liver and spleen, as in the first and second mechanisms, hemolysis is *extravascular*. When red cells rupture within the vascular system, as by the third mechanism, the process is known as *intravascular* hemolysis.

Loss of Red Cell Deformability

During its 120-day life span, the erythrocyte travels 100 to 300 miles, traversing high-pressure arterial systems and squeezing through capillaries and sinusoidal walls that are only 1 to 3 μm in diameter. To negotiate its 7- to 8-μm diameter through spaces one third its size, the red cell must be extremely flexible (Fig. 6-2). Flexibility plays a critical role in red cell survival and in its ability to deliver oxygen.

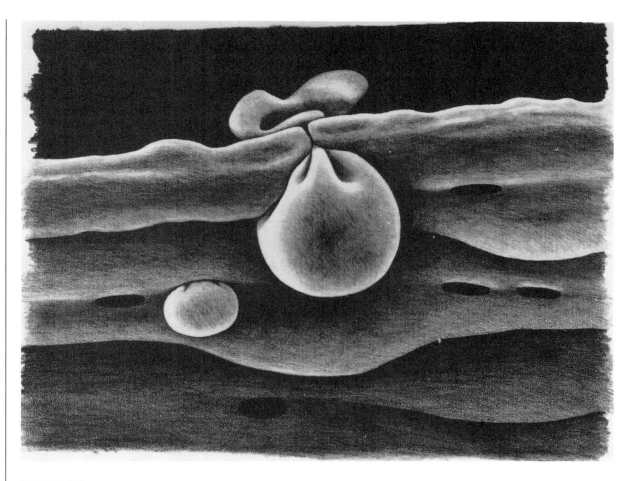

FIGURE 6-2.
Red cells squeezing through a rat spleen sinusoidal slit. Redrawn from a scanning electron micrograph. (From Mohandas N, et al. Red blood cell deformability and hemolytic anemias. *Semin Hematol* 16:103.)

Flexibility or deformability of the red cell is dependent on four variables:

- The viscoelastic properties of the membrane, which in turn are dependent mainly on the integrity of the spectrin-actin cytoskeleton.
- The surface-to-volume (S:V) ratio of the cell (the more spherical the cell, i.e., the lower its S:V ratio, the less deformable it is).
- The mean corpuscular hemoglobin concentration of the erythrocyte (an increase in intracellular hemoglobin concentration decreases deformability).
- The physical state of the hemoglobin within the cell (polymerization or precipitation of intracellular hemoglobin, as seen in sickle cell anemia, glucose-6-phosphate dehydrogenase [G6PD] deficiency, or thalassemia, impairs red cell flexibility).

Any process that decreases a red cell's deformability impedes its passage through the tiny slits in the splenic sinusoidal walls. Macrophages surrounding the sinusoids phagocytize the trapped cell, causing extravascular hemolysis.

Phagocytosis of Antibody- and Complement-Coated Red Cells

IgG and IgM antibodies that attach to red cell membrane antigens cause phagocytosis of red cells by macrophages of the liver and spleen (see Chapter 10 for more details).

Disruption of Membrane Integrity: Intravascular Hemolysis

Intravascular hemolysis occurs when holes appear in the red cell membrane. Membrane leaks are made when:

- Hemolytic complement (C5–C9) is fixed to the membrane as in ABO-mismatched transfusion reactions, or paroxysmal nocturnal hemoglobinuria (PNH).
- Membrane sulfhydryl groups are oxidized as in severe G6PD deficiency.
- Bacterial toxins alter membrane lipids (*Clostridium perfringens* lecithinase).
- A parasite invades and subsequently emerges from a red cell (malaria).
- The erythrocyte is mechanically cut or abraded within the vascular system by fibrin (microangiopathic hemolytic anemia or abnormal heart valves).
- The temperature exceeds 49° C. (burns).
- A hypotonic solution is infused.

Pores with an effective diffusion radius greater than 32.5 angstroms (Å) allow hemoglobin to leak out of the red cell. Smaller holes allow water to move in to equalize the osmotic gradient produced by the high concentration of intracellular hemoglobin. In either case, the red cell bursts, and hemoglobin and red cell membrane fragments are released directly within the vascular space, a process called **intravascular hemolysis**.

Normal Pathway of Red Cell Breakdown

Two possible mechanisms explain how macrophages recognize and destroy aged normal red cells: (1) the development of spherocytosis and (2) the attachment of antibody. The activities of various intracellular enzymes are known to decrease as a red cell ages. ATP concentration consequently decreases, depriving the calcium pump of its energy source, and intracellular calcium levels rise. The increase in intracellular calcium may activate a cross-linking enzyme (transglutaminase), which causes covalent linkages of membrane proteins. The result is fragmentation and loss of bits of the cell membrane, spherocytosis, decreased deformability, and ultimate entrapment by spleen and liver macrophages.

A second line of evidence suggests that with normal red cell aging there is an alteration of membrane sialoglycoproteins. An IgG autoantibody present in normal human serum progressively attaches to these altered membrane proteins. When a sufficient level of antibody coating is reached, macrophages recognize the red cell as foreign and phagocytize it.

When the red cell is engulfed by a macrophage, the red cell membrane is digested, and hemoglobin is broken into its three component parts—globin, iron, and protoporphyrin (Fig. 6-3). The globin chains are degraded, and their amino acids recycled in the body's amino acid pool. The iron is zealously conserved. Serum transferrin carries it from the macrophage back to the marrow for hemoglobin synthesis, or to macrophage storage sites in the liver, spleen, and marrow. The protoporphyrin moiety is converted to bilirubin, which diffuses out of the macrophage and complexes with serum albumin, now called "indirect" or "unconjugated" bilirubin. The bilirubin-albumin complex is transported to the liver hepatocyte, where the bilirubin is conjugated with glucuronide (direct or conjugated bilirubin) by the enzyme glucuronyl transferase. Water-soluble

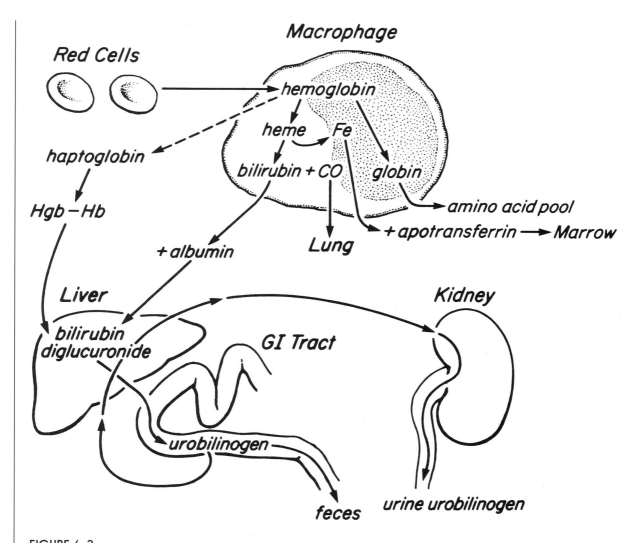

FIGURE 6-3.
Extravascular hemolysis. Almost all hemoglobin is degraded intracellularly and its products recycled. Traces of hemoglobin are bound to haptoglobin. The bilirubin pathway uses both bowel and kidney for excretion of the residual porphyrins.

bilirubin diglucuronide then is excreted via the bile into the gastrointestinal tract, where it is reduced by bacteria to fecal urobilinogen. Some urobilinogen is reabsorbed from the gut by the enterohepatic circulation and then is excreted in the urine. During the conversion of 1 mole of protoporphyrin to bilirubin, there is oxidative cleavage of the methene bridge of the protoporphyrin ring, with release of 1 mole of carbon monoxide, which is expired in the lungs. This is the principal reaction producing carbon monoxide in the body.

Extravascular versus Intravascular Hemolysis

In *extravascular* hemolysis, destroyed red cells are processed by the spleen and liver in the same manner as that of normal senescent red cells. However, because of the rapid breakdown of red cells during hemolysis, the capacity of the liver to conjugate the increased burden of bilirubin may be exceeded, and serum levels of unconjugated (indirect) bilirubin may rise. Increased levels of fecal and urinary urobilinogen also can be measured during hemolysis.

During *intravascular* hemolysis, hemoglobin is degraded by different pathways (Fig. 6-4). Normal plasma contains **haptoglobin**, an α_2-globulin that can bind 100 to 140 mg/dL of free hemoglobin or about 1% of the hemoglobin in red cells. The α-globin chain of free plasma hemoglobin binds to haptoglobin to form a complex that is rapidly cleared by the hepatocytes. Serum haptoglobin levels therefore are very low or absent in those with intravascular hemolysis. Even in brisk extravascular hemolysis, enough hemoglobin leaks out of the

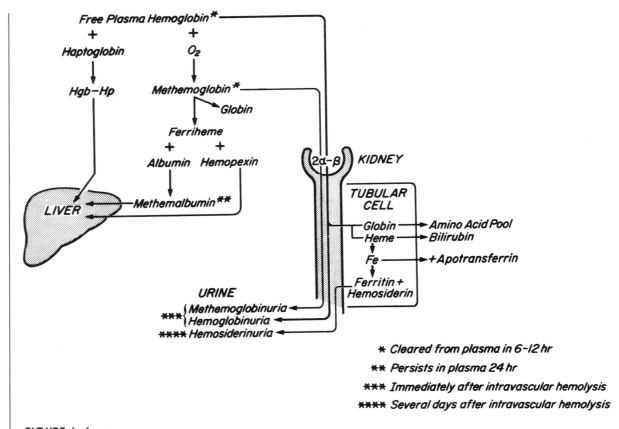

FIGURE 6-4.

Intravascular hemolysis. The time of appearance and clearance of hemoglobin and its products is indicated by asterisks.

macrophages to bind with and deplete haptoglobin. Therefore, a low serum haptoglobin concentration is a good test of hemolysis, but is not specific for intravascular hemolysis.

After saturating haptoglobin, some of the remaining free hemoglobin is oxidized to methemoglobin. Part of the methemoglobin dissociates into globin and ferriheme. The ferriheme combines with albumin to form methemalbumin, giving the plasma a brown color. A third plasma protein, **hemopexin**, also binds ferriheme. The hemopexin-ferriheme complexes are cleared by the hepatocytes.

The remaining free intravascular hemoglobin dissociates into dimers that are filtered in the urine. A portion of this filtered hemoglobin is reabsorbed by the renal tubular cells, where globin is degraded to amino acids and protoporphyrin converted to bilirubin. Most of the iron remains in the tubular cell in the form of ferritin or hemosiderin. When the tubular cell exfoliates into the urine, the iron is lost with it and may be seen in urine sediments stained for iron with Prussian blue. Thus, hemosiderinuria is a strong indicator of intravascular hemolysis. When intravascular hemoglobin release is brisk, the hemoglobin filtered by the glomerulus cannot all be reabsorbed by the tubular epithelium. Free hemoglobin appears immediately in the urine, producing a red-brown color.

In conclusion, in chronic extravascular hemolysis iron is tenaciously conserved; in chronic intravascular hemolysis, large amounts of iron are lost in the urine as free hemoglobin, methemoglobin, and hemosiderin, and the patient may become iron-deficient. Other complications of hemolysis are covered later in this chapter.

Role of the Spleen in Hemolysis

The spleen is an organ with both lymphoid and macrophage functions. Because of its unique "open" circulation, it acts as an efficient filter to remove even minimally defective red cells from the circulation. The spleen has a capsule from which trabeculae extend inward. Arterial vessels enter these trabeculae, branch repeatedly, and finally reach the white pulp (Fig. 6-5). There, the artery is surrounded by a sleeve of T lymphocytes. Embedded in this periarterial lymphatic sheath are lymphoid follicles composed of B lymphocytes. The artery then continues into the red pulp, ultimately terminating in the splenic cords. These cords are bands of tissue lying between the splenic sinuses containing double layers of macrophages monocytes, and lymphocytes.

Although most of the blood flowing through the red pulp of the spleen travels rapidly, as if in enclosed vessels, a smaller portion travels slowly. The slower-moving red cells are deposited in the splenic cords, where they meander across the cords and then insinuate themselves through the 1- to 3-μm slits in the sinus wall. The sinuses anastomose freely and then empty into the splenic veins. If an erythrocyte is stiff and cannot pass through the sinus wall slits, the cord macrophage phagocytizes it.

The metabolic environment of the spleen "conditions" slightly abnormal red cells, making them even more rigid. As blood passes the white pulp, plasma is skimmed off so that blood entering the cords has a high red cell concentration, sluggish flow, and a decreased supply of substrates. *The splenic cord is hypoxic, acidotic, and hypoglycemic.* A red cell caught in this environment is less able to generate ATP, may become spherocytic, may be unable to transverse the sinuses, and may be phagocytized. Red cells with only minor abnormalities, as in hereditary spherocytosis, can successfully pass through the circulation in every part of the body except the spleen (the body's fine filter). Splenectomy in such patients eliminates the hemolysis. More seriously deformed red cells, such as sickled cells, are also removed by the macrophages of the liver (the body's

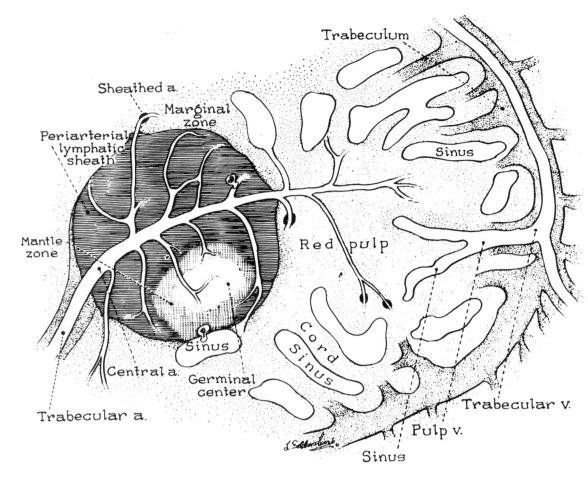

FIGURE 6-5.

Diagram of the organization of blood vessels in the spleen. (From Weiss L. The spleen. In: Greep RO, Weiss L, eds. *Histology*. New York: McGraw-Hill, p. 445.)

coarse filter), and splenectomy is ineffective in such diseases (see Chapter 15 for more details).

Role of Antibody and Complement in Hemolysis

Immune hemolysis is discussed in detail in Chapters 9 and 10. In this chapter, only a few preliminary points will be made. Antibodies that attach to red cell surface antigens may be of the immunoglobulin classes IgG or IgM. The antibody may not fix complement at all, fix complement only through C3b, or bind to completion through C9. Bound IgG antibodies that do not fix complement attach to Fc receptors on splenic macrophages, and the red cell is preferentially removed in the spleen. This clearance is inefficient, requiring hundreds or even thousands of IgG molecules per red cell, depending in part of the subtype of IgG. IgG antibodies that fix complement through C3b attach to C3b receptors on splenic macrophages. The presence of C3b as well as IgG on the red cell surface markedly augments clearance by the spleen. Therefore, splenectomy may be of benefit in patients with IgG autoimmune hemolytic anemias. However, if a red cell is very heavily coated with IgG antibody, even in the absence of C3b, the liver rather than the spleen will be the main site of hemolysis. Splenectomy would be less likely to produce significant improvement.

IgM antibodies must bind complement to the red cell membrane to effect red cell clearance. When complement is bound through C3b by an IgM antibody, there is attachment to a C3b receptor on liver macrophages (Kupffer's cells). Splenectomy will be of little benefit. When an IgM antibody fixes complement on the red cell membrane through C9, complement complexes are generated that penetrate the lipid bilayer, forming pores of a size sufficient to cause intravascular hemolysis (Fig. 6-6).

Marrow Response to Hemolysis

Erythroid hyperplasia is seen in the marrow within 2 days of an acute hemolytic episode. The reticulocyte count begins to rise in 3 to 4 days, but a new steady state is achieved only after 2 to 3 months of chronic hemolysis. The normal marrow is capable of increasing its daily output of red cells at least fivefold in response to chronic hemolysis. Thus, a red cell life span as short as 20 days may be associated with a normal hematocrit. This is called **compensated hemolysis**. Further decreases in life span are accompanied by anemia. Under intense stimulation, the marrow becomes very hypercellular, erythroid elements replace marrow fat, and active marrow expands in the axial skeleton, long bones, and skull {#106}. The cause of red cell hyperplasia in hemolysis is not clear. Erythropoietin concentration is not increased when hemolysis is compensated, suggesting that other factors also may stimulate red cell production.

In children with severe hereditary hemolytic anemias, hematopoiesis may resume in organs such as the liver and spleen that produced red cells in the embryo. Tumor-like masses of erythropoietic cells also may develop along the vertebrae, representing extensions of marrow through the thin vertebral bony cortex. Production of blood cells outside the marrow cavity is known as **extramedullary hematopoiesis**.

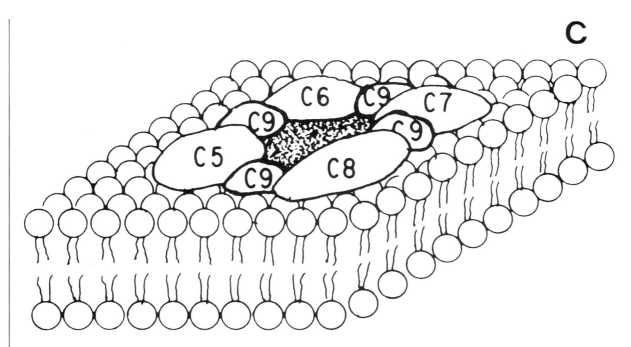

FIGURE 6-6.
Diagram of electron micrograph of holes in the red cell membrane created by complement. (From Rosse W. Interactions of complement with the red cell membrane. *Semin Hematol* 16:133.)

When hemolysis is extravascular, iron released from the broken-down red cells is efficiently shuttled back to the erythroid marrow for the manufacture of new hemoglobin. The expansion of marrow mass and the efficient recycling of iron account for the ability of the marrow to increase red cell production from the normal rate of 2.5×10^{11} cells daily to as much as 2×10^{12} cells per day.

Complications of Hemolysis

Anemia

If the red cell life span is less than 20 days, anemia results. Symptoms of weakness, fatigue, and shortness of breath may ensue.

Aplastic Crisis

In association with parvovirus B19 infections, anyone may have a temporary, selective failure of red cell production {#90}. This is a self-limited red cell aplasia lasting about 1 week, associated with a flu-like illness. The normal person replaces 1/120 of the red cells daily. If the normal marrow shuts down for 7 days, there is a trivial fall in hematocrit of 7/120, from 45% to approximately 42.5%. On the other hand, a patient whose red cell survival is only 10 days destroys and replaces 1/10 of the cells daily. If erythrocyte production ceases for a week while destruction continues at the previous rate, approximately 7/10 of the red cells will be destroyed and the hematocrit will fall to perhaps 13.5%. Such an aplastic crisis may occur in any chronic hemolytic anemia and is recognized by the disappearance of reticulocytes from the blood and normoblasts from the marrow. Transfusions are required until the patient's own red cell production resumes.

Folic Acid Deficiency

Folic acid requirements are increased in chronic hemolysis and may exceed the amounts supplied by a normal diet. The occurrence of folate deficiency is marked by worsening anemia, decreasing reticulocyte counts, hypersegmented neutrophils and macrocytes on peripheral smear and megaloblastic changes in the marrow. All patients with chronic hemolysis should be given a daily folic acid supplement of 1 mg.

Skeletal Abnormalities

When the marrow space is massively expanded, it can deform surrounding bones. This is especially notable in the skulls of growing children, producing the "hair on end" appearance of the skull x-ray—a combination of trabecular bone striations and thinning of the outer table. Forehead bossing, broad cheek bones, and protruding maxillae produce a characteristic hemolytic or "chipmunk" appearance in patients with severe hereditary hemolytic anemia.

Kernicterus and Gallstones

The enormous increase in bilirubin production due to rapid heme degradation in hemolysis may have untoward effects. In the newborn, hemolysis (Rh incompatibility, hereditary enzyme defects) is particularly hazardous. Hepatic glucuronyl transferase activity is low, and unconjugated bilirubin accumulates in the plasma and gains access to the brain. Basal ganglia are vulnerable because they are incompletely myelinated at birth. Serious neurologic sequelae including seizures, choreoathetosis, and mental retardation may ensue. Kernicterus may be prevented by performing exchange transfusions when serum indirect bilirubin levels approach 20 mg/dL or by exposing the infant to ultraviolet light.

Gallstones are a common finding in patients with chronic hemolytic disorders. These are black, bilirubin-containing stones and may occur even in children and young adults with hereditary hemolytic disorders. Gallstones in older adults do not suggest hemolysis.

Iron Overload

Patients with extravascular hemolysis retain all the iron liberated during red cell degradation. Furthermore, they absorb more dietary iron than normal, especially when ineffective erythropoiesis (as in thalassemia) is also present. If the patient also requires red cell transfusions to grow and function, body iron stores rapidly increase. The excess iron is initially deposited in macrophages, but with accumulations of 25 to 50 g of iron in adults (100 to 250 transfusions), deposition occurs in parenchymal cells of the heart, pancreas, liver, and endocrine glands, leading to fibrosis of these organs. Transfusion hemochromatosis is an important cause of death in thalassemia major. Most other chronic hemolytic anemias are less severe and require transfusion only during aplastic crises or surgery, and hemosiderosis only rarely develops. Patients with chronic intravascular hemolysis (e.g., PNH) lose large amounts of iron in the urine and are not at risk for iron overload.

Complications Peculiar to Intravascular Hemolysis

During acute intravascular hemolysis, large amounts of free hemoglobin and red cell membrane fragments are liberated in the blood. Free hemoglobin itself probably is not harmful, but membrane lipids such as phosphatidylserine and phosphatidylethanolamine can activate clotting factors and initiate disseminated intravascular coagulation (DIC). If an antigen-antibody reaction causes the intravascular hemolytic episode (ABO-incompatible blood transfusion), complement activation occurs, with the liberation of C3a and C5a. These small polypeptides act directly on vascular smooth muscle and also release vasoactive substances from mast cells, thus producing renal vasoconstriction and shock. Acute intravascular hemolytic reactions, therefore, may be associated with DIC, acute renal failure, shock, and death (see Chapter 9 on hemolytic transfusion reactions and Chapter 18 on DIC).

Diagnosis of Hemolysis

Peripheral Smear

The peripheral smear is very valuable for the detection and evaluation of hemolysis. Large numbers of polychromatophilic macrocytes or shift cells {#17}, spherocytes {#26}, elliptocytes {#25}, spur cells {#28}, target cells {#34}, sickled cells {#35}, or helmet cells {#44} and fragments {#30} may immediately suggest the correct diagnosis (see Appendix I). A supravital stain may reveal Heinz bodies {#40} (precipitated hemoglobin or globin chains) in addition to reticulocytosis, suggesting the diagnosis of G6PD deficiency, oxidant injury, unstable hemoglobins, or thalassemia.

Reticulocytosis

A persistently high reticulocyte index is the best clinical test of hemolysis {#31}. Obviously, if the patient is in aplastic crisis or is folate-depleted or if the hemolytic episode has occurred so recently that the marrow has not had time to increase production, the reticulocyte index will not be elevated.

Measurement of the Products of Red Cell Destruction

Increased indirect (unconjugated) bilirubin and low or absent serum haptoglobin levels are found in most patients with brisk hemolysis. Elevated serum levels of the enzyme lactic dehydrogenase (LDH) also are common. This enzyme, present in high concentration in normal red cells, is released when the red cell is destroyed.

Transiently, hemoglobin, methemoglobin, and methemalbumin are found in the plasma after intravascular hemolysis. Methemoglobinuria and hemoglobinuria may be seen immediately after intravascular hemolysis, and hemosiderinuria follows the episode in a few days and may still be detected 2 to 4 weeks later.

The peripheral smear and reticulocyte count are the best screening tests to detect hemolysis. The indirect bilirubin, haptoglobin, and LDH are also useful. More specific tests, such as osmotic fragility, hemoglobin electrophoresis, and Coombs' (antiglobulin) test, will be described subsequently.

Chromium-51 Survival

The gold standard for the diagnosis of hemolysis is the documentation of a short red cell life span in a patient who is not bleeding. An aliquot of the patient's red cells is incubated with radioactive chromate ($^{51}CrO_4^-$) which binds to β chains of hemoglobin. The

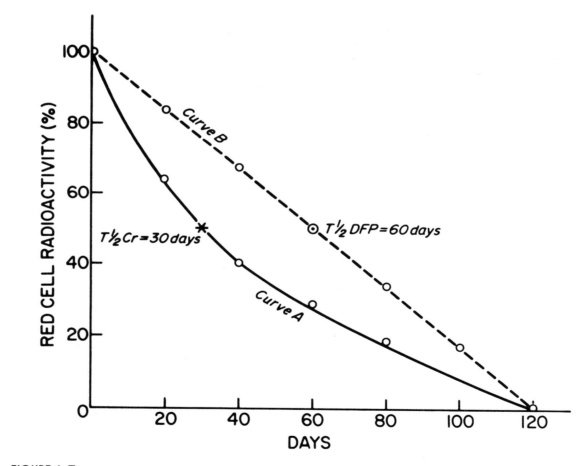

FIGURE 6-7.
Red cell (RBC) survival in normals. Curve A = chromium-51 RBC survival. Half-life by this method is 30 days because of a 1% daily elution of chromium from the red cell. Curve B = diisopropyl fluorophosphate (^{32}P) RBC survival. Half-life by this method is the expected 60 days because there is no elution.

labeled cells are reinfused into the patient, blood samples are taken at intervals for 1 to 3 weeks, and a survival curve is plotted. Results are expressed as half-life. Because of a 1% daily elution of ^{51}Cr from the red cells, the normal half-life by this method is 30 days rather than the expected 60 days (Fig. 6-7). In extreme hemolysis, half-lives shorter than 24 hours have been measured. In addition to half-life determination, the site of red cell destruction can be ascertained by placing scintillation counters over the liver and spleen. If radioactivity is heavily concentrated in the spleen (spleen-to-liver ratios greater than 5:1), the hemolysis may be ameliorated by splenectomy. Chromium survival studies, however, are rarely performed as simpler methods of detecting hemolysis are available (e.g., reticulocyte index, peripheral smear, LDH).

Classification of Hemolytic Disorders

Several classifications have been proposed, none of which is completely consistent. Disorders have been grouped according to whether they are hereditary or acquired, intravascular or extravascular, and whether the abnormality resides within the cell itself (intracorpuscular) or in the environment of the cell (extracorpuscular). Table 6-1 contains a list of hemolytic diseases. Many anemias, such as iron deficiency and the megaloblastic anemias that have only a slight decrease in life span, are not listed because hemolysis, though present, is a minor mechanism in these disorders.

DISORDERS OF THE RED CELL MEMBRANE

Abnormalities of Structural Proteins

The red cell membrane consists of an asymmetric lipid bilayer that is traversed by a number of different transmembrane receptor and antigen-bearing proteins. On the inner aspect of the lipid bilayer is the spectrin-actin cytoskeleton, which controls the shape and deformability of the red cell. Since membrane skeletal proteins are linked to some of the transmembrane receptor proteins, the skeletal proteins may also be responsible for transmitting signals from growth factors and hormones into the cytoplasm of the red cell.

The major proteins that are found in the cytoskeleton are spectrin, actin, protein 4.1, and ankyrin.

- Spectrin, the major skeletal protein, is a long flexible molecule composed of two similar spaghetti-like chains, called α and β, which are aligned in parallel and twist around each other (Fig. 6-8). In the membrane, most are organized as tetramers linked head to head (α-chain head to β-chain head). The tails of spectrin are attached to protein 4.1, which facilitates the attachment of the tail of spectrin to actin.
- Actin forms a junction from which spectrin molecules branch into a two-dimensional complex anastomosing web under the lipid bilayer (Fig. 6-8).
- Ankyrin attaches to spectrin near the head of the β chain and then attaches to the transmembrane protein called band 3 (the anion channel).
- Protein 4.1 at the tail of spectrin attaches to transmembrane protein band 3 and possibly to glycophorin C. The ankyrin and protein 4.1 attachments are not static but can break and reform thus contributing to the deformability of the membrane.

From the complex nature of the spectrin-actin-4.1-ankyrin transmembrane protein interactions, it is easy to see opportunity for error. In fact, a variety of such defects do occur causing the clinical disorders hereditary spherocytosis and hereditary elliptocytosis.

TABLE 6-1. Classification of Hemolytic Disorders

I. Intracorpuscular Abnormalities
  A. Membrane
    1. Hereditary: hereditary spherocytosis, hereditary elliptocytosis, hereditary stomatocytosis
    2. Acquired: paroxysmal nocturnal hemoglobinuria
  B. Hereditary defects of globin synthesis
    1. Hemoglobinopathies—SS, SC, CC, unstable hemoglobins, and so on
    2. Thalassemias*
  C. Hereditary enzyme defects
    1. Glycolytic pathway
      • Pyruvate kinase hexokinase
      • Triose isomerase
      • Glucose phosphate isomerase
    2. Pentose phosphate pathway: glucose-6-phosphate dehydrogenase (G6PD) deficiency
    3. Miscellaneous intracellular enzyme deficiencies
      • Glutathione reductase
      • Glutathione peroxidase
      • ATPase deficiency
      • 5'-Pyrimidine nucleotidase deficiency

II. Extracorpuscular Abnormalities
  A. Associated with antibodies (acquired)
    1. Isoantibodies: erythroblastosis fetalis, transfusion reactions
    2. Autoantibodies:
      • Warm-reacting (idiopathic or associated with lymphoma, chronic lymphocytic leukemia, systemic lupus erythematosus)
      • Cold agglutinin disease (idiopathic or associated with *Mycoplasma* pneumonia, infectious mononucleosis, lymphoma)
      • Cold hemolysin (paroxysmal cold hemoglobinuria)
      • Drug-induced antibodies
  B. Unassociated with antibodies
    1. Disorders of serum lipids:
      • Hereditary; abetalipoproteinemia
      • Acquired: spur cell anemia (liver disease)
    2. Traumatic (microangiopathic) hemolysis (acquired)
      • Disseminated intravascular hemolysis
      • Thrombotic thrombocytopenic purpura
      • Hemolytic uremic syndrome
      • Preeclampsia
      • Malignant hypertension
      • Cardiac valvular abnormalities or prostheses
      • March hemoglobinuria
    3. Infectious agents (acquired)
      • Bacterial toxins (*Clostridium welchii, Bacteroides*)
      • Parasites (malaria, *Bartonella*)
    4. Chemical, physical toxins (acquired)
      • Heavy metals
      • Arsine
      • Naphthalene
      • Intravenous distilled water
      • Burns

TABLE 6-1. Classification of Hemolytic Disorders (Continued)

III. Interaction of Intracorpuscular and Extracorpuscular Defects (Hereditary Intracorpuscular

Defects Requiring an Environmental Exposure to Induce Hemolysis)
  A. G6PD deficiency
  B. Favism
  C. Certain unstable hemoglobins

In thalassemia, the main mechanism of anemia is ineffective erythropoiesis, with hemolysis a major secondary mechanism.
(Adapted from Harris JW, Kellermeyer RW: The Red Cell, rev. ed. Harvard University Press, 1970:540–541.)

Hereditary Spherocytosis

Hereditary spherocytosis (HS) is a spectrum of hemolytic disorders produced by several genetic abnormalities. The common form of HS is an autosomal dominant hemolytic disease that affects approximately 1 in 5000 in the US population. Although found in all races, it is most prevalent among northern Europeans. HS is frequently associated with defects of chromosome 8 at the site of the ankyrin gene. Abnormalities or deficiencies of ankyrin are believed to lead to a deficiency of spectrin (Fig. 6-9). Spectrin deficiency causes loss of membrane with formation of small spherical red cells termed **microspherocytes** or spherocytes {#26} (Fig. 6-9).

   A direct relation between the degree of spectrin deficiency and the severity of the disease exists. The spherocyte also has a high intracellular hemoglobin concentration (MCHC, 36 to 37 g/dL). The low S:V ratio and the high MCHC make the spherocyte poorly deformable. In addition, the HS cell membrane is excessively permeable to sodium. To overcome this increased permeability, the cell

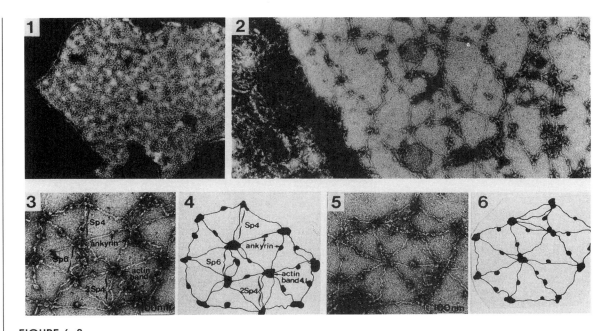

FIGURE 6-8.
Ultrastructure of the red cell membrane. 4 and 6 are schematic representations of 3 and 5. The knitted lattice is made up of pentagons, hexagons and heptagons with spectrin, tetramers (Sp4), hexamers, (Sp6) and double tetramers. (2Sp4) linked to actin-band 4.1 junctions. Ankyrin globules are seen in the middle of the spectrin threads. (From Palek J, Lambert S. Genetics of the red cell membrane skeleton. *Semin Hematol* 27:290.)

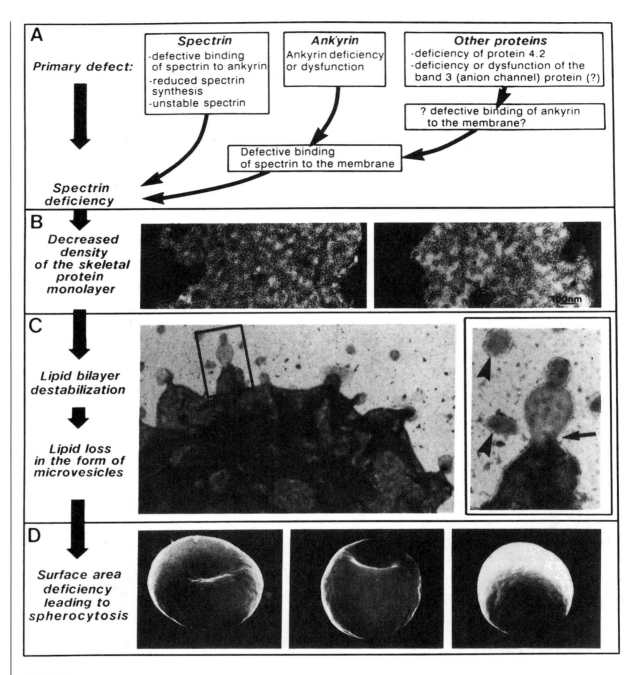

FIGURE 6-9.

Pathophysiology of the red cell defect in hereditary spherocytosis. B shows the reduced density of the hereditary spherocytosis cytoskeleton on the right compared with the normal one on the left. C shows the lipid layer separating from the abnormal skeleton (*arrow on left*) with micro-vesicles free in the medium (*arrowheads*). (From Palek J, Lambert S. Genetics of the red cell membrane skeleton. *Semin Hematol* 27:290.)

requires extra glucose to maintain its Na$^+$-K$^+$ pump activity. Because of lack of flexibility of the spherocyte and its dependence on accelerated glycolysis to compensate for the membrane sodium leak, the spleen presents the main threat to its survival.

When the spherocyte enters the spleen, it is detained in the splenic cord, where glucose levels are very low and intracellular ATP falls rapidly. Na$^+$-K$^+$

pump activity cannot be sustained, and sodium and water enter the cell, causing further sphering. After several passes through the spleen, the cell becomes hyperspheroidal; it cannot negotiate the sinusoidal slits, and it is phagocytized by splenic macrophages.

CLINICAL PICTURE

The clinical spectrum in HS is variable. Patients may have a mild anemia, splenomegaly, and jaundice, but many are asymptomatic and undiagnosed, even in old age. A newborn may require exchange transfusion to prevent kernicterus. Bilirubin gallstones occur in a large proportion of patients, even in childhood, and cholecystitis may be the first clinical evidence of the disease. As in other hemolytic disorders, aplastic crises and folic acid deficiency may occur.

LABORATORY FINDINGS

The peripheral smear is the key to diagnosis. Spherocytes, small dark cells without central pallor, make up at least 20% of the cells {#26}. However, in some proven cases, spherocytes are not conspicuous and other tests must be used. As in other causes of hemolysis, there is reticulocytosis and this is a simple test for screening family members. Elevated serum indirect bilirubin is found in only 70% of patients with HS. Typical abnormalities should be found in one parent and about half the patient's siblings.

OSMOTIC FRAGILITY TEST

The osmotic fragility test is helpful in the diagnosis of HS. It indirectly measures the S:V ratio of the cells by determining how much water the cells can accommodate before they rupture. A spherocyte, with its low S:V ratio, can accumulate less water than a biconcave disc. Red cells from the patient and a normal control are suspended in varying concentrations of saline, from 0.85% (isotonic saline) to distilled water. HS cells usually begin to lyse at 0.65%, whereas normal cells do not hemolyse until 0.5% concentrations of saline are reached (Fig. 6-10). Since one third of patients have a normal test, the osmotic fragility has been made more sensitive by preincubating the cells for 24 hours, during which glucose supplies are used up and the increased Na^+-K^+ pump activity cannot be sustained.

Immunoassays for spectrin and other proteins may replace fragility studies in the diagnosis of this curable disease.

TREATMENT

Because spherocytes are trapped only by the spleen, splenectomy eradicates the hemolysis and anemia resolves, except in the most severe cases of spectrin deficiency. The basic membrane defect persists, however, and microspherocytes are still present in the blood. Because the spleen has a critical role in phagocytosis of encapsulated bacteria, especially in children, splenectomy should be delayed at least until age 5 years. After this, the small risk of overwhelming *Streptococcus pneumoniae* sepsis can be reduced by the administration of pneumococcal vaccine, given several weeks before surgery.

Hereditary Elliptocytosis (Ovalocytosis)

Similar to HS, hereditary elliptocytosis is also inherited as an autosomal dominant. Again, its genetics and clinical features are quite heterogeneous, but the most common variety is due to a defect in spectrin spectrin self-association. The

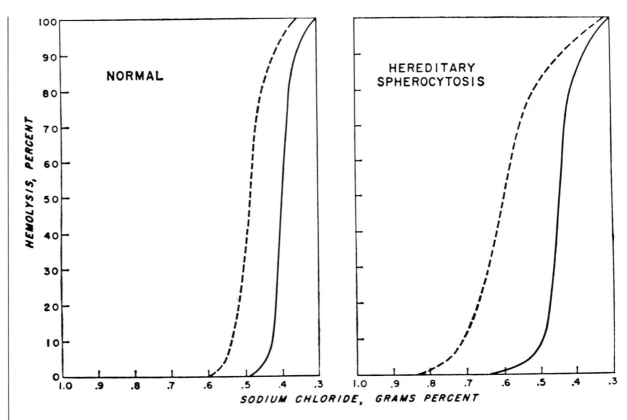

FIGURE 6-10.

Osmotic fragility curves of normal red cells (*left*) and red cells of hereditary spherocytosis (*right*). Curves depict the percentage of red cells hemolyzed after incubation in various concentrations of NaCl. Solid lines depict results with freshly drawn red cells. Dashed lines depict results after 24 hours of aseptic incubation at 37° C. Isotonic NaCl solution is 0.85%.

abnormal cells are cigar-shaped {#25} and have increased osmotic fragility. Although more common than HS (1 per 2,500 US population), only 15% of patients have overt hemolysis. Hemolysis, where present, is eliminated by splenectomy.

Hereditary Stomatocytosis

Hereditary stomatocytosis is a rare autosomal dominant disorder in which the red cell membrane is unusually permeable to Na$^+$, and the red cells gain Na$^+$ and H$_2$O. On peripheral smear, the cells have a slit or mouth-shaped area of central pallor {#29}. The cells maintain a 15- to 30-fold increase in Na$^+$-K$^+$ pump activity in a vain effort to compensate for the sodium leak. Clinically, affected patients have anemia, reticulocytosis, jaundice, and splenomegaly, and they show improvement, but not cure, after splenectomy. The absence of an integral membrane protein called **stomatin** is the putative cause.

Abnormalities of Membrane Lipids

Spur Cell Anemia

Red cell membrane lipids are exchangeable with plasma lipids. Spur cell anemia is an acquired disorder of plasma lipoprotein metabolism seen in patients with severe liver disease. In these patients, plasma low-density lipoproteins have a high cholesterol-to-phospholipid ratio. The erythrocyte membrane accumulates cholesterol and develops a bizarre spiculated appearance (acanthocyte) {#28}. Severe hemolysis occurs, primarily in the spleen.

Hereditary Abetalipoproteinemia (Acanthocytosis)

Hereditary abetalipoproteinemia is a rare autosomal recessive disorder in which the patient produces no plasma β-lipoproteins. As a result, plasma triglyceride, cholesterol and phospholipid levels are very low. Despite the overall decrease in plasma phospholipids, the sphingomyelin-to-lecithin ratio is increased in the plasma and in the red cell membrane. These lipid alterations produce the acanthocyte. Although mild hemolysis occurs in such patients, the concurrent diffuse nervous system abnormalities and malabsorption syndrome are responsible for most of the morbidity.

Students evaluating blood smears should be wary of overinterpreting cells with irregular projections; these are common artifacts of slide preparation, and can be confused with acanthocytes or spur cells.

Hemolysis Due to Fragmentation of the Membrane: The Traumatic Hemolytic Anemias

Hemolysis due to intravascular trauma to red cells may occur in the heart, the large vessels, or the microvasculature. Fibrin is believed to be the cause of the red cell injury. Abnormal or prosthetic heart valves or arterial grafts accumulate fibrin, which may cause the red cells to shear as they pass these shaggy, roughened surfaces. Microvascular endothelial damage, as seen in malignant hypertension or vasculitis, may cause fibrin strands to be deposited across small arterioles and capillaries. As the erythrocyte traverses these small vessels, it is sliced by the fibrin strand like a pancake hitting a wire (Fig. 6-11). The membrane of the fragment may reseal, producing the schistocyte. Some of the fragments do not reseal, and hemoglobin is released intravascularly.

The blood smear is diagnostic. The hallmark of the traumatic hemolytic anemias is the appearance of schistocytes, or red cell fragments {#30} in the peripheral blood. Helmet shapes, triangles, spherocytes and other small pieces may be seen. Hemolysis is primarily intravascular with consequent hemosiderinuria and negative iron balance.

Traumatic Cardiac Hemolytic Anemia

Most patients with prosthetic aortic and mitral valves have chronic, mild, well-compensated intravascular hemolysis. However, severe hemolysis may occur when an edge of an aortic prosthesis separates from the root of the aorta. Blood passing through the roughened slit at systolic velocity and pressure may be badly fragmented. Treatment is iron therapy, transfusion if needed and, for severe hemolysis, removal and replacement of the prosthetic valve.

Microangiopathic Hemolytic Anemias

In the group of disorders known as microangiopathic hemolytic anemias, fibrin strands are strung across the microvasculature or there is severe endothelial

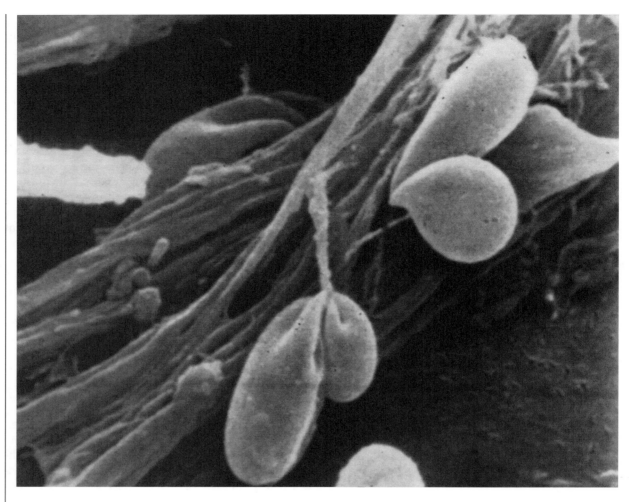

FIGURE 6-11.

An erythrocyte being cut by a fibrin strand in an in vitro model of microangiopathic hemolytic anemia. (From Bull BS, Kuhn IN. The production of schistocytes by fibrin strands: a scanning electron microscope study. *Blood* 35:104.)

damage in the small vessels and red cells fragment as they pass. One condition in which microangiopathic hemolytic anemia occurs is thrombotic thrombocytopenic purpura (TTP). In TTP, platelet thrombi occlude the microvasculature. These thrombi are believed to cause the clinical pentad of renal failure, fluctuating neurologic signs (seizures, paresthesias, coma), fever, thrombocytopenia, and microangiopathic hemolytic anemia.

A similar disorder of small children is called the hemolytic uremic syndrome. It differs from TTP in that neurologic disease is rare, it often follows a viral upper respiratory infection or a *Shigella* or *Escherichia coli* gastroenteritis, and it is only rarely fatal. DIC (Chapter 13), vasculitis, malignant hypertension, disseminated carcinoma, and several complications of pregnancy (preeclampsia, abruptio placentae) also may produce microangiopathic hemolytic anemia.

March Hemoglobinuria

With jogging a national obsession, we must mention march hemoglobinuria, a transient intravascular hemolysis with hemoglobinuria following strenuous running or long-distance walking. The disorder is caused by the pounding of the soles of the feet against a hard surface, with mechanical trauma to the red cells. Hemoglobinuria clears 6 to 12 hours after exercise, and the condition is benign, though

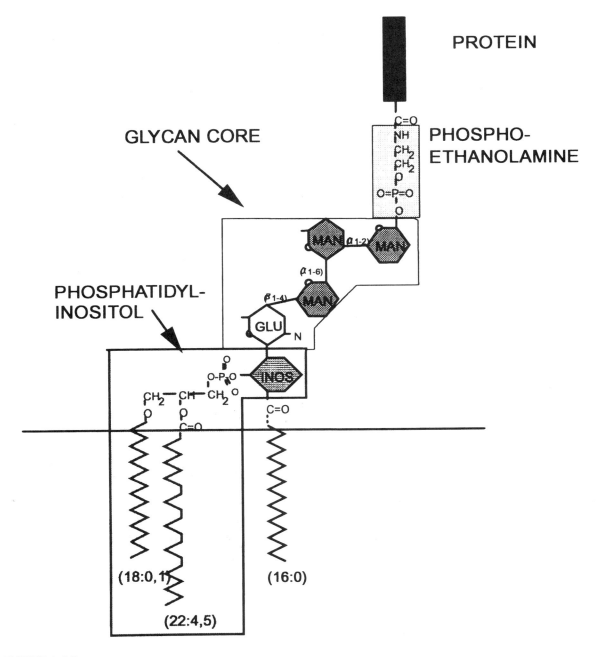

FIGURE 6-12.
The molecular defect in paroxysmal nocturnal hemoglobinuria. Fatty acids below the heavy line are intracellular. The glycan core, phosphoethanolamine, and protein are lost when the glucose-phosphatidylinositol bond is not made by PIG-A. Many different proteins depend on this bond. (From Rosse WF, Ware RE. The molecular basis of paroxysmal nocturnal hemoglobinuria. *Blood* 86:3278.)

frightening. Treatment consists of retraining the runner to alter his or her pounding gait, adding padded insoles to the shoes, or switching to bird watching. (Too much bongo drumming may also result in hemoglobinuria.)

Hemolysis Due to Excessive Sensitivity of the Membrane to Complement: Paroxysmal Nocturnal Hemoglobinuria

PNH is a fascinating acquired membrane disorder characterized by intravascular hemolysis and hemoglobinuria, especially during sleep. Although rare, it has been an important model for the study of the mechanisms of intravascular hemolysis, the pathways of intravascular hemoglobin clearance, and the alternate pathway of complement activation.

PNH is caused by a somatic mutation of the pluripotent marrow stem cell; thus platelets and white cells as well as red cells are affected. The defect is in a gene on the X chromosome called PIG-A. This results in the loss of the glycophosphatidylinositol anchor from the cell membrane. This anchor ordinarily attaches a variety of proteins to the bilayer (Fig. 6-12).

At least 18 red cell membrane proteins are markedly decreased on PNH cells, of which three seem important in the pathogenesis of the disease. These are decay accelerating factor; membrane inhibitor of reactive lysis, and C8-binding protein, all of which normally inactivate complement. When these proteins are reduced or absent, the cells become unable to resist complement attack and intravascular hemolysis ensues. No antibody is needed to evoke the cell destruction.

Patients with PNH have two or three populations of red cells with differing degrees of complement sensitivity. The most sensitive (PNH III cells) have no decay-accelerating factor, are 20 to 30 times more vulnerable than normal, and have a half-life of approximately 6 days, whereas PNH I cells have a normal life span. The degree of hemolysis depends on the proportion of PNH III cells present in the individual. Hemolysis occurs maximally at night and also occurs after exercise, but the mechanism is uncertain. A low pH enhances lysis of PNH cells in vitro, and the small pH changes that occur under these in vivo conditions may be sufficient to activate the system.

The patient with PNH usually has an aplastic or hypoplastic marrow with anemia, leukopenia, and thrombopenia. This has led to the theory that the primary event is marrow damage, followed by the selection of a mutant PNH stem cell clone. As in other marrow stem cell disorders, patients have an increased risk of developing acute leukemia.

In addition to chronic anemia, PNH patients have a high incidence of venous thrombosis, often involving the hepatic veins and portal system. This is thought to be due to the release of red cell membrane lipids during intravascular hemolysis, with activation of the coagulation system. Since PNH platelet membranes also are complement-sensitive, they may contribute to the hypercoagulable state.

Diagnosis

The sucrose hemolysis test suspends red cells in an isotonic low-ionic-strength medium, which aggregates serum globulins onto the red cell surface. This activates small amounts of complement, causing PNH cells, but not normal cells, to lyse. In the acid-serum lysis test (Ham's test), PNH cells lyse in fresh complement-containing serum acidified to a pH of 6.4, whereas normal cells do not."Flow cytometry has replaced the other tests."

Treatment

In intravascular hemolysis, iron in the form of hemosiderin and free hemoglobin is lost in the urine, and the patients are chronically iron-deficient. However, iron replacement in PNH may intensify hemolysis by increasing production of the complement-sensitive red cell population. Iron can be administered safely after the patient has been transfused to normal.

Transfusions are the mainstay of therapy and may be given indefinitely without fear of iron overload. Corticosteroids in doses of 15 to 30 mg every other day may ameliorate hemolysis.

SUMMARY POINTS

The red cell membrane is a very complex structure which evolved in response to the need for increased oxygen carrying capacity. Many different abnormalities of this membrane exist, some hereditary, some acquired. All may result in premature destruction of red cells with subsequent anemia.

CASE DEVELOPMENT PROBLEM: CHAPTER 6

History: A 25-year-old man was referred for evaluation of an enlarged spleen and mild scleral icterus (jaundice) noted on a routine physical examination. The patient's sister was told that she had anemia and a big spleen and had had a splenectomy 2 years earlier.

Laboratory values: HCT 43%; hemoglobin 15.5 g/dL; RBC count $5.1 \times 10^6/\mu L$; reticulocyte count 5%; bilirubin 2.2 mg/dL;.3 mg/dL direct, 1.9 mg/dL indirect; peripheral smear, small cells with loss of central pallor; marrow hyperplastic with G/E = 1:2, but otherwise normal.

1. Calculate the mean corpuscular volume (MCV) and the mean corpuscular hemoglobin concentration (MCHC).
2. Calculate the effective production (reticulocyte) index.
3. Assuming that the patient is in a steady state, what is the destruction index?
4. Describe this process in kinetic terms.
5. (a) What is your tentative hematologic diagnosis? (b) Cite the evidence.
6. What further studies would you want to confirm your diagnosis?
7. An osmotic fragility curve was obtained (**Fig. 6-13**). (a) How do you interpret this? (b) How would this curve change if the cells were incubated for 24 hours at 37° C before doing the osmotic fragility? Why?
8. Why does the patient have an elevated indirect (unconjugated) bilirubin level?
9. (a) Would the patient benefit from splenectomy? (b) Are there any risks associated with splenectomy?
   The patient was advised to have a splenectomy, but he postponed it because of business problems. Four months later, he had an acute onset of right upper quadrant pain, fever, and vomiting. On admission, he had right upper quadrant guarding and tenderness. A gallbladder ultrasonogram revealed multiple stones. A diagnosis of acute cholecystitis was made.
10. What is the likely cause of gallstones in this 25-year-old-man?
    When the acute cholecystitis subsided, the patient had surgery with removal of his gallbladder and spleen.
11. Review the pathophysiology of this anemia and how splenectomy affects the expression of the disease.

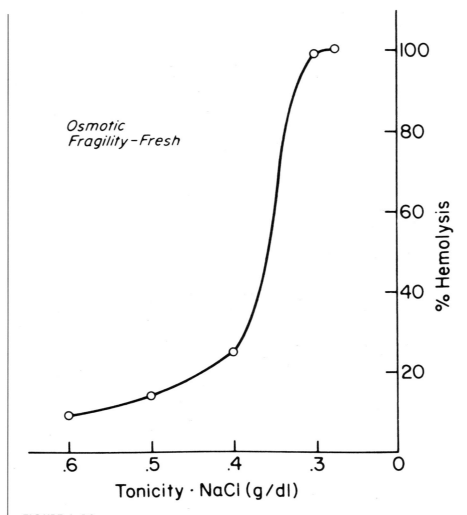

FIGURE 6-13.
Osmotic fragility curve of fresh erythrocytes in a 25-year-old man with an enlarged spleen and mild scleral icterus.

CASE DEVELOPMENT ANSWERS

1 . MCV = $\dfrac{43\%}{5.1}$ × 100 = 84 fL   (normal)

   MCHC = $\dfrac{15.5}{43\%}$ = 36 g/dL (elevated)

2.   RI = 5% × $\dfrac{5.1 \times 10^6/\mu L}{50,000/\mu L}$ × $\dfrac{1}{1}$ = 5 = approximately 5 times normal

3. Five times normal.
4. Compensated hemolysis.
5. (a) Hereditary spherocytosis. (b) Spherocytes are seen in the blood. A sister has had splenectomy, suggesting that she is similarly afflicted.
6. Osmotic fragility test; blood smears, and reticulocyte counts on the patient's parents, siblings, and children.
7. (a) Approximately 25% of the patient's red cells are more sensitive than normal to lysis in hypotonic solutions, due to decreased S:V ratio. (b) After 24 hours of incubation, even more of the patient's cells will lyse prematurely.

They will have metabolized all the available glucose; thus, ATP cannot be generated, and the sodium pump will be unable to extrude the sodium and water that are leaking into the cell.

8. This is due to extravascular hemolysis, with increased production of bilirubin from hemoglobin. The relatively small increase in direct bilirubin attests to the ability of the normal liver to handle a fivefold increase in bilirubin conjugation.

9. (a) The spleen has 1- to 3-μm slit-like spaces in the walls of the sinusoids, which trap the undeformable spherocyte, preventing the spherocyte from returning to the circulation. Splenectomy is curative in all but the most severe cases. (b) There is an increased incidence of overwhelming bacterial infection (septicemia, meningitis), especially in young children. Pneumococcal, meningococcal, and *Haemophilus influenzae* vaccines should be given before splenectomy.

10. The gallstones are probably bilirubin stones caused by the increased load of bilirubin processed by the liver over the years. The risk of gallstones in patients younger than 40 years with hereditary spherocytosis is markedly increased.

Disorders of Globin Synthesis

Edwin A. Azen

OUTLINE

OBJECTIVES

- Understand the basic biochemical differences between the thalassemias and the hemoglobinopathies.
- Explain why babies with β-chain abnormalities are not symptomatic at birth.
- Describe two pathophysiologic processes that underlie sicklemia.
- Describe the vicious cycle of sickle cell disease.
- Explain the properties of globin learned from its disorders.
- Describe three pathophysiologic processes that underlie thalassemia major.
- Explain why α-thalassemia has four degrees of severity.

Normal adult human hemoglobin contains four globin chains, two α and two β. Each globin chain carries a heme group attached at a specific site on the globin molecule (Fig. 7-1). The four globin chains and their four heme groups make up the complete hemoglobin molecule. The other two minor adult human hemoglobins have identical α chains, whereas their non-α chains give them their distinctive properties. The α chains and non-α chains occur as identical pairs. Thus, the chemical structures of the normal adult hemoglobins can be represented as $\alpha_2\beta_2$ [hemoglobin A], $\alpha_2\gamma_2$ [hemoglobin F], and $\alpha_2\delta_2$ [hemoglobin A$_2$].

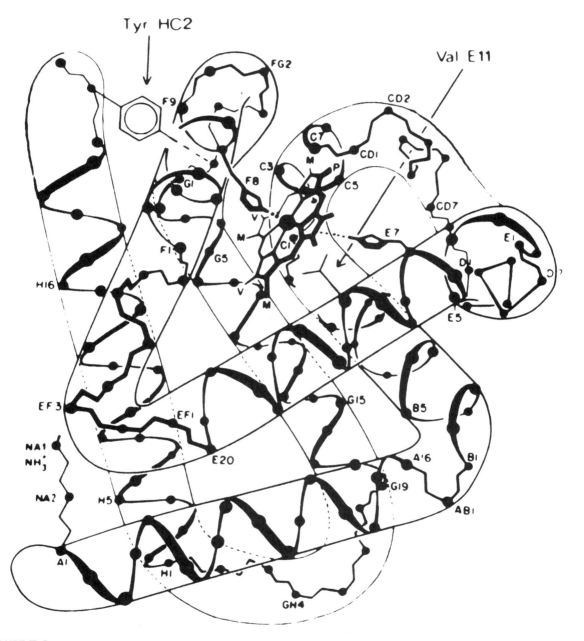

FIGURE 7-1.
Tertiary structure of a globin chain. Globin folds into a tertiary structure such that polar or charged amino acids are located on the exterior of the molecule and the heme ring resides in a hydrophobic niche between the E and F helices. Heme is linked to the proximal (F8) histidine and the distal (E7) histidine. (From Hoffman R, Benz EJ, Jr et al. *Hematology*, 2nd ed. Edinburgh: Churchill Livingstone, p. 460, with permission.)

The value of the detailed chemistry of the hemoglobins is not only what we learn about the pathophysiology of important diseases and their prevention by genetic screening, but also the analogies that can be made among the hemoglobins and many other human proteins. Hemoglobin is probably the best studied of all proteins. The smooth functioning of the synthetic process, the interaction of the subunits, the tertiary structure, and the effect of alterations on the function of heme are understood in great detail. One would predict that all the kinds of errors, and perhaps the numbers, in the synthesis of hemoglobin will be found in other proteins. Proteins such as the clotting factors that may have half concentration by both antigenic and functional methods are analogous to thalassemia, in which defects in synthesis are responsible. Proteins that have full concentration by antigenic methods but poor functional activity are like a hemoglobinopathy in which an amino acid substitution causes altered function.

SYNTHESIS AND GENETIC EXPRESSION OF GLOBINS

Globin-chain genetic loci usually occur in duplicated nonallelic pairs, which differ in their expressions at different stages of development. Most humans have two α genes and an embryonic ζ gene on chromosome 16. The order of the genes from 5' to 3' is ζ-α_2-α_1. Two adult β-type genes, β and δ, two fetal γ-type genes, Gγ- and Aγ- and an embryonic ϵ gene are located on chromosome 11. The order of genes from 5' to 3' is ϵ-Gγ-Aγ-δ-β. The two types of γ-globin genes are distinguished by one amino acid difference, glycine (Gγ) for alanine (Aγ), at the same amino acid position (136). In diploid cells, therefore, there are four α genes, four β-type genes (two β and two δ genes), and four γ genes.

Hemoglobin F ($\alpha_2\gamma_2$) is the major hemoglobin of the fetus; the major hemoglobin of the adult is hemoglobin A ($\alpha_2\beta_2$). δ Chains are produced at a low level in adults (Fig. 7-2). The mechanism of the switch from γ- to β-chain synthesis, which occurs near the time of birth, is not well understood (Fig. 7-3). It probably involves the interaction of cell-specific and ubiquitous transcription factors with promoter and enhancer regions of DNA surrounding the globin genes. This interaction leads to the formation of protein-protein complexes at the promoter region, which enhance gene-specific transcription. The globin genes are transcribed into nuclear RNA, which is subsequently modified by RNA processing. The globin-gene sequences include both those required for encoding the amino acid sequences for the globin and others that are not encoded into the mature mRNA. The latter intervening sequences of DNA (introns), which are encoded in nuclear RNA, are excised in the formation of mature mRNA.

There are two major categories of autosomally inherited abnormalities of globins. In one type, the **hemoglobinopathies**, there are qualitative changes in the globin. This is usually due to a single nucleotide change in the DNA, leading to a single amino acid change. Sickle cell anemia in which there is a change in codon 6 of the β chain to form β^S and hemoglobin S ($\alpha_2\beta_2^S$) is a good example of this type. Hemoglobinopathies are common in populations from regions endemic for malaria, presumably because the abnormal hemoglobins are in some way protective and selective for survival. Other less common qualitative changes include elongated globins and globins that are a product of the fusion of two globin genes.

Hemoglobins S, C, D, Punjab, and E are the common hemoglobin variants. Most of the many hemoglobin variants are rare and often have been discovered by electrophoretic screening. The variants usually cause no hematologic abnormality in the heterozygous state, and the true homozygous (as opposed to mixed heterozygous) state is not often seen because of the rarity of the variant gene. In other hemoglobinopathies, the heterozygotes may be sick owing to the nature of the abnormal globin.

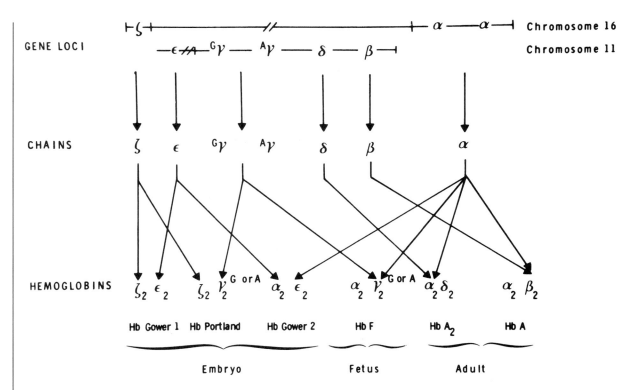

FIGURE 7-2.
The human hemoglobins in the embryo, fetus, and adult. The hierarchy of chromosomes, gene loci, chain monomers, and final products is indicated. (From Weatheral DJ, Clef JB. *The Thalassemia Syndromes*, St. Louis: Blackwell, p. 29.)

The second type of inherited globin abnormality is characterized by decreased amounts of normal globin. These disorders are called **thalassemia syndromes**. In some cases, globin-chain production may be virtually absent.

HEMOGLOBINOPATHIES

Detection of Abnormal Hemoglobins

The abnormal globins are usually detected in the clinical laboratory by electrophoresis of hemoglobin. The different hemoglobins migrate with characteristic mobilities because of differences in charge at the pH of the electrophoretic media. An example of electrophoresis of hemoglobins on cellulose acetate at pH 8.6 is shown in Figure 7-4. More sophisticated biochemical studies of the hemoglobin may be required in selected cases to characterize the hemoglobinopathy; these may include studies of oxygen binding properties, solubility and stability properties, chromatographic isolation, peptide maps, and amino acid sequencing. Polymerase chain reaction (PCR) amplification combined with specific oligonucleotide hybridization and restriction enzyme analysis are being widely applied to prenatal diagnosis and carrier detection.

Hemoglobins that Polymerize (Hemoglobin S)

Mechanism of Aggregation

The hemoglobin S abnormality provides one of the best examples of how an inherited single-point mutation in the DNA can lead to a devastating disease.

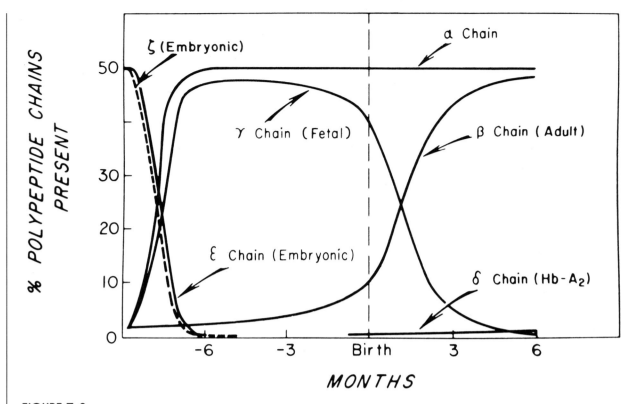

FIGURE 7-3.

Changes in human globin synthesis during prenatal and neonatal development. (From Bunn FH, Forget BG, Ranney HM. *Human Hemoglobins.* Philadelphia: WB Saunders, p. 107.)

Sickle β globin results from a single-point mutation in the sixth codon of the β globin, which leads to the substitution of a hydrophobic valine residue for a negatively charged glutamic acid. The abnormal β S-globin chains then complex with normal α chains to form the hemoglobin S tetramer ($\alpha_2\beta_2^S$). Having the valine on the surface of hemoglobin affects interactions with other hemoglobin molecules without disturbing internal molecular movements related to O_2 binding. The nonpolar valine fits like a lock and key with a hydrophobic pocket of another hemoglobin molecule.

Oxygenated solutions of hemoglobins S and A show similar solubilities, although there are subtle differences in susceptibility to denaturation, and in spectroscopic and optical activities. However, concentrated deoxygenated hemoglobin S and A solutions show strikingly different physical and chemical properties. Deoxygenated hemoglobin S is relatively insoluble compared with hemoglobin A and aggregates into long polymers (Fig. 7-5).

According to a physical model, aggregation occurs in stages. First, in the nucleation stage, hemoglobin S units associate to form aggregates of two, three, and successively larger forms. The early nucleation phase is the rate-limiting step in polymer formation and is sensitive to small changes in temperature, pH, and hemoglobin S concentration. Thus, therapeutic agents that cause only small changes in solubility of hemoglobin S may have profound effects on the rate of gel formation. At some critical stage of growth, further addition of hemoglobin units becomes more favorable energetically. This growth phase represents the formation of the long polymers, which align themselves into tactoids (paracrystalline gels). Studies suggest that the initial polymer consists of two spirally wound linear chains, which later form linear aggregates of 14 laterally interacting polymer chains. The tetramer is oriented so that in one of the two β subunits $\beta6$,

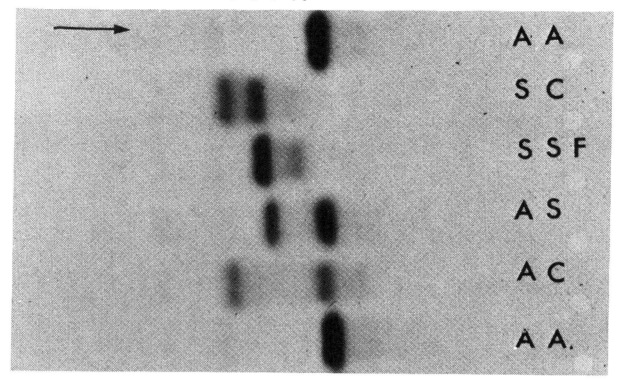

FIGURE 7-4.

Separation of various hemoglobins with electrophoresis on cellulose acetate, pH 8.6. Hemolysates represented are AA (normal adult), SC (hemoglobin SC disease), SSF (homozygous sickle disease, SS, with increased F), AS (sickle trait), and AC (C trait). (From Miale JB. *Laboratory Medicine.* St. Louis: CV Mosby, p. 857.)

valine forms a hydrophobic contact with a complementary site on the β subunit of the partner strand. Viewed on end, the polymers resemble spirals of hemoglobin tetramers stacked on top of each other. Hemoglobin F inhibits polymerization owing to a glutamine residue at $\gamma87$, which prevents a critical lateral contact of the double strand of the sickle fiber.

The most important factor affecting polymerization of hemoglobin S is *oxygen.* Only deoxyhemoglobin S aggregates; other forms of hemoglobin S, such as oxyhemoglobin, carboxyhemoglobin, and methemoglobin, do not aggregate. The process of polymerization is not fully understood, but deoxygenation leads to formation of a sufficient number of intermolecular bonds to stabilize the polymer. The incorporation of hemoglobin S into polymers favors a decrease in oxygen affinity of hemoglobin S, further favoring aggregation. However, nonpolymerized hemoglobin S does not have a decreased binding affinity compared with that of hemoglobin A.

The *concentration* of hemoglobin S is also very important in aggregation. If other factors are held constant, higher concentrations of hemoglobin S lead to striking enhancement of aggregation. Other hemoglobins interact with hemoglobin S either to enhance or to inhibit aggregation. In mixtures of two hemoglobins, hybrid forms may arise. Thus, in a mixture of hemoglobins S and F, intact tetramers ($\alpha_2\beta_2^S$ and $\alpha_2\gamma_2^F$) as well as the hybrid form ($\alpha_2\beta^S\gamma^F$) occur. The intact tetramers of deoxyhemoglobin A and F, as well as hybrids, do not participate in the sickle polymer and reduce the sickling effect by dilution. Hemoglobin F inhibits sickling more than does hemoglobin A; patients with high hemoglobin F have less sickling for the same amount of S hemoglobin than patients with low

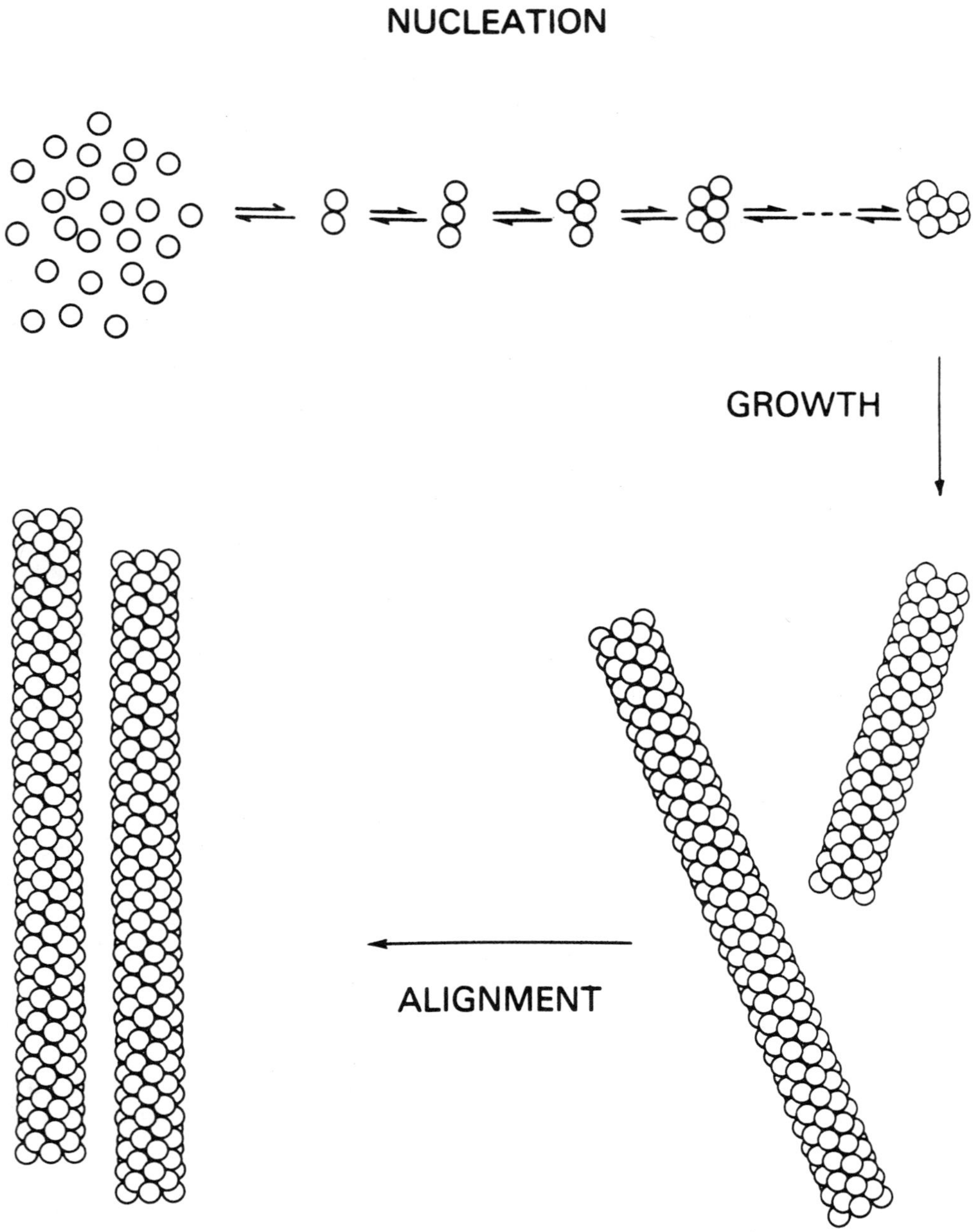

NUCLEATION

FIGURE 7-5.

Possible mechanism of deoxyhemoglobin S polymerization. The hemoglobin S tetramers, represented as spheres, aggregate in solution by multiple steps to form nuclei, which undergo rapid growth and alignment to form the paracrystalline gel. (From Dean J, Schechter AN. Sickle cell anemia: molecular and cellular bases of therapeutic approaches, *N Engl J Med* 299:761.)

hemoglobin F. Further, increased hemoglobin F is accompanied by a poorly understood decrease in hemoglobin S. The sparing effect of hemoglobin F on sickling is the basis for current treatment efforts.

The sickling of the intact red cell is primarily due to polymerization of hemoglobin S and not to alterations of the cell membrane, although secondary changes occur in the membrane. Intracellular polymerization deforms the red cell membrane into the characteristic sickle forms (Fig. 7-6). Pure deoxyhemoglobin S in solution behaves the same as it does in the cell.

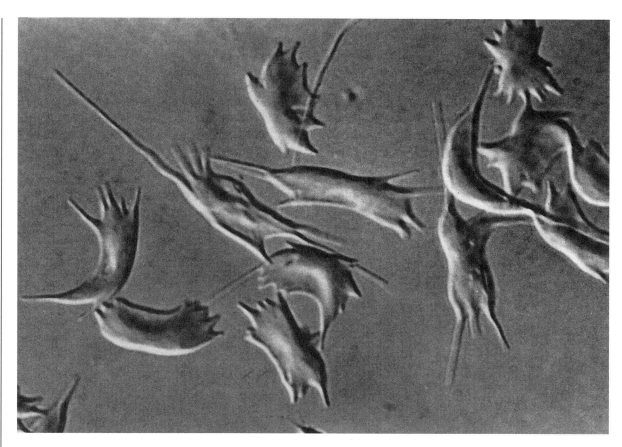

FIGURE 7-6.

Sickle cells seen with the interference microscope. (From Bessis M. *Living Blood Cells and Their Ultrastructure*. New York: Springer-Verlag, Fig. 19-6.

Another factor affecting aggregation is pH. Lowering the pH from 8.5 to 6.5 decreases oxygen affinity by the Bohr effect, which increases the amount of deoxyhemoglobin and promotes aggregation. The low pH in the renal medulla makes the kidney subject to damage from sickling. Increase in *2,3-bis-phosphoglycerate* (2,3-BPG) also stabilizes the deoxygenated structure and promotes aggregation.

Two secondary changes occur in the red cell membrane because of repeated sickling: one leads to increased viscosity; the other to increased adherence to endothelium. The red cell membrane is damaged and fragments are lost when the cell is sickled. There is also an influx of calcium, activating K^+-specific channels in the membrane with enhanced loss of K^+ and water, probably associated with an influx of Na^+. Cell dehydration enhances further sickling. In addition, there is adenosine triphosphate (ATP) depletion.

Sickle erythrocytes also have an affinity for endothelium, which in some cases leads to attachments that exceed the shear forces found in the circulation. Microvascular endothelial cells and subpopulations of sickle reticulocytes express CD36, which binds to thrombospondin secreted by platelets and endothelial cells. Thus, thrombospondin can act as a bridging molecule between sickle red cells and endothelium. The state of *endothelial cell activation* is important for adhesion of sickle cells. Inflammatory cytokines such as tumor necrosis factor (TNF)-α are generated by infections, trauma, or stress. These cytokines act on endothelium to increase the expression of endothelial adhesion factors (e.g., ICAM-1 [intercellular adhesion molecule-1]). Sickled cells have increased receptors for these adhesion factors (e.g., $\alpha_4\beta_1$, an integrin molecule) (Fig. 7-7).

Transit time through the tissues is also important. Erythrocytes must be exposed to low oxygen tension for more than 60 seconds for sickling to occur. The normal circulation time is less than 60 seconds. However, a fall in blood pressure, prolonged inactivity, a clot, or a local pileup of sickle cells all lead to delay in return of blood to the lung. There is also a population of dense cells high in hemoglobin S released from the marrow. Some of these cells are already irreversibly sickled. Moreover, in some tissues such as the spleen, long circulation times are normal. Thus, the protective effect of rapid transit back to the lung may be thwarted.

In summary, sickling is enhanced by the following:

- Decreased oxygen
- Increased 2,3-BPG
- Increased intracellular hemoglobin S concentration
- Decreased pH
- Endothelial adhesion
- Slowed transit time through the circulation

Physiologic Consequences

The physiologic consequences of sickling are many. There is a constant baseline level of sickling. These sickle cells are unable to easily navigate through the small pores and channels of the spleen and are sequestered there and destroyed,

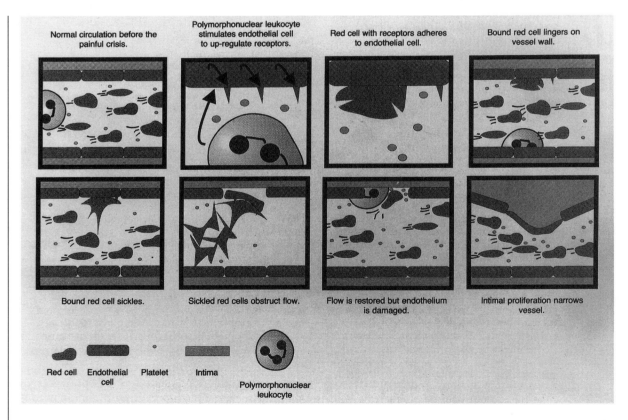

FIGURE 7-7.
Sequence of proposed interactions between endothelium and SS red cells in painful crises. (From Platt OS. *N Engl J Med* 330:783.)

leading to hemolytic anemia. In adults, the spleen is often infarcted by this sickling process (autosplenectomy), and sequestration of red cells may occur in other organs, especially the liver. When four or five of the factors that enhance sickling come into play, as when the patient has pneumonia, increased numbers of sickles form, and blood viscosity increases dramatically. Sickled cells stick to endothelium and jam like barbed wire in the capillaries (Fig. 7-7). This may lead to loss of the endothelial cell or delay in red cell transit. The flow of blood in the microcirculation slows, and more oxygen is extracted from the red cells by the metabolic needs of the tissues, thus starting the "vicious viscous sickle cycle." Sickle cell blockage of vessels accounts for the clinical manifestations of pain and tissue necrosis.

Sickling Diseases

The term "sickle cell disease" indicates a genetic disease with symptomatic sickling. Although the sickle diseases often lead to increased mortality, there is evidence that the sickle gene protects against malaria. The sickle cell gene is found mainly in people from sub-Saharan Africa, but also is found among Greeks, Italians, Saudis, Israeli Arabs, and Veddoids of southern India. The major sickle cell diseases include sickle cell anemia S/S disease (β^S/β^S); in addition, people who are mixed heterogeneous for β^S and β^C (lysine at position 6) or β^S and β^T (β-thalassemia) are prone to sickling. The β^C and β^T genes probably also provide a selective advantage against malaria. By one estimate, the incidences of the three most common sickle cell diseases in the African-American population are S/S (1 in 1875); S/C (1 in 1250); and S/thal (1 in 3333). The other sickle cell diseases are much rarer.

There is a wide spectrum of clinical severity among the sickling disorders. Hemoglobin S/S disease tends to be the most severe, and S/C disease the least severe, although many exceptions occur. The textbook description of S/S disease is that of a very severe disorder with early death; however, many cases in the population are mild or virtually asymptomatic. Fifty percent of patients survive beyond the fifth decade. Early mortality is highest among symptomatic patients. The sickle cell mutation is thought to have occurred at least four times, that is, in four different genetic backgrounds. Modifying genetic factors, such as a high concentration of fetal hemoglobin or the presence of coexisting α-thalassemia, are thought to diminish the severity of the disease. Often the reason why the disease is mild is not known.

The manifestations of sickle cell disease can be divided into two pathophysiologic processes: hemolytic anemia and microinfarction of tissues. The anemia is due to increased red cell destruction (hemolysis). Anemia leads to markedly increased erythropoiesis in the bone marrow. Enlarged marrow cavities deform the bones in extreme cases {#106}. Temporary decline in erythropoiesis due to infection (aplastic crisis) may lead to severe anemia and heart failure. The greatly increased erythropoiesis increases the requirement for folic acid.

The patient with sickle disease is subject to a lifelong body-wide destructive process caused by occlusion of the microvasculature with ischemic death (infarction) of tissue. Clinical expressions of the organ damage are complex. Microinfarctions in tissues lead to chronic pain, impaired growth and development, and increased susceptibility to bacterial infections. The susceptibility to infections is related to impaired splenic function due to sickle cell thromboses in the spleen, monocyte-macrophage blockade from cell debris, and decreased opsonization of bacteria. Very severe pleural, abdominal, bone, and muscular pains are common. These are called "painful crises."

In sickling disease, any tissue of the body may be affected. Brain infarcts may result in strokes and seizures. There may be blindness due to retinal infarcts {#107}, detachment, and vitreous hemorrhages. Pulmonary infarctions and infections lead to lung destruction, pulmonary hypertension, and subsequent cardiac failure {#108}. Splenic sequestration crisis in babies may be fatal. This is a syndrome of pneumococcal sepsis and a rapidly enlarging spleen, resulting in acute severe anemia and shock. In adults, the spleen is frequently infarcted, atrophic, and nonfunctional. The liver may be severely damaged by infarction, and there is increased gallbladder disease due to bilirubin stones {#109}. Acute abdominal pain often mimics a surgical emergency. Hematuria, inability to produce concentrated urine, and renal failure are also seen. Painful swelling of the hands and feet (dactylitis) is seen in early childhood {#111}. Bone infarctions occur in many long bones, especially the femurs {#109}. Patients are peculiarly susceptible to *Salmonella* osteomyelitis {#110}. Acute monoarticular or polyarticular arthritis may occur. Aseptic necrosis of the femoral head leads to permanent crippling {#112}. Chronic leg ulcers are seen {#113}, especially around the ankles. Priapism {#114} often leads to impotence. Many deaths occur among those who have had no previous organ failure during an acute episode of pain, respiratory failure, or stroke.

The heterozygous A/S (β^A/β^S) trait found in 10% of African Americans is asymptomatic and should not be considered a disease. In special situations, however, such as flying at high altitudes in unpressurized aircraft, A/S individuals may have splenic infarction. Commercial flights do not create a hazard, but it is prudent for those with the sickle cell trait to avoid exposure to low ambient oxygen. In addition, persons with sickle cell trait may have painless hematuria and an impairment in the ability to produce concentrated urine owing to renal medullary vascular abnormalities. *The renal medulla is hypoxic, acidic, and hyperosmolar*—conditions that are ideal for sickling. Denial of employment or of life or health insurance to those with sickle cell trait on the grounds of increased risk of illness or death is not justified and is illegal under the laws of several states.

DIAGNOSIS OF SICKLE DISORDERS

The available screening tests for sickle hemoglobin include solubility tests, techniques to induce sickling, and hemoglobin electrophoresis. Several solubility tests are commercially available for detection of sickle hemoglobin; these depend on the decreased solubility of deoxygenated hemoglobin S in phosphate buffer solutions. In these tests, more hemoglobin precipitates from a solution containing hemoglobin S than from the control solution containing hemoglobin A. Solubility tests do not reliably distinguish the sickle trait from the various sickle diseases. A less common screening test is the sodium metabisulfite test. When this agent is added to red cells, it induces sickling by reducing oxygen tension {#36} It also does not distinguish the sickle trait from the sickle diseases.

The most reliable clinical test for sickling disorders is hemoglobin electrophoresis, which identifies sickle cell disease and many related disorders. In hemoglobin S/S disease, hemoglobin electrophoresis shows 80% to 95% hemoglobin S, 0% to 20% hemoglobin F, and a normal amount of hemoglobin A_2. In hemoglobin A/S trait (β^A/β^S), electrophoresis shows about 35% hemoglobin S and 60% hemoglobin A. In hemoglobin S/β–thalassemia (β^S/β^T), most of the hemoglobin is S, and hemoglobin A is low or even absent. Hemoglobin A_2 may be increased. In some doubly heterozygous states, such as in hemoglobin S/C {#39} (β^S/β^C) disease, both hemoglobins are present in about equal proportions.

The blood smear in sickle trait (β^A/β^S) is normal; sickled cells are not seen. In homozygotes (β^S/β^S), the major features of the blood smear are irreversibly sickled forms and polychromatophilia {#35}. The sickled forms usually are seen only after a child reaches 5 years of age, after splenic atrophy from infarction. In hemoglobin S/β thal (β^S/β^T), the blood smear shows hypochromic and microcytic red cells, polychromatophilia, target cells, and sickle cells.

PREVENTION AND TREATMENT OF SICKLING DISEASES

All newborns in most states are screened for sickle hemoglobin (and some other hemoglobinopathies) by electrophoresis of hemoglobins. Public education, screening, and genetic counseling should play an important role in preventing sickle cell anemia. There is a 25% chance that offspring will have S/S disease if both parents are carriers. Diagnosis of the S/S disease is now possible early in pregnancy. DNA from fetal amniotic fluid cells (at 16 to 18 weeks) or chorionic villi (at 10 to 12 weeks) is directly studied for the β-globin gene.

Treatment for sickle cell disease is directed at the patient's symptoms. The painful crises may be triggered by chilling, infections, acidosis, or dehydration. Often the precipitating cause is unknown. Intravenous fluids and narcotics are usually necessary. Acidosis or hypoxia, when present, needs prompt attention. Since affected patients have an increased susceptibility to bacterial infections, any infection must be treated early and vigorously with antibiotics. Blood transfusions are seldom indicated for anemia, but extensive transfusions may be necessary during aplastic crisis. Sometimes exchange transfusions are used in preparation for surgery. Folic acid supplementation is often helpful.

There are a number of novel approaches to prevent and treat the sickle cell crisis, but few have been shown clinically applicable. Some agents can inhibit hemoglobin S polymerization. However, these antisickling drugs are too toxic for clinical use. Some treatments can lower intracellular hemoglobin concentration, such as induction of hyponatremia with osmotic swelling of red cells, but the treatment is too cumbersome for clinical use. Progress has been made in using certain agents as clotrimazole and Mg^{2+} to retard K^+ and water loss from SS red cells, and clinical evaluations are just beginning.

Since evidence is abundant that hemoglobin F inhibits sickling, drugs that increase production of hemoglobin F might benefit patients with sickle cell disease. Among these drugs, hydroxyurea is in widespread use to stimulate hemoglobin F production. A national multicenter clinical trial showed the drug to be relatively nontoxic and effective in reducing the frequency and severity of painful crisis. Bone marrow transplantation may be curative but is rarely applicable.

Hemoglobins That Crystallize (Hemoglobin C)

Hemoglobin C disease is found in people of African descent and is clinically important mainly when combined with hemoglobin S, as in hemoglobin SC disease. About 3% of African Americans are A/C heterozygotes, and 1 in 10,000 is a CC homozygote. The C trait (A/C) is asymptomatic with a normal red blood count. In the blood smear of the homozygote, most red cells are target cells, and there are rare intraerythrocytic crystals. The mechanism of target cell formation is unknown. In hemoglobin C, lysine replaces glutamic acid in the sixth position of the β chain.

Patients who are homozygotes (β^C/β^C) have mild to moderate hemolytic anemia. The shortened life span of C/C red cells is due to their increased rigidity, leading to splenic sequestration, and crystallization of hemoglobin C {#33}. Crystallization of hemoglobin occurs in the red cell and is enhanced if the cells are deoxygenated or dehydrated.

Red cells of people with compound heterozygosity (β^S and β^C) will sickle. Indeed, hemoglobin S/C disease is more prevalent than S/S disease in older adults, even though the gene frequency for S is higher than that for C at birth.

This is because S/C disease is milder and causes fewer deaths in the younger age groups. The spleen is usually enlarged in the adult with S/C disease, but infarcted in S/S disease. The peripheral blood smear in S/C disease reveals numerous target and sickle cells and polychromatophilia. Sometimes intracellular crystals are seen.

Hemoglobins That Denature (Hemoglobin Köln)

An unstable hemoglobin should be suspected if the patient has a congenital hemolytic anemia. Hemoglobin Köln, one of the more common abnormalities, has been described repeatedly in different families around the world. In this abnormality, amino acid mutations and deletions often occur in the vicinity of the heme pocket and disrupt the stability of the heme-globin linkage. These abnormalities lead to precipitation of the abnormal hemoglobin within the red cells. The hemoglobin precipitates and "Heinz bodies" are detected by supravital stains as 1- to 2-μm particles, often attached to the membrane. The Heinz bodies usually are not seen except after splenectomy. Although these are rare disorders, more than 60 different types have been seen.

Electrophoretic separation of the variant hemoglobin from hemoglobin A may be difficult. The severity of the hemolysis is variable, and many persons do not require treatment. In severe cases, splenectomy may lead to improvement in the anemia.

Hemoglobins That Alter Iron Valence (Hemoglobin M)

Congenital methemoglobinemia is very rare and is a cause of familial cyanosis. Most of these variant hemoglobins (e.g., hemoglobin M Milwaukee) have substitution of a tyrosine for the proximal or distal heme-associated histidines in α or β chains. It is postulated that the tyrosine forms a covalent link with the heme iron, stabilizing it in the ferric, non–oxygen-combining form. The presumptive diagnosis of M hemoglobins is made from abnormal absorption spectroscopy and hemoglobin electrophoresis.

The patient with hemoglobin M appears cyanotic (blue) and the blood is brown, but no treatment is required or available for this benign condition. It is important to diagnose this rare disorder, however, to reassure the patient and prevent the mistaken impression that the patient has cyanosis due to some other disorder, such as heart or lung disease. (Note the other causes of methemoglobinemia in Chapter 8).

Hemoglobins That Alter Oxygen Affinity (Hemoglobin Chesapeake)

The uncommon disorders that alter oxygen affinity actually shift the oxygen dissociation curve to the left, resulting in impaired release of oxygen to the tissues. The amino acid substitutions lead to impaired heme-heme interactions during oxygenation. If there is no interaction between the heme groups, as is the case in myoglobin, the oxygen dissociation curve is a rectangular hyperbola.

In familial erythrocytosis due to abnormal globin (e.g., hemoglobin Chesapeake), mean hemoglobin values are about 20 g/dL. The elevated hematocrit causes increased blood viscosity and increases the risk of strokes and myocardial infarction. Phlebotomy may be required to reduce the viscosity, but this treatment should be used sparingly, since the increased red cell mass is compensating for tissue hypoxia. The concentration of hemoglobin varies inversely with the $P_{50}O_2$ (partial pressure of oxygen at 50% saturation). Hemoglobin electrophoresis frequently fails to separate the abnormal hemoglobin from hemoglobin A. Therefore, measurement of the oxygen affinity of the hemoglobin is necessary to confirm the diagnosis.

THE THALASSEMIAS

Geography and Genetics

The thalassemias are hereditary dysfunctions in the synthesis of normal globin polypeptide chains. These disorders primarily affect Southern European, African and Asian peoples. Heterozygous thalassemia, like heterozygous β^S and β^C, is believed to protect the heterozygote against malaria. Other blood abnormalities associated with increased resistance to malaria include glucose-6-phosphate dehydrogenase (G6PD) deficiency, ovalocytosis, and absence of the Duffy a and b (Fy^a, Fy^b) erythrocyte membrane antigens. About 10% of Sicilian and Greek populations are heterozygous for β-thalassemia. In some areas of Greece and Sardinia, the incidence may be as high as 20%. α-Thalassemia genes are common in East Asian and African American populations.

Pathophysiology

The thalassemias have several different molecular mechanisms but are discussed together because of the common feature of unbalanced globin synthesis. In β-thalassemia syndromes, there is a marked decrease of β-chain synthesis compared with α-chain synthesis. α–Thalassemia is different in that there is a deficit of α chains and a relative excess of β chains.

The three major causes of anemia in thalassemia are (1) decreased globin synthesis, (2) ineffective erythropoiesis, and (3) hemolysis. There are also three minor contributions to the anemia: splenic pooling of blood, interference with heme synthesis by excess iron, and folic acid deficiency.

First, reduced synthesis of globin blocks hemoglobin production, resulting in hypochromic microcytic erythrocytes. This is true for all homozygous and some heterozygous states. Heme synthesis also is impaired by accumulation of heme intermediates as a consequence of decreased globin synthesis. Second, the imbalance of globin-chain production leads to accumulation of free globin chains in red cells and their marrow precursors. In homozygous β-thalassemia (thalassemia major; Cooley's anemia), excess normal α chains accumulate in marrow normoblasts and circulating red cells because there are virtually no β-globin chains to oligomerize with them. The α chains aggregate and precipitate within the cells and attach to the cell membranes. These precipitated α-chain bodies (Heinz bodies) lead to membrane damage and premature destruction of red cells and their precursors. By contrast, in α-thalassemia, excess β and γ chains form soluble tetramers as well as precipitates. $\beta4$ is hemoglobin H, and $\gamma4$ is hemoglobin Bart's. Because of their high oxygen affinity, hemoglobins H and Bart's do not deliver oxygen to the tissues. Hemoglobin H is also unstable and forms inclusion bodies (hemoglobin H bodies), which the spleen removes.

The inclusion body formation in α- and β-thalassemia is largely responsible for the markedly ineffective erythropoiesis (intramedullary destruction of red cells) and hemolytic anemia that are seen. Since α chains precipitate more readily than β and γ chains, ineffective erythropoiesis is much more a characteristic of β- than α-thalassemia. Because the spleen removes inclusion bodies from red cells, inclusions virtually never are seen in the presence of the spleen. Ineffective erythropoiesis leads to massive expansion of erythroid precursors in the bone marrow. The bone marrow cavity expansion leads to thinning and deformity of bones.

In β-thalassemia, hemoglobin F is irregularly distributed in the red cells. The cells that have the most hemoglobin F have the least excess of α chains, since the γ chains combine with the α chains to form hemoglobin F ($\alpha_2\gamma_2^F$). Thus, red cells that contain a larger amount of hemoglobin F survive longer than those with less hemoglobin F. The large spleen associated with homozygous thalassemia destroys red cells and other blood elements and also is a large pool for erythrocytes, thus contributing to the anemia.

The anemia of thalassemia is aggravated by folic acid deficiency because of the high folic acid requirement of the hyperplastic marrow. Iron overload is another problem in thalassemia. Iron stores accumulate because of increased gastrointestinal absorption of iron and numerous blood transfusions. Excess iron in the mitochondria of erythroid precursor cells leads to decreased functioning of mitochondrial heme-synthesizing enzymes.

β-Thalassemia

Molecular Pathology

Two major types of β-thalassemia abnormalities, β^+ and β^0, are recognized. Most thalassemias are due to mutations near or within the β-globin gene and affect the β-gene complex on the same (*cis*) chromosome. These mutations lead to decreased (β^+) or absent (β^0) β-globin synthesis. The classification of thalassemia genetic abnormalities is as follows:

- Transcription mutants. There are nucleotide substitutions in the important DNA sequences (TATA box and CAT box) located upstream (5') from the start of the RNA transcription (Cap) site. These sequences normally set the level of RNA transcription and the actual start of RNA synthesis.
- Deletions and crossovers of β-globin–like genes. Deletions may rarely occur at the locus-controlling regions located many kilobases upstream from their regulated globin genes and lead to complete transcription silencing of these genes. Although most β-thalassemias are not associated with obvious gene deletions, δ-/β-thalassemia is an example of extensive deletion in the β-gene cluster. Hemoglobin Lepore, in which there is unequal crossing-over between β and δ genes, leads to a decrease in β-globin RNA synthesis .
- Splice junction mutants that occur at the invariant nucleotides at the splice sites (GT—AG).
- Other splice junction mutants that occur at the splice sites but not in the invariant nucleotides.
- Internal intervening sequence mutants, which involve nucleotide changes at sites that generate new splicing signals.
- Coding region mutants that affect RNA processing, which may activate nearby cryptic donor-like sites.
- Mutations within the sequence AATAAA at the 3' end of the gene, which signals RNA cleavage and addition of the poly A tail.
- Mutations affecting mRNA function, which occur within β-gene coding sequences and render the final mRNA nonfunctional; these include nonsense mutations, small deletions, or insertions with frame shifts.

Since there is genetic heterogeneity of the globin abnormalities with many different molecular defects and varying degrees of functional impairment, symptoms are variable. Different molecular defects may sometimes produce similar clinical manifestations. Thus, there may be absent or mild clinical effects (thalassemia minor), disease of intermediate severity (thalassemia intermedia), or severe disease with early death (thalassemia major).

Clinical Features

HETEROZYGOUS β-THALASSEMIA (THALASSEMIA MINOR)

Thalassemia minor is usually not a disease. The patients are likely asymptomatic, and the disorder may be suspected when there is mild anemia with low mean corpuscular volume (MCV) on routine blood counts. Hemoglobin levels are usually 10 to 11 g/dL. The MCV is typically 55 to 70 fL. The mean corpuscular hemoglobin concentration (MCHC) is not usually as low as in iron deficiency, despite microcytosis. The peripheral smear shows microcytosis, hypochromia, and anisocytosis and poikilocytosis, with targeting and basophilic stippling of red cells. Erythroid hyperplasia is found in the marrow. Splenomegaly occurs in about one third of cases.

It is important to distinguish iron deficiency from thalassemia trait. Use of iron therapy in thalassemia is ineffective and may be harmful by contributing to the excess iron in the body. Features of thalassemia and iron deficiency are compared in Table 7-1. Accurate diagnosis depends on determination of hemoglobin A_2 levels and the measurement of serum iron and iron-binding capacities. A combination of hematologic and genetic analysis of the patient and family members may be necessary. Finally, because heterozygous β-thalassemia and iron deficiency are both common, a patient may have both.

Several types of heterozygous β-thalassemias can be distinguished on the basis of hemoglobin electrophoresis and quantitative assays of the hemoglobins. $β^+$-thalassemia characteristically shows increased hemoglobin A_2 (4% to 6%) and F (2% to 5%) and a variable amount of hemoglobin A. In the uncommon $δ$-/$β$-thalassemia (F-thalassemia), hemoglobin F is increased (5% to 20%) and A_2 is normal or decreased.

HOMOZYGOUS β OR COMPOUND HETEROZYGOUS THALASSEMIA

In many cases the clinical course of thalassemia major is severe, although the disease is not evident at birth because of the preponderance of hemoglobin F. A few months after birth, abnormalities gradually appear: hypochromic microcytic anemia, splenomegaly, hepatomegaly, prominent frontal, and maxillary bone enlargement (bossing). The skull x-ray demonstrates expansion of the marrow cavity. Infections, pathologic bone fractures, splenomegaly with associated leukopenia and thrombopenia, and impaired growth and development occur. Iron

TABLE 7-1. Differentiation of β-Thalassemia From Iron Deficiency Anemia

	β-Thalassemia Minor	Iron Deficiency
Definitive Tests		
Hemoglobin electrophoresis		
Hemoglobin A_2	Increased	Decreased
Hemoglobin F	± Increased	Normal
Serum iron	Normal	Decreased
TIBC	Normal	Increased
Associated Findings		
MCV/red cell (RBC) ratio	<13	>13
RBC protoporphyrin	Normal	Increased
RBC morphology	Very abnormal	Minor changes
Serum ferritin	Normal–high	Low
Bilirubin	Increased	Decreased
Dominant inheritance	Yes	No

MCV, mean corpuscular volume; RBC, red blood cell; TIBC, total iron-binding capacity.
From Bunn FH, Forget BG, Ranney HM: Human Hemoglobins. Philadelphia: WB Saunders, p. 169.

overload damages the heart, liver, pancreas, and other organs. Death may occur in childhood or early adulthood.

The anemia is usually severe. The peripheral blood is marked by erythrocyte hypochromia, anisocytosis and poikilocytosis, target cells, polychromasia, and basophilic stippling {#38}. Normoblasts may also be present. The bone marrow shows erythroid hyperplasia, and supravital stain {#39} shows inclusion bodies (α-chain aggregates) in the normoblasts.

On hemoglobin electrophoresis of the usual high A_2, β^+-thalassemia, a variable amount of hemoglobin A is found. Hemoglobin F is elevated from 10% to 90% of the total hemoglobin and is irregularly distributed in the red cells. The ratio of hemoglobin A_2 to hemoglobin A is higher than the normal ratio of 1:40. Hemoglobin A is totally absent in β^0-thalassemia.

In the uncommon homozygous form of δ-/β-thalassemia, affected persons have mild anemia (9 to 10 g/dL). This is mainly because the synthesis of γ chains is more efficient than in the β^+ and β^0 forms of thalassemia. Because there is no δ- and β-chain synthesis, patients have 100% hemoglobin F and no hemoglobin A or A_2.

α-Thalassemia

Molecular Pathology

The α-globin genes are tandemly duplicated such that the genes and flanking sequences are highly homologous. The high homology predisposes the α-globin gene cluster to unequal crossover events, deletions, and reduplications. There are also nondeletion mutations similar to those described for β-thalassemia.

Because there are four α-globin genes, there are four potential α-thalassemia syndromes compared with two for β-thalassemia. In East Asian populations, both α genes are commonly deleted from the same chromosome. Thus, the combination of two of these chromosome defects would allow fetal death. In contrast, it is uncommon for two α genes to be deleted from one chromosome in Mediterranean and African American populations; it is more common in these populations for one α gene to be deleted from a chromosome. Thus, the incidence of α-thalassemia trait ($\alpha\alpha^T/\alpha\alpha^T$, α thal 1) and the silent carrier trait ($\alpha\alpha/\alpha\alpha^T$, α thal 2) is significant in these groups, whereas the incidence of hydrops fetalis $\alpha^T\alpha^T/\alpha^T\alpha^T$) and hemoglobin H ($\alpha\alpha^T/\alpha^T\alpha^T$) disease is negligible. In southeast Asia, both types of chromosomes are common and thus α-thalassemia is characterized by a deletion of one to four α-globin gene loci.

In some populations, an α-gene termination mutant determines hemoglobin Constant Spring (CS), which for unknown reasons is produced in small amounts. Hemoglobin CS contains two normal β chains and two elongated α chains, which have 31 additional amino acids at their C-terminal ends. Thus, CS disease behaves like an α-thalassemia defect. For example, when a *CS* gene is combined with two α-thalassemia genes of the usual type, hemoglobin H disease is produced. In some populations (as in Saudi Arabia and the Mediterranean region), the α genes are present, but their control or function is impaired. This also leads to decreased α-globin production.

Clinical Features

As with β-thalassemia, there is great genetic heterogeneity with many different defects of the α-globin genes that lead to a variety of clinical types, as described below.

α-THALASSEMIA 2

When one α-chain gene is thalassemic ($\alpha\alpha/\alpha\alpha^T$), the affected person is not sick and diagnosis is usually inferred from a family study. In the cord blood of neonates, there are increased γ chains forming Bart's hemoglobin (γ4), which disappear after 6 months of life.

α-THALASSEMIA 1

When two α-chain genes are thalassemic ($\alpha\alpha^T/\alpha\alpha^T$), there is microcytosis and hypochromia of the red cells, with mild anisocytosis and poikilocytosis and hemoglobin that is mildly depressed (10 to 12 g/dL). Bart's hemoglobin (γ4) is increased in the cord blood of neonates but disappears after 6 months of life.

HEMOGLOBIN H DISEASE

When three α-chain genes are thalassemic ($\alpha\alpha^T/\alpha^T\alpha^T$), there is a chronic hemolytic anemia with a hemoglobin level usually about 8 to 10 g/dL. In the newborn, 20% to 40% of hemoglobin is Bart's, and this is replaced in older children and adults by hemoglobin H (β4), which varies between 5% and 30%. As many as 50% of East Asians with hemoglobin H disease also have 3% to 5% hemoglobin CS.

The peripheral blood smear shows hypochromia, microcytosis, poikilocytosis, polychromasia, and targeting of red cells. When the blood is incubated with brilliant cresyl blue, there is in vitro precipitation of excess β chains (hemoglobin H; β4) as multiple speckled bodies. Anemia may become more severe after ingestion of oxidant drugs that accelerate oxidation and precipitation of hemoglobin H. The diagnosis is confirmed by hemoglobin electrophoresis.

HYDROPS FETALIS

When four α-chain genes are thalassemic ($\alpha^T\alpha^T/\alpha^T\alpha^T$), the affected fetus is stillborn prematurely or dies at birth. The peripheral blood smear shows hypochromia and nucleated red cells. Hemoglobin electrophoresis shows hemoglobin Bart's (γ4) predominantly. Hemoglobin Bart's, like Hemoglobin H, has a very high oxygen affinity and cannot deliver oxygen to the tissues. The cause of death is liver failure, however, rather than heart failure as was previously thought. The liver is engorged with nucleated red cells (extramedullary hematopoiesis). Hypoxia no doubt contributes to the death of the fetus.

Prevention and Treatment of Thalassemia

Prenatal diagnosis of thalassemia is possible in a limited number of medical centers. To prevent the occurrence in children of severe homozygous α- or β-thalassemia, high-risk populations should be screened to detect thalassemia trait. If both prospective parents show the β-thalassemia trait, they should be informed that the chance of having a severely affected child is one in four.

In recent studies, the diagnosis of many types of thalassemia can be made by studying the DNA of fibroblasts cultured from fetal amniotic fluid cells. It is easier and safer to aspirate amniotic fluid cells rather than obtain blood cells from the placenta. Chorionic villus sampling permits DNA analysis in the first trimester of pregnancy. Oligonucleotide probes that are specific for thalassemia mutations are hybridized to PCR-amplified DNAs from the globin genes and thus permit accurate prenatal diagnosis. Also, hydrops fetalis, hereditary persistence of fetal hemoglobin, and δ-/β-thalassemia, characterized by DNA deletions, were readily diagnosed using molecular techniques. Screening programs have greatly reduced the incidence of β-thalassemia major in several populations, including Sardinian, Greek, Turkish, and Italian.

The treatment of the severely affected homozygous thalassemia patient is mainly supportive. Regular transfusions are given to reduce the severe effects of the anemia on bone structure, spleen size, and growth and development. Although general health is much improved with regular transfusion, the accumulation of excess iron from the transfusions must be counteracted. This has led to successful programs to remove the excess iron from the tissues. Currently, patients are treated by continuous subcutaneous infusions (8 to 12 hours/day for life) of deferoxamine, a potent chelator of iron, which facilitates urinary excretion of iron (Fig. 7-8). Vitamin C also appears to enhance urinary iron excretion.

Because of the intense erythroid hyperplasia, patients with thalassemia are maintained on folic acid supplements. Splenectomy may be required to relieve massive splenomegaly, especially when the transfusion requirement becomes excessive. Splenectomy is hazardous for patients younger than 5 or 6 years because of the risk of gram-positive septicemia. A butyrate compound has been used to increase the fetal hemoglobin and improve the anemia, but the results

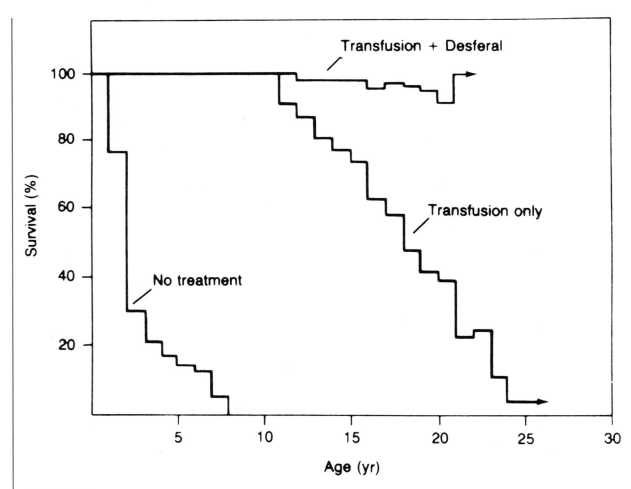

FIGURE 7-8.
Improved life expectancy with transfusion and iron chelation (deferoxamine [Desferal]). (From Cao A, et al. A short guide to the management of Cooley's anemia. The Cooley's Foundation, p. 650.)

have been disappointing. Allogeneic bone marrow transplantation can also be done. A dream for the future is to manipulate the patient's hematopoietic stem cells and repair the genetic defect.

SUMMARY POINTS

The genetic diseases of hemoglobin evidently became prevalent because they protected against malaria. Genetic counseling has markedly reduced the incidence of thalassemia in some places, such as Sicily. Sickle cell disease continues to be a source of great suffering. The research team that can safely and effectively put an end to the infarctions and painful crises will be medical heroes.

SUGGESTED READINGS

Platt O. The adhering sickled cells may mechanically injure endothelial cells, leading to repeated areas of vascular injury and repair. (Easing the suffering caused by sickle cell disease.) *N Engl J Med,* 330:783.

Setty BNY, Stuart MJ. Vascular cell adhesion molecule-1 is involved in mediating hypoxia-induced sickle red blood cell adherence to endothelium: potential role in sickle cells disease. *Blood,* 88:2311.

CASE DEVELOPMENT PROBLEMS: CHAPTER 7

Problem I

History: A 25-year-old African American school teacher was brought to the emergency room after 6 hours of severe pain in the back, knees, and ankles. She had had occasional attacks of this type in the past. Her brother had similar episodes and was believed to have a positive sickle preparation. Her parents were entirely well.

Physical examination: The patient was slightly jaundiced and pale, with a spleen palpable 4 cm below the left costal margin.

Laboratory values: hemoglobin 9.9 g/dL; RBC 3.2 million/μL; hematocrit (HCT) 30%; WBC 12,000/μL with normal differential; reticulocytes 13%; serum bilirubin 3.2 mg/dL indirect.

1. Calculate the reticulocyte index (production index).
2. Describe this anemia in kinetic terms.
   Examination of the woman's peripheral smear revealed many shift cells, many targets, occasional sickled cells, anisocytosis, and poikilocytosis.
3. Which of the following is the most likely diagnosis? Defend your choice: sickle cell anemia (S/S), sickle cell trait (A/S), sickle C disease (S/C).
4. What test would you order to make a definitive diagnosis?
5. Explain the pathophysiology of the "painful crisis."
   The patient recovered after 48 hours and returned to work. Two years later, her hematocrit was noted to be gradually falling to a level of 23%, with a decrease in reticulocyte count from her usual 18% to 20%, to 4%. A peripheral smear revealed the target cells and sickled cells as before, but also an increase in hypersegmented polys (polymorphonuclear leukocytes) and some oval macrocytes. A bone marrow aspirate was performed.
6. (a) Predict the findings on marrow. (b) Explain the probable cause of the falling hematocrit.
   The patient was treated appropriately, and her hematocrit returned to its previous level of 30%.

Six months later, she was readmitted 5 days after the onset of fever, cough, muscle aches, and malaise during a flu-like illness. Her hematocrit, which had been 30% 1 week before, was now 18%, with a reticulocyte count of 0.5%.

7. (a) How do you explain the fall in hematocrit and reticulocyte count? (b) Why would a flu-like illness not have a similar effect on a normal person?

The patient did well over the next 5 years, with only an occasional pain crisis. She was then admitted because of dyspnea on exertion and ankle swelling. Her physician determined that she was in congestive heart failure.

8. What factors contribute to the heart failure in this patient?
9. Review the pathophysiology of S/S and S/C disease.

Problem II

History: A 23-year-old woman came to her physician for prenatal care 2 months after her last period. She had no complaints.

Physical examination: An enlarged uterus was found estimated at 8 weeks' gestation.

Laboratory values: HCT 32%, hemoglobin (Hb) 10.5 g/dL, RBC 5.25 million/μL; smear revealed hypochromia and microcytosis, shift cells, and anisocytosis and poikilocytosis.

1. What are the red cell indices?
2. Is the hematocrit abnormal at 8 weeks' gestation? What happens to the hematocrit during pregnancy? The red cell mass? The plasma volume?
3. What is the differential diagnosis of a microcytic anemia?
4. (a) What is the most likely cause of this anemia? (b) What further history would you need to help you make a choice?

The physician prescribed oral iron and asked her to return in 4 weeks. Her hematocrit was unchanged at that time.

5. How much should the hematocrit rise after 4 weeks of iron treatment?
6. What are the most common reasons for failure to respond to iron therapy?

The physician obtained the following lab data: serum iron/total iron binding capacity 170/380 μg/dL; reticulocytes 1.8%; bone marrow erythroid hyperplasia with G/E of 1.5:1; stool guaiacs × 3-negative. The hemoglobin and other red cell values were unchanged.

7. What is the kinetic classification of this anemia?
8. What is your tentative diagnosis now?
9. How would you confirm your diagnosis?

The patient's iron therapy was discontinued, and she uneventfully delivered a normal infant at 40 weeks' gestation. The infant's hematocrit was normal at birth. At age 6 months, however, the infant began to become progressively irritable and listless. Examination at 8 months revealed splenomegaly and pallor, HCT 16%, and Hb 4.8 g/dL. The peripheral smear showed extreme hypochromia, poikilocytosis, nucleated red cells, and many target cells.

10. What is your diagnosis? How would you prove it?
11. Why wasn't the anemia manifest in the infant at birth?

The child required frequent transfusions to maintain hematocrit at 18% to 20%. His activities were limited. At age 16, onset of heart failure and diabetes mellitus were noted, and liver function tests were abnormal.

12. What is the cause of the diabetes, cardiac failure, and liver disease in this child?
13. What should the original physician have done when the diagnosis of β-thalassemia minor was made in the pregnant mother?
14. Review the pathophysiologies of β-thalassemia minor and major.

CASE DEVELOPMENT ANSWERS

Problem I

1. $RI = \dfrac{0.13 \times 3.2 \times 10^6/\mu L}{50,000/\mu L} = $ approximately $8 \times$ normal
2. This is a high reticulocyte index (RI) for the degree of anemia and suggests chronic hemolysis.
3. The patient probably has S/C disease because of splenomegaly and the large number of target cells on smear. Patients with S/S disease usually have infarcted, shrunken spleens by the time they reach adulthood. Patients with sickle trait (S/A) are not anemic and do not have symptoms.
4. Hemoglobin electrophoresis.
5. Cells sickle, occluding small blood vessels to bones, joints, liver, and spleen and causing microinfarcts and pain. The circulation in these areas stagnates and causes a further drop in oxygen tension and further sickling—the "vicious viscous sickle cycle."
6. (a) The G/E was 1:1; there were giant bands and metamyelocytes, and megaloblastic maturation in the red cell series was noted. (b) Folic acid deficiency is the cause of falling hematocrit and bone marrow findings. This is thought to be due to the excessive utilization of folate by the marrow over a period of years and may occasionally be seen in any patient with longstanding hemolytic anemia.
7. (a) This is an aplastic crisis. During parvovirus infections, the marrow may stop producing red cells transiently. This occurs in healthy persons as well as in those with hemolytic disorders. (b) If we assume that all production stops; that production = destruction; that the rate of destruction in the patient is eight times normal, then in 5 days, 8%/day × 5 days = 40% of her cells will be destroyed; 40% × HCT 30% = 12% HCT will be lost. Therefore, the patient's hematocrit will fall precipitously from 30% to 18% in 5 days. The marrow will recover spontaneously when the viremia subsides, but transfusion may be required in the interim.
8. The heart failure is due to chronic intrapulmonary sickling and thrombosis, causing pulmonary hypertension and right-sided failure. Chronic sickling in small coronary vessels causes diffuse myocardial fibrosis, which contributes to the heart failure.

Problem II

1. MCV 61 fL, MCHC 33%, MCH 20 pg.
2. Beginning at week 6 of pregnancy, the plasma volume begins to rise, reaching its peak at 24 weeks, at which time there is approximately a 40% increase in plasma volume. An increase in red cell mass of 17% to 25% occurs during pregnancy. Therefore, a mild "dilutional" anemia usually occurs with hematocrits of 32% to 34% at 24 weeks and thereafter. A hematocrit of 32% at 8 weeks' gestation is abnormally low.
3. (a) Iron deficiency. (b) Anemia of chronic inflammation. (c) Thalassemia minor. (d) Lead poisoning. (e) Sideroblastic anemia.
4. (a) The most likely cause of a microcytic anemia in a woman of childbearing age is iron deficiency. (Review the iron losses in pregnancy and during normal period.) In this patient, however, the indices suggest that something else may be the cause of the anemia. The MCHC is normal although the MCV is very low. (b) Number of previous pregnancies, menorrhagia, iron supplements during previous pregnancies, other sources of possible bleeding, that is, gastrointestinal tract. Has the patient ever had normal blood counts? Any family history of anemia? Is patient of Mediterranean origin?

Any underlying chronic illnesses, that is, rheumatoid arthritis? Pica? Does the patient work in industries using lead?

5. Production can increase to three times normal after a lag of about 1 week. In 4 weeks, the replacement should be approximately $21/100 \times HCT\ 42\% =$ approximately 8%.

6. (a) Not taking the iron. (b) Continued bleeding. (c) Failure to absorb the iron. (d) The wrong diagnosis—patient is not iron-deficient at all.

7. RI = $0.018 \times 5.25 \times 10^6/50,000 \times 1/1.5 = 1.3$. The low RI and the erythroid hyperplasia in the marrow indicate that ineffective erythropoiesis is occurring.

8. The patient has a low MCV, indicating a cytoplasmic maturation defect— and ineffective erythropoiesis. She probably has thalassemia minor.

9. Hemoglobin electrophoresis on starch block revealed a 6% hemoglobin A_2 (normal = 2.5% to 3%); hemoglobin F was normal, confirming the diagnosis of heterozygous thalassemia.

10. Thalassemia major. Check the father for heterozygous thalassemia and the infant for hemoglobin F.

11. At birth, the infant has γ chains primarily. The adult complement of β chains is not reached until the infant is about 6 months of age.

12. These changes are probably due to iron deposition in the pancreas, liver and heart. The causes of this hemosiderosis are the repeated blood transfusions (about 250 mg of iron in each 500 mL of blood) and the increased gastrointestinal absorption of iron associated with ineffective erythropoiesis.

13. The physician should have checked the father to determine whether he had thalassemia trait, since this genetic defect has a significant incidence in people from Mediterranean countries. This would have allowed the patient to have prenatal testing of the fetus.

Red Cell Metabolism, Enzyme Deficiencies, and Hemoglobin Function

Nasrolla T. Shahidi, Donald R. Harkness, Robert D. Woodson, Timothy Cripe

OUTLINE

OBJECTIVES

- Know the importance of the glycolytic pathway in red cell function and the roles of adenosine triphosphate (ATP), 2,3-bisphosphoglycerate (BPG), NADH in the red cell.
- Describe the metabolic effects and clinical consequences of pyruvate kinase deficiency.
- Know the different clinical syndromes observed in patients with different variants of glucose-6-phosphate dehydrogenase (G6PD).
- Describe fetal X chromosome inactivation and its significance.
- Explain how oxygen and 2,3-BPG interact with hemoglobins A, S, and F.
- Explain the cause, clinical manifestations, and therapy of methemoglobinemia.

The red cell is the only cell in the body without a nucleus and mitochondria, yet it is able to function for 4 months without new protein synthesis or the Krebs cycle. It metabolizes glucose, its basic fuel, to produce adenosine triphosphate (ATP), maintain iron in the ferrous state, and prevent denaturation of its proteins and lipids. In this chapter, we review the red cell's metabolic features, examine four common enzymatic abnormalities, and explore the way in which the red cell regulates oxygen delivery.

Glucose enters the red cell by a facilitated transport system that is independent of insulin. The hexokinase reaction phosphorylates glucose at the sixth carbon atom. Glucose-6-phosphate dehydrogenase (G6PD) is then metabolized in the red cell by both the glycolytic and the hexose monophosphate pathways.

GLYCOLYTIC PATHWAY

Adenosine Triphosphate

Figure 8-1 shows the glycolytic (Embden-Meyerhof) pathway, which generates 2 moles of red cell adenosine triphosphate (ATP) per mole of glucose consumed. ATP is used by the erythrocyte to power the ATPase sodium-potassium pump and to maintain the erythrocyte membrane in a flexible, highly deformable state. When ATP production is inadequate, the erythrocyte loses potassium and gains sodium and calcium. The membrane becomes so stiff that it no longer can squeeze through pores in the spleen. Enzymatic defects in the glycolytic pathway typically produce nonspherocytic hemolytic anemia. Older cells are more subject to destruction because the activity of many enzymes normally declines during red cell aging. If an enzyme has rapid decay (decreased half-life) or altered kinetics, metabolic insufficiency may occur well before the cell's usual 120-day expiration time.

2,3-Bisphosphoglycerate

Figure 8-1 shows that the glycolytic intermediate 1,3-BPG may alternatively pass through a side pathway known as the Rapoport-Luebering shunt, in which 2,3-BPG formerly known as 2,3 DPG is formed. When this occurs, there is no net synthesis of ATP, but the compound formed, 2,3-BPG, plays an important role in regulation of hemoglobin function and oxygen transport.

NADH

Hemoglobin is normally oxidized to methemoglobin ($Fe^{2+} \rightarrow Fe^{3+}$) at a rate of 1% to 3% per day, and it must be continuously reduced to functional form by nicotinamide adenine dinucleotide hydrogenase (NADH). Certain drugs and toxins enhance methemoglobin production. Provision of NADH for methemoglobin reduction is the third major function of the glycolytic pathway. This reaction is coupled to glyceraldehyde phosphate dehydrogenase. NADH can then transfer an electron to iron via NADH methemoglobin reductase (also termed NADH diaphorase) and cytochrome b5 to reduce methemoglobin (ferrihemoglobin).

HEXOSE MONOPHOSPHATE PATHWAY

The major function of the hexose monophosphate shunt is to protect the red cell from direct damage by oxygen radicals. Under normal circumstances, approximately 95% of glucose is metabolized through the glycolytic pathway; the

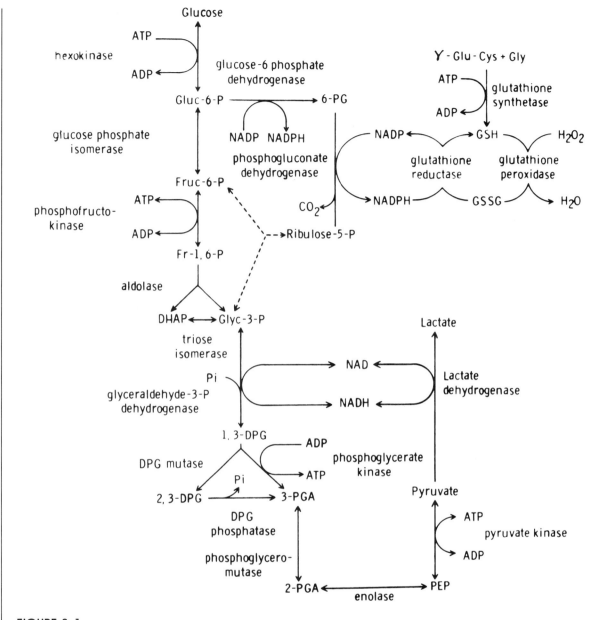

FIGURE 8-1.

Glycolytic, hexose monophosphate and Rapoport-Luebering pathways in the red cell. NADPH for glutathione reduction is produced by both glucose-6-phosphate dehydrogenase and phosphogluconate dehydrogenase. Triosephosphate isomerase is abbreviated triose isomerase. ADP, adenosine diphosphate; ATP, adenosine triphosphate; 2,3-DPG, 2,3-diphosphoglycerate = 2,3-bisphosphoglycerate (2,3-BPG); 3-phosphoglycerate (PGA). (From Harkness DR. Hereditary disorders of red cells. In: Harrington WM, Reiss E, eds. *Fundamentals and Clinical Aspects of Internal Medicine*. Miami: University of Miami, p. 69

remaining 5% is metabolized in the oxidative hexose monophosphate shunt pathway (Fig. 8-1). In this pathway, glucose-6-phosphate is first converted by G6PD to 6-phosphogluconate. This compound is then oxidized at the first carbon, producing the five-carbon compound ribose-5-phosphate, and carbon dioxide. A series of molecular rearrangements ultimately yields fructose-6-phosphate and glyceraldehyde-3-phosphate, which are then metabolized in the glycolytic pathway.

Unlike the glycolytic pathway in which NAD is a coenzyme, the hexose monophosphate pathway requires nicotinamide adenine dinucleotide phosphate(NADP). NADPH serves as an electron donor for the reduction of oxidized glutathione (GSSG), a reaction catalyzed by glutathione reductase. Reduced glutathione (GSH), a tripeptide composed of γ-glutamic acid, cysteine, and glycine, is present in red cells in high concentration (approximately 2 mM, which is nearly half the molar concentration of hemoglobin). It serves the critical function of protecting other proteins and lipids of the red cell from oxidant denaturation.

Oxidants (superoxide and hydrogen peroxide) are common products of biologic processes. They can result from normal oxidation reactions (including the reactions of molecular oxygen with hemoglobin), drug metabolism, ionizing irradiation, and the killing of bacteria by leukocytes. If unopposed, these reactive species attack hemoglobin, enzymes, and cell membranes, causing irreversible damage. As shown in the following series of reactions, however, glutathione reduces peroxides, thus protecting other cellular constituents.

$$O_2 + e^- \rightarrow O_2 \bullet \text{ (superoxide)}$$

$$2\,O_2 \bullet + 2\,H^+ \xrightarrow[\text{Dismutase}]{\text{Superoxide}} H_2O_2 + O_2$$

$$H_2O_2 + 2\,GSH + \xrightarrow[\text{Peroxidase}]{\text{Glutathione}} GSSG + 2\,H_2O$$

$$GSSG + 2\,NADPH + \xrightarrow[\text{Reductase}]{\text{Glutathione}} 2\,GSH + 2\,NADP$$

When the oxidation products, GSSG or mixed disulfides (protein-S-SG), are reduced by glutathione reductase, NADPH is depleted. This temporarily increases the flow of glucose-6-phosphate into the hexose monophosphate pathway to replenish NADPH. NADH generated from the glycolytic pathway cannot substitute for NADPH. This protective mechanism is jeopardized by abnormalities in the hexose monophosphate pathway. NADPH also reduces catalase, another important red cell enzyme, which breaks down hydrogen peroxide. Catalase may be more important than glutathione peroxidase in detoxifying reactive oxidants.

NADPH produced by this pathway also can reduce methemoglobin. This reduction occurs only when an intermediate electron acceptor is provided. The best-known drug for this purpose is methylene blue, which is used to treat chemically induced methemoglobinemia.

ENZYME DEFICIENCIES OF THE GLYCOLYTIC PATHWAY

Pyruvate Kinase Deficiency

The second most common erythrocyte enzyme deficiency is pyruvate kinase (PK) deficiency. This enzyme catalyzes the conversion of 2-phosphenolpyruvate to pyruvate with production of ATP. Its deficiency causes decreased consumption of glucose and subnormal ATP production. The partial block at this point in the glycolytic pathway leads to increased concentrations of intermediates proximal to the block, particularly 2,3-BPG, 2-phosphenolpyruvate, and 3-phosphoglycerate. The decrease in ATP synthesis adversely affects cation transport, causing PK-deficient red cells to lose potassium and gain sodium at an accelerated rate. The increase in 2,3-BPG levels markedly decreases the affinity of hemoglobin for oxygen, facilitating oxygen delivery. Patients with PK deficiency therefore have greater tolerance for anemia than do persons with other anemias of equal severity.

PK deficiency is an autosomal recessive trait. Over 300 cases have been described, mostly in northern Europeans. The deficiency is effectively limited to red cells, since other cells have a second PK enzyme, which is the product of a different gene. The primary clinical manifestation in homozygotes is chronic hemolytic anemia. Even reticulocytes are somewhat vulnerable to the metabolic stress (low PO_2 and pH) imposed by the spleen. In most patients, anemia, jaundice, or both are noted in infancy or in early childhood. In severe cases, hemolysis may produce neonatal jaundice requiring exchange transfusion. As in other chronic hemolytic anemias, transient aplastic crises, probably the result of certain viral infections, may be observed.

Examination of peripheral blood in PK deficiency often shows only polychromatophilic macrocytes (young reticulocytes). Occasionally, patients display irregular-shaped red cells (poikilocytes). Definitive diagnosis is made by demonstration of abnormal activity of the PK enzyme. No specific treatment is available for patients with PK deficiency. Splenectomy in persons with severe enzyme deficiency has proved beneficial and may obviate or lessen the need for transfusions. In milder cases, however, splenectomy is not advisable.

Other Glycolytic Enzyme Deficiencies

Deficiencies of most of the other enzymes in the glycolytic pathway have been reported, but they are relatively uncommon. The typical finding is chronic hereditary nonspherocytic hemolytic anemia. Inheritance of all but one of the glycolytic pathway enzyme deficiencies (phosphoglycerate kinase deficiency, an X-linked abnormality) is autosomal recessive. Some deficiencies are present simultaneously in white cells, platelets, and other tissues, which may have abnormal functions. In triosephosphate isomerase deficiency, neurologic abnormalities and defective erythrocytes lead to early death. Phosphoglycerate kinase deficiency causes neurologic abnormalities in hemizygotes. Phosphofructokinase deficiency in muscle leads to muscle fatigue and cramping with exercise.

A deficiency of NADH-methemoglobin reductase (diaphorase) causes congenital methemoglobinemia, but not hemolytic anemia. This enzyme is also normally low in neonates, so that they are susceptible to the effects of drugs and toxins that produce methemoglobinemia. One natural toxin is nitrate in well water, which is converted to nitrite in the gut.

DEFECTS OF THE HEXOSE MONOPHOSPHATE PATHWAY

Glucose-6-Phosphate Dehydrogenase Deficiency

G6PD deficiency is the most common red cell enzyme deficiency. According to the World Health Organization (WHO) reports, more than 100 million people in the world have G6PD deficiency. The incidence is particularly high in the Mediterranean basin. In some areas of Sardinia, 30% of males are affected. Among African Americans, the incidence is about 11% and among Saudi-Arabians about 13%. The geographic distribution of this deficiency coincides with that of malaria. The malaria parasite cannot grow as well in G6PD-deficient red cells as it can in normal cells, suggesting that G6PD deficiency protects the host against malaria.

The gene for the G6PD enzyme is located on the X chromosome. Either the normal X chromosome or the G6PD mutant-containing X chromosome is randomly inactivated during fetal life (Fig. 8-2). Females are therefore heterozygous carriers, and males are hemizygotes. The wide range of erythrocyte G6PD values in female heterozygotes is due in part to varying proportions of normal and G6PD-deficient somatic cells, and females with G6PD deficiency are therefore mosaics. Mosaicism among individual erythrocytes can be documented by an elution staining method for G6PD enzyme activity {#41}. This technique depends on the ability of normal red cells, but not G6PD-deficient red cells, to reverse hemoglobin oxidation. Because the same G6PD isoenzyme is found in all tissues, mosaicism, when present, is found throughout the body. The enzyme has therefore been used as a tumor marker. In the heterozygote with G6PD deficiency, the demonstration that all cells in a tumor have the same G6PD enzyme is strong evidence that the tumor arose from a single cell.

More than 440 G6PD variants have been described to date, and WHO has given them four classes of clinical severity (Table 8-1). Many of these have normal or only slightly reduced enzyme activity and are not associated with clinical manifestations. The normal G6PD isoenzyme, designated B, migrates as a slow band on electrophoresis. A mutant isoenzyme with normal function, designated A+, occurs in about 30% of African Americans and migrates as a fast band. Another variant of this isoenzyme, designated A–, possesses approximately 10% of the activity of the normal A+ enzyme and does not cause symptoms unless

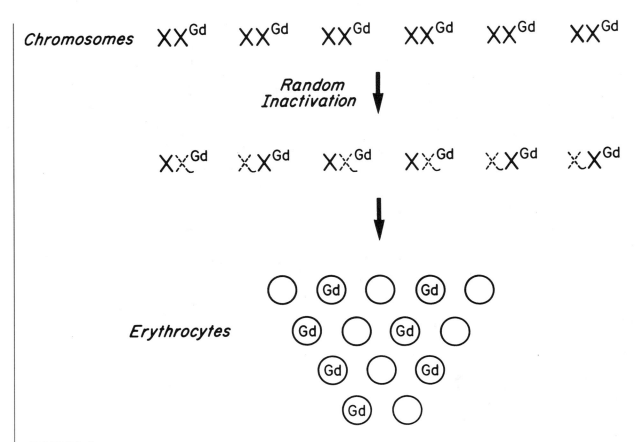

FIGURE 8-2.
Random inactivation of the X chromosome during fetal life.

TABLE 8-1. Classification of G6PD Variants

WHO Class	Clinical Severity	Example
1	Severe*	Campinas
2	Moderate	Mediterranean
3	Mild	A–
4	None	A+

G6PD, glucose-6-phosphate dehydrogenase; WHO, World Health Organization.
*Congenital nonspherocytic hemolytic anemia.

there is an oxidant stress. G6PD A– occurs in 11% of African Americans. A severely defective enzyme, G6PD Mediterranean, occurs in Italians, Greeks, Sephardic Jews, and other peoples of Mediterranean countries.

The clinical picture is variable. In most people with G6PD deficiency, the life span of the red cell is virtually normal. Some people with G6PD Mediterranean have chronic low-grade hemolysis.

G6PD activity declines as red cells age. The half-life for activity of the common B isoenzyme is 62 days. This level of activity is sufficient to sustain the red cell for its normal 120-day life span. In contrast, the half-life for the activity of the A– variant is 13 days, and the half-life for the Mediterranean variant is a matter of hours. Since platelets and granulocytes have much shorter circulation times, decay of G6PD activity is apparently too slow to disturb their functions, although granulocytes with severely deficient activity appear to have a defective oxidant pathway and poor bacterial killing power.

As previously discussed, maintenance of glutathione reductase and catalase in the reduced form is a major function of the hexose monophosphate pathway. When the red cell is compromised by a deficiency of NADPH, reactive species are then free to attack sulfhydryl groups. The oxidation of the exposed SH group at the $\beta93$ position of hemoglobin alters the tertiary configuration of the molecule and predisposes it to denaturation. Heme and globin then dissociate, and the insoluble denatured globin (Heinz body) is prone to form disulfide bridges to the red cell membrane. Although the resulting hemolysis is usually extravascular, the red cell membrane may be so disturbed that lysis occurs intravascularly.

G6PD deficiency may be expressed as one of five different syndromes:

- Drug-induced hemolysis
- Infection-induced hemolysis
- Favism
- Neonatal jaundice
- Hereditary chronic nonspherocytic hemolytic anemia

Drug-Induced Hemolysis

Drug-induced hemolysis has been known since the end of the last century. The hemolytic activity of acetylphenylhydrazine on normal red cells was first described in 1888. Smillie reported severe hemolytic anemia in a small percentage of his patients who were treated for hookworm with betanaphthol. Similar observations have been made after use of 8-aminoquinoline derivatives as antimalarial agents. The latter observations led to the discovery of an intrinsic abnormality of red cells and low concentration of reduced glutathione (GSH), which was later shown to be due to a deficiency of erythrocyte G6PD.

When a person with A– type G6PD deficiency ingests therapeutic daily doses of the antimalarial drug, primaquine, moderately severe hemolysis accompanied by hemoglobinuria begins at 1 to 3 days (Fig. 8-3). The delay is required for metabolic activation of the drug. Increased reticulocytes and Heinz bodies are seen in

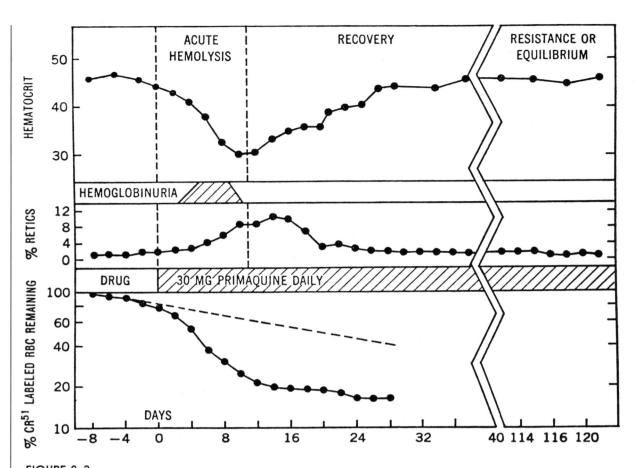

FIGURE 8-3.

Course of experimentally induced hemolytic anemia in primaquine-sensitive person. Note the evidence for intravascular hemolysis. Observe the changes in the slope of the red cell (RBC) survival curve. (From Alving AS, et al. Mitigation of the haemolytic effect of primaquine and enhancement of its action against erythrocytic forms of the chessen strain of *Plasmodium vivax* by intermittent regimens of drug administration. *Bull WHO* 22:621.)

supravital stains. The hematocrit drops owing to loss of older erythrocytes, but recovery is spontaneous despite continuation of the drug.

The self-limited nature of hemolysis is due to emergence of younger red cells, which have sufficient enzyme activity to resist oxidant stress. The individual eventually achieves a state of compensated hemolysis (continuing hemolysis without anemia) in which production of cells accelerates to match the continuing premature loss of older cells. The presence of many young red cells during a hemolytic crisis can mask the diagnosis because measurement of G6PD activity in these cells may be near normal. If G6PD deficiency is suspected but a normal value is obtained, a second test is warranted several weeks after hemolysis has resolved. By contrast, in individuals with the Mediterranean variant most of their erythrocytes may be destroyed in the course of a hemolytic episode, thus requiring emergency transfusion. In such cases, the diagnosis is *not* masked even during hemolysis.

A number of drugs and compounds cause hemolysis in G6PD-deficient persons. These are shown in Table 8-2. In general, these drugs are quinones or are activated to quinones by the liver. The variability of a given drug's effect on different patients depends not only on the nature of the enzyme defect, but also on the rate of oxidation and acetylation of the drug by the liver.

TABLE 8-2. Compounds Associated With Hemolysis in G6PD-Deficient Patients

Drug Class	Agent
Antibacterial	Sulfamethoxazole (Gantanol, Septra, Bactrim)
	Nitrofurantoin (Furadantin)
	Nalidixic acid (NegGram)
Sulfones	Thiazolesulfone
	Diphenylsulfone (DDS, Dapsone)
Antimalarial	Primaquine
	Pamaquine
	Pentaquine
Other agents	Doxorubicin
	Methylene blue
	Trinitrotoluene (TNT)
	Phenylhydrazine

GP6D, glucose-6-phosphate dehydrogenase.

Drugs that are now known to be safe include other sulfas such as sulfisoxazole (Gantrisin), antituberculous drugs such as isoniazid, antipyretic and anti-inflammatory drugs including phenylbutazone and acetaminophen, antimalarial drugs such as chloroquine and camoquin, chloramphenicol, ascorbic acid, and quinidine. Some of these drugs, however, are known to cause hemolysis and other hematologic problems not associated with redox reactions.

Infection-induced Hemolysis

Infection is probably the common cause of hemolysis in G6PD deficiency. It may be confused with drug-induced hemolysis because antibiotics and antipyretics are so commonly used to treat infection. Acute hemolytic anemia may be associated with bacterial or viral infections. The presumed mechanism is generation of hydrogen peroxide and superoxide by neutrophils and macrophages.

Favism

Some G6PD-deficient persons develop severe, occasionally fatal, hemolytic anemia after ingesting fava beans. The factor present in the fava bean can be transmitted to a nursing infant by the mother's milk. Oxidant compounds have been isolated from the fava bean, but these cause oxidant injury to normal cells as well. Patients with favism usually have the Mediterranean type of G6PD deficiency. The deficiency of this enzyme, however, is not alone sufficient for the production of fava bean–induced hemolysis, since only some persons with G6PD deficiency are susceptible. A second factor, as yet unknown, is also required. People of African descent with the A– type of G6PD deficiency do not have favism.

Neonatal Jaundice

In the newborn with G6PD deficiency, severe jaundice may lead to kernicterus. In the Mediterranean basin, particularly in Greece, deficiency of G6PD is the major cause of neonatal jaundice, requiring exchange transfusion. The pathophysiology may be related to G6PD deficiency in the liver, since hemolysis is not a major factor.

Hereditary Nonspherocytic Hemolytic Anemia

Approximately 30% of chronic hereditary nonspherocytic hemolytic anemia is due to G6PD deficiency. This type of G6PD deficiency differs from the more common A– variant, in which enzyme activity, though abnormal, still permits normal erythrocyte life span in the absence of drugs or infection. Persons with chronic hemolytic anemia due to G6PD deficiency are clinically indistinguishable from those with hemolytic anemia due to glycolytic enzyme deficiencies. Their red cells are normochromic and normocytic, and the osmotic fragility of the red cells is normal. Splenectomy is of no benefit.

Other Hexose Monophosphate Pathway Deficiencies

Although deficiencies of other enzymes in this pathway might be expected to produce hemolysis similar to G6PD deficiency, this is generally not the case. Deficiency of 6-phosphogluconate dehydrogenase does occur, but it is not known to cause abnormalities. This is also true of glutathione peroxidase and glutathione reductase. Although activities of both are significantly decreased by the dietary deficiency of necessary cofactors—selenium in the case of the peroxidase and riboflavin in the case of the reductase—in neither instance is there a documented association of decreased enzyme activity with hemolysis. Rare cases of chronic hemolytic anemia and sensitivity to oxidant drugs have been observed in patients with low glutathione levels due to a deficiency of either of the two enzymes necessary for synthesis of this tripeptide, γ-glutamylcysteine synthetase and glutathione synthetase.

Pyrimidine-5'-Nucleotidase Deficiency

Patients who are homozygous for this enzyme deficiency have life-long hemolytic anemia and may have mental retardation. It is probably the third most common cause of hereditary enzyme-mediated hemolysis. The enzyme degrades RNA. When the enzyme is deficient, ribosomal aggregates persist and are seen in Wright's stain as basophilic stippling {#38}. Pyrimidine-5'-nucleotidase is very sensitive to inhibition by lead. In fact, its inhibition is thought to cause the basophilic stippling and hemolysis seen in lead poisoning. The exact manner in which its deficiency causes hemolysis is unclear.

HEMOGLOBIN FUNCTION, 2,3-BISPHOSPHOGLYCERATE, AND REGULATION OF OXYGEN RELEASE

Molecular Physiology

Normal adult hemoglobin contains four globin chains: two α and two β. A heme group (see Chapter 2) is attached at a specific site on each globin chain. One hemoglobin molecule combines reversibly with four molecules of oxygen to form oxyhemoglobin. One gram of hemoglobin can bind a maximum of 1.39 mL of oxygen at standard temperatureand pressure.

A plot of the partial pressure of oxygen against the percentage of hemoglobin saturated with oxygen is sigmoid in shape (Fig. 8-4). This shape is of great physiologic importance. Its upper flat portion allows the blood to become virtually saturated with oxygen at the PO_2 in the pulmonary alveoli; its steep down-slope permits release of a great deal of oxygen with only a modest drop in PO_2 as blood flows through tissue. The sigmoid shape of the oxygen equilibrium curve is a consequence of heme-heme interaction, or "subunit cooperativity," with oxygen

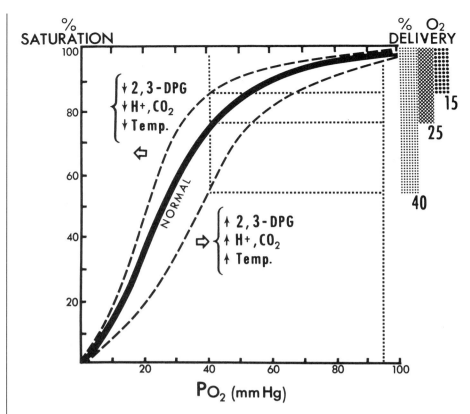

FIGURE 8-4.

The normal blood-oxygen equilibrium curve (*middle curve*) under standard conditions (pH 7.4, 37° C, PCO_2 40 mm Hg) with left- and right-shifted curves. At a given PO_2 (40 mm Hg in this example), the percentage of oxygen released (*bars at right*) varies appreciably. 2,3-DPG = 2,3-BPG, bisphosphoglycerate. (From Harkness DR. Hereditary disorders of red cells. In: Harrington WM, Reiss E, eds. *Fundamentals and Clinical Aspects of Internal Medicine*. Miami: University of Miami, p. 976.)

binding to the first heme increasing the strength of its binding by the second, the second increasing the strength of binding by the third, and so on. This characteristic of hemoglobin depends on its tetrameric structure and on the presence of dissimilar chains in the tetramer (two α and two β chains in the case of normal adult human hemoglobin). Thus, monomers such as myoglobin or isolated α or β chains yield an oxygen equilibrium curve, which is a rectangular hyperbola; so does a tetramer containing only β chains (hemoglobin H). An elegant explanation has been devised to account for this shape of the oxygen equilibrium curve. There are ionic bonds within and between the α and β chains, which stabilize the molecule. These bonds are broken sequentially as each heme group is oxygenated. This causes the subunits to move significantly with respect to one another. Rupture of salt bonds also causes subtle movement within the adjacent subunit such that the affinity of its iron for oxygen increases. The hemoglobin molecule, like the lung, thus "breathes" as oxygen comes and goes (Fig. 8-5).

The middle curve of Figure 8-4 depicts the normal blood-oxygen equilibrium curve under standard conditions (pH 7.4, 37° C, PCO_2 40 mm Hg). The PO_2 at 50% saturation is termed the P_{50}; its average value is 27 mm Hg in normal persons under standard conditions. When shifted to the right (Fig. 8-4), blood-oxygen affinity is reduced, P_{50} is higher, and more oxygen is released from blood at any given pressure. The opposite is true when the curve is shifted to the left;

Oxyhemoglobin

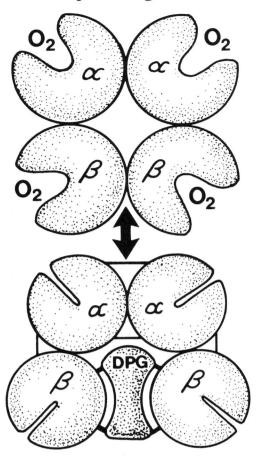

Deoxyhemoglobin

FIGURE 8-5.
In the deoxygenated state, the hemoglobin molecule opens to accept a single 2,3-diphosphoglycerate (DPG) = 2,3-bisphosphoglycerate (BPG), and hydrogen ions establish salt bridge between individual chains. With oxygen uptake, the salt bridges are ruptured, 2,3-BPG and CO_2 expressed, and the heme groups open to receive molecules of oxygen. (From Hillman R, Ault K. *Hematology in Clinical Practice.*
New York: McGraw Hill, p. 6.)

blood PO_2 must fall farther for a given amount of oxygen to be released. Several factors normally regulate the position of the oxygen equilibrium curve. These are pH, PCO_2, temperature and 2,3-BPG.

Bohr Effect

In 1906, Christian Bohr discovered that the hemoglobin-oxygen equilibrium was sensitive to the partial pressure of carbon dioxide in blood. The effect of carbon dioxide, largely due to the associated change in pH, can be expressed qualitatively by the reaction:

$$HbH + O_2 \longleftrightarrow HbO_2 + H^+$$

The protons liberated or consumed by this reaction are called **Bohr protons**. Several important physiologic consequences follow from this relationship, some of which are covered in detail in other disciplines: (1) acidification of blood shifts the oxygen equilibrium curve to the right, (2) oxygenation of hemoglobin decreases intraerythrocytic pH (by a few hundredths), (3) the increase in H^+ with oxygenation requires simultaneous movement of anions (chloride and bicarbonate) across the red cell membrane to maintain electroneutrality, and (4) red cells swell slightly with acidification to maintain osmotic equilibrium.

Carbon Dioxide, Nitric Oxide, and Temperature

Carbon dioxide also has a smaller direct effect on the hemoglobin-oxygen-equilibrium. In addition to its effect on pH, carbon dioxide binds directly to the N-termini of α and β chains of hemoglobin, and this binding produces a right shift of the curve. Increased temperature also shifts the curve to the right.

These effects of pH, PCO_2, and temperature on the oxygen-binding curve are biologically important. For example, during vigorous exercise, muscles produce lactic acid, carbon dioxide, and heat, all of which enhance oxygen release at the site where the oxygen is needed. On return to the lung, PCO_2 falls, pH rises, and the blood is cooled, all of which promote oxygen binding by hemoglobin.

2,3-Bisphosphoglycerate

In 1925, an organic phosphate, 2,3-BPG, was found in high concentration in red cells. The function of this high 2,3-BPG concentration remained unknown for 40 years. In 1967, two groups of investigators demonstrated that 2,3-BPG has a profound effect on the binding of oxygen by hemoglobin; it decreases hemoglobin-oxygen affinity, thus facilitating release of oxygen from hemoglobin to tissue. ATP has a similar effect on hemoglobin-oxygen affinity, but it has little effect in vivo because of its low concentration in erythrocytes. By contrast, 2,3-BPG concentration in normal human erythrocytes is about 4.5 mM—nearly equimolar with hemoglobin (5.3 mM). The oxygen equilibrium curve shifts progressively to the right as erythrocytic 2,3-BPG concentration rises.

2,3-BPG exerts its effect by combining with deoxyhemoglobin and appreciably lowering the oxygen affinity (raising the P_{50}; see Fig. 8-5). With oxygenation, 2,3-BPG is expelled. Thus, it dissociates from and reassociates with hemoglobin during oxygenation and deoxygenation:

$$Hb(2,3\text{-}BPG) + 4O_2 \leftrightarrow Hb(O_2)_4 + 2,3\text{-}BPG$$

The γ chains of fetal hemoglobin ($\alpha_2\gamma_2F$) do not bind 2,3-BPG. This explains why the oxygen equilibrium curve of the fetus and neonate lies to the left of the adult curve despite similar 2,3-BPG levels.

Although the saturation of hemoglobin with oxygen is changing continuously in the circulation, synthesis of 2,3-BPG is enhanced if the average fraction of deoxyhemoglobin to oxyhemoglobin is increased. Thus, 2-3-BPG rises when there is hypoxia of any cause. The facilitation of oxygen delivery by the resultant shift of the oxygen equilibrium curve is an important adaptive mechanism. This adaptation, however, works against the sicklemia patient, in whom a high oxygen saturation rather than deoxygenation is preferred.

PHYSIOLOGIC AND PATHOPHYSIOLOGIC CONDITIONS ASSOCIATED WITH CHANGES IN 2,3-BPG

The fraction of oxygen released from blood in the tissues depends on blood flow rate, hemoglobin concentration, arterial blood oxygen saturation, and tissue oxygen consumption. The position of the oxygen equilibrium curve, in concert with these factors, determines the PO_2 in the microvessels. This pressure gradient enables oxygen to diffuse from blood to adjacent cells. Adaptive changes in oxygen transport occur in different clinical situations. For example, conditions that increase the amount of deoxygenated hemoglobin in the red cell stimulate synthesis of 2,3-BPG and therefore result in a right shift of the oxygen dissociation curve. Any cause of hypoxia exhibits this effect, including anemia, cardiac failure, and cyanotic heart disease (mixing of deoxygenated venous blood with arterial blood). Acidosis also shifts the curve to the right (Bohr effect); alkalosis shifts the curve to the left. In these cases, levels of 2,3-BPG change to compensate for the pH effect, although more slowly. Finally, high serum phosphate levels also stimulate 2,3-BPG synthesis and cause a right shift and vice versa. This may account in part for the lower hematocrit in children who have higher serum phosphate levels than adults.

Fetal Blood-Oxygen Affinity

A left shift of the blood-oxygen equilibrium curve is present in the fetus of virtually every species. This allows the fetal blood to bind more oxygen in the placenta, where PO_2 is lower than it is in the lung. In humans, this is accomplished by fetal hemoglobin, which has a low affinity for 2,3-BPG, whereas other mechanisms for increasing oxygen affinity are used in other species.

Stored Blood

When blood is stored in standard blood bank medium for later transfusion, 2,3-BPG decreases to negligible levels after 2 weeks, and the oxygen dissociation curve shifts to the left. Upon transfusion, 2,3-BPG is regenerated, approaching normal levels after about 24 hours. Thus, hemoglobin release of oxygen is impaired for the first day after transfusion. The temporary left shift is a disadvantage for seriously ill patients receiving multiple transfusions but is little consequence to most transfused patients.

ACQUIRED ABNORMALITIES OF HEMOGLOBIN

Carboxyhemoglobin

Carboxyhemoglobin is hemoglobin that is combined with carbon monoxide. A small amount of carbon monoxide is produced endogenously as a result of heme catabolism (see Chapter 4). This generates a carboxyhemoglobin level of about 0.4% (of total hemoglobin), although normal persons usually have a level of 0.5% to 1% as a result of low level environmental exposure. Higher levels most often result from smoking (2% to 15%) or exposure to incompletely burned carbon or hydrocarbon fuels. Toxic levels also result commonly from inhalation and metabolism of methylene chloride, a major component of most paint strippers and a common industrial solvent. Carboxyhemoglobin imparts a bright red color to the blood. This is sometimes visible as a bright cherry-red color of skin and mucous membranes in patients with carbon monoxide poisoning. Common manifestations are shown in Table 8-3. Note that modest carboxyhemoglobin levels, commonly found in environmental exposure (cigarette smoke, heavy traffic), cause subtle changes in neurologic and intellectual function.

The major effect of carbon monoxide is disruption of oxygen transport owing to displacement of oxygen from hemoglobin. Significant binding of carbon monoxide to hemoglobin occurs at low PCO values, since the affinity of hemoglobin for carbon monoxide is 236 times greater than its affinity for oxygen. Approximately 50% of hemoglobin is saturated at a PCO of 0.1 mm Hg. One result of this high affinity is that carbon monoxide is released from hemoglobin and exhaled slowly, the half-life being about 4 hours. However, carbon monoxide and oxygen binding are competitive; exposure to 100% oxygen decreases the half-life to about 1 hour.

A reduction in blood oxygen capacity due to anemia is known to be far better tolerated than an equivalent reduction due to carbon monoxide. This is due mainly to two factors. First, the binding of carbon monoxide shifts the oxygen equilibrium curve of the remaining non-carbon monoxide–liganded hemoglobin appreciably to the left (Fig. 8-6). This significantly lowers the gradient for oxygen diffusion in tissue. Second, anemia sharply reduces whole blood viscosity, a built-in compensation that increases blood flow. By contrast, viscosity is unchanged in carboxyhemoglobinemia. For further discussion of viscosity, see Chapter 9.

Methemoglobin

Methemoglobin refers to hemoglobin in which the iron has been oxidized to the ferric state. This occurs to the extent of 1% to 3% daily, and small amounts of methemoglobin (less than 1%) are present normally. Increases in methemoglobin may occur as a result of a hemoglobinopathy (hemoglobin M; Chapter 7), diaphorase deficiency, or exposure to drugs and other chemicals. These toxins do not cause gross methemoglobinemia until the capacity of the NADH methemoglobin reductase system is exceeded (Table 8-4). This is more likely to occur in babies, because of the low activity of this system in infancy, or in persons heterozygous for methemoglobin reductase deficiency.

The effect of methemoglobin on oxygen delivery is similar to that of carboxyhemoglobin. The oxygen binding capacity is reduced, and the oxygen equilibrium curve of the remaining normal hemoglobin is shifted to the left. Symptoms, however, are milder and do not occur until the concentration reaches about 30%. Methemoglobin turns blood brown. Cyanosis is apparent in whites when 1.5 to 2 g/dL of hemoglobin has been converted to methemoglobin. This level differs from that in cyanosis due to deoxygenated hemoglobin (blue), in which about 5 g/dL of deoxyhemoglobin is required to produce a visible change in skin color.

TABLE 8-3. Acute Toxicity of Carbon Monoxide

Carboxyhemoglobin Saturation (%)	Effect
3–10	Subtle alteration of vision, hearing, and response times
10–20	Headache, exertional dyspnea
20–40	Fatigue, altered judgment, dizziness
40–60	Confusion, collapse
>60	Coma, convulsions, death

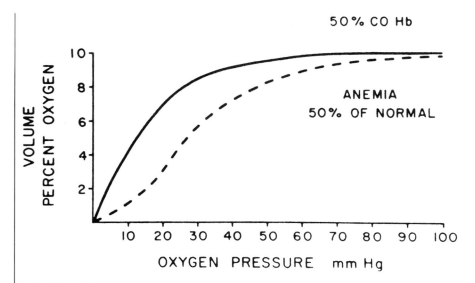

FIGURE 8-6.
Effect of carbon monoxide on the position of the oxygen equilibrium curve in comparison with anemia. In both instances, the oxygen content of arterial blood is reduced by 50%, but much more oxygen can be released at a given tissue PO_2 in anemia.

Sulfhemoglobin

Sulfhemoglobin is a hemoglobin derivative or derivative with a specific absorbance. It does not transport oxygen under physiologic conditions. Its formation is usually associated with a drug, especially phenacetin, acetanilid, or sulfonamide, and is irreversible. The factors predisposing certain persons to the development of sulfhemoglobin are unknown.

SUMMARY POINTS

Although the red cell lacks a nucleus and mitochrondria, it is a metabolically active cell. Glucolytic metabolism generates ATP, which powers the Na^+-K^+ pump and helps maintain membrane flexibility. Through the hexose monophosphate shunt, glutathione is able to protect the cell from oxidative damage. Deficiences of critical enzymes in these pathways result in accelerated or drug-induced red cell destruction, causing hemolytic anemia. X-linked G6PD deficiency is the most common red cell enzyme deficiency worldwide.

TABLE 8-4.   Some Agents Causing Acquired Methemoglobinemia

Direct Oxidants	Indirect Oxidants
Amyl nitrite	Sulfonamides
Silver nitrate	Aniline dyes
Bismuth subnitrate	Phenacetin
Nitroglycerin	Acetanilid
Nitrates in water or food	Phenazopyridine (pyridium)
Nitrous gases	

Microenvironmental conditions also affect the binding of oxygen to hemoglobin, including the presence of fetal hemoglobin, pH (Bohr effect), temperature, and exposure to other ligands, such as carbon monoxide, sulfur-containing compounds, and agents that change the oxidation state of iron.

SUGGESTED READINGS

Beutler E. G6PD deficiency. *Blood* 1994;84(11):3613-3636.

Williams WJ, Beutler E, Ersler AJ, Lichtman MA. *Hematology*. New York: McGraw-Hill, 1995.

CASE DEVELOPMENT PROBLEM: CHAPTER 8

History: A 22-year-old African American male army sergeant was admitted to a field hospital in Korea in 1959 with weakness, malaise, back pain, and dark urine of 3 days' duration. He had arrived from the United States 7 days earlier. He had no fever.

Physical examination: Temperature was 38° C, and physical examination negative except for slightly yellow sclerae. The spleen was not palpable.

Laboratory data: HCT 38%; RBC 4.2 million/μL; WBC 2800 μL, with 40% segmented neutrophils. Smear was unremarkable except for a few spherocytes, "bite cells" and burr cells. The urine was dark brown; specific gravity, 1.024. The specimen was negative for bile but positive for hemoglobin. There were 1 to 2 white cells per high-power field; no red cells seen.

1. What is the single most important piece of laboratory data?
2. How do you interpret this positive piece of information?
3. List tests and results that would confirm your impression.
4. What etiologic factors would you consider in the differential diagnosis?
5. What further investigations would you perform?

While you are in the laboratory reviewing the blood smears, you note amorphous bodies in the red cells on the reticulocyte smear. These bodies are not visible in the red cells on the Wright-stained smear.

6. What particles can be found in red cells? Which of these particles are found only on supravital stains? What is the biochemical composition of these particles? Make a small table naming all the red cell particles, their composition, and staining characteristics.
7. Under what conditions are insoluble protein granules found in red cells?
8. Which category seems most likely?
9. What do you postulate caused the episode in this patient?
10. What further history would you request?
11. Why did the patient have hemoglobin in the urine when the spleen and liver should be the sites of the removal of Heinz bodies?
12. What treatment do you offer?

CASE DEVELOPMENT ANSWERS

1. The urine was positive for hemoglobin.
2. It is an indication of intravascular hemolysis.
3. Elevation of plasma hemoglobin. Absence of haptoglobin from plasma.
4. Malaria ("black water fever"), because the patient is an endemic area; however, the patient does not have fever. Drugs or infection in a susceptible individual. Traumatic damage to red cells (march hemoglobinuria in this case).

5. (a) Blood smear for malaria parasites: negative. (b) Obtain drug history: The patient has been given pills by a medical corpsman. He does not know the name of the pills. He has not been on a long march.
6. Heinz bodies. See Appendix I.
7. (a) Red cells exposed to oxidant stress. (b) Red cells with excess β chains (hemoglobin H disease) or excess α chains (β-thalassemia major) have similar-appearing particles produced by another mechanism. (c) Unstable hemoglobins (hemoglobin Köln).
8. Red cells exposed to oxidant stress.
   Further questioning revealed that the patient had been given primaquine 45 mg daily for the prophylaxis of malaria for the preceding 7 days (for a controlled clinical trial). No one else in the patient's squad had reported illness during the previous several months of the drug trial.
9. G6PD deficiency with hemolysis due to the drug.
10. Family history: The patient's brother once became jaundiced after receiving a sulfa preparation.
11. Cells may lyse in the circulation when membrane lipids are oxidized, but the mechanism is not more clearly understood.
12. No specific treatment is required.

One month later, the patient was given prophylaxis with chloroquine 0.5 g and primaquine 45 mg once weekly without recurrence. It has been determined that G6PD A– subjects can tolerate small doses of primaquine for malarial prophylaxis.

PART II
BLOOD BANKING

Blood Transfusion

Karl V. Voelkerding

OUTLINE

OBJECTIVES

- Identify the antigens present on red cell types A, B, AB, and O and their frequency in United States.
- Define the relationship of the precursor chain to the H chain; the H chain to the A and B chains.
- Note the cells on which AB and H antigens are found.
- State the risk of reaction if random donor blood is given to a recipient of unknown blood type.
- Understand how two linked genes determine the complex CDE haplotype.
- Know the phenotypic frequency of RhD-positive (+) and RhD-negative (−)
- Describe how a patient is classified as RhD+.
- Name two processes by which Rh antibodies can be induced.
- Define naturally occurring, immune, complete, saline-reacting, irregular, incomplete, cold-reacting antibodies, warm antibodies.
- Understand the importance of so-called minor antigens.
- Be able to describe the risks of transfusion and obtain informed consent.
- Learn ABO and Rh typing techniques. Estimate the time required for a crossmatch.
- Know the rationale for the antibody screen.
- Outline the pathophysiology of acute intravascular hemolysis.
- Explain delayed transfusion reactions.
- Know the most common kind of transfusion reaction.

A donation of blood is a tithe of one's vital essence—10% of the life's blood to some anonymous sick person who cannot pay it back. It is a conspicuous demonstration of altruism and human goodness. It is also the basis of a huge industry. Fourteen million pints (units) of blood are processed from 8 to 10 million donors in this country yearly to meet patient needs. Similar programs are carried out in most Western countries. Blood supply, however, is uncertain in Third World countries and nonexistent in rural areas. Although the blood itself is free, the cost of processing makes it an expensive commodity, so that the cost to the patient is about $70 per unit. Much of this chapter is devoted to explaining the processing and testing of blood as well as detailing the risks of its use.

HISTORY

A brief history of blood banking is instructive.

1628—William Harvey discovered the circulation of blood.
1665—Shortly thereafter, Richard Lower, in England, tried the first transfusions in modern times. He kept dogs alive by transfusion from other dogs.
1667—J. Denis in France and Lower in England transfused blood from lambs to humans. The next year, animal-to-human transfusion was outlawed, and advances were delayed for 150 years.
1818—J. Blundell in England performed the first direct transfusion for postpartum hemorrhage.
1900—Carl Landsteiner in Austria discovered the ABO blood group.
1915—R. Lewisohn in New York City used citrate to anticoagulate blood, making storage possible.
1930—The first blood bank was established in England.
1937—The first blood bank in this country was started at Cook County Hospital in Chicago.
1940—The Rh blood group was discovered.
1941—The American Red Cross established a national blood program.
1952—Plastic bags were introduced, replacing glass bottles.
1961—Platelet transfusion was recognized to stop bleeding in aplastic anemia and acute leukemia.
1962—Antihemophilic factor was commercially fractionated.
1967—Rh immune globulin was introduced to prevent immunization of pregnant women.
1971—Hepatitis B testing began.
1972—Apheresis was used to extract single components from blood, returning the remainder to the donor.
1985—HIV was recognized as a new hazard of blood transfusion, and testing was introduced.
1988—The etiologic agent for hepatitis C was identified, and testing was introduced.

American Association of Blood Banks

BLOOD COMPONENTS

The purpose of transfusion is to replace missing components of blood without undue risk. In current practice, whole blood is rarely given. The blood is fractionated in the blood bank laboratory into separate components. Some components, such as plasma, albumin, and clotting factor VIII, can be frozen or lyophilized and kept indefinitely. Others, such as platelets, must be used within a few days. The most common component transfused is the red cell, followed by platelet, plasma, immunoglobulins, and clotting factor VIII (antihemophilic factor). White blood cells are rarely transfused. The unit of transfused material is based on the amount donated—450 mL. Thus, a unit of red cells, platelets, white cells, or plasma is the amount recovered from a donated "pint" of 450 mL of blood.

When blood is donated, a plastic bag containing 65 mL of citrate/dextrose/phosphate/adenine (CPDA) mixture is filled to volume. The blood is centrifuged, and the plastic bag is squeezed to force the plasma and platelets into a second bag, leaving behind packed red cells. The bag with plasma and platelets is then centrifuged, and the plasma is squeezed into a third bag, yielding plasma and a platelet concentrate. If all the components of whole blood are required for replacement of massive hemorrhage, red cells, plasma, and platelets would be given as separate components.

Red cells survive up to 35 days at 4° C in CDPA solution. Citrate prevents clotting; dextrose is used for glycolysis; and phosphate and adenine help replenish adenosine triphosphate (ATP). In spite of these nutrients, potassium is lost from red cells, the 2,3-bisphosphoglyceric acid (BPG) concentration declines, and lactate accumulates (the storage "lesion"). The biochemical abnormalities are corrected after a day in the circulation. Red cells in storage are lost at the rate of 1% per day as they are in the body, so that at 35 days, only 70% of the red cells are intact. On average, 1 unit of packed red cells raises the hematocrit 3%. Patients who need blood replacement over months and years (e.g., those with aplastic anemia or thalassemia major) must be given preference for freshly drawn units.

Red Cells

The primary indication for red cell transfusion is to establish adequate oxygen carrying capacity in the individual patient setting. Red cell transfusions are most commonly given in the setting of symptomatic anemia, hemorrhage, or surgical blood loss. The hazards of receiving blood are iron accumulation, antigenic stimulation, and risk of infection. These risks are taken up separately later in the chapter.

Platelets

The second most important component of blood is the platelet. *The primary indication for platelet transfusion is to establish adequate numbers of platelets to prevent spontaneous hemorrhage or to prevent excessive bleeding during invasive procedures.* Each unit of blood yields about 5×10^{10} platelets. Platelet concentrates can be stored at room temperature for up to 5 days without loss of survival. Thrombocytopenia requiring platelet transfusion is commonly encountered in patients with hematologic or other malignancies who undergo chemotherapy. A single unit of platelets transfused normally raises the platelet count 6000 to 8000/μL. Platelet cross-matching is not yet developed.

A special problem for the patient who must receive platelets over a long period of time is the risk of developing antibodies that will destroy the platelets and make the transfusion ineffective. These antibodies may be directed against human leukocyte antigens (HLA) or other antigens on the platelet surface. About 40% of patients who receive platelets repeatedly over the course of a month will develop platelet refractoriness. In addition to antibody formation, splenomegaly, fever and sepsis as well as platelet storage contribute to shortened platelet ssurvival in the patient.

Fresh Frozen Plasma

The next most frequently used blood product is fresh frozen plasma. It is valued because most of the clotting factors are retained. The primary indication for transfusion of fresh frozen plasma is to achieve hemostasis by increasing the concentrations of circulating clotting factors in patients with compromised liver function. If expansion of the blood volume is needed, purified albumin or the less pure plasma protein fraction is preferred.

γ-Globulin

The next most commonly used plasma component is the immunoglobulin fraction, intravenous immunoglobulin, used to treat a variety of immune disorders. It confers passive immunity and is used to maintain patients with common variable immunodeficiency. It also interferes with macrophage functions, so that autoimmune destruction of platelets can be temporarily halted.

BLOOD GROUPS

The science of blood banking is built around the immunology of blood antigens and the system of procuring and fractionating the blood into its components. Therefore, most of this chapter is devoted to understanding the immunology of the red cell.

Blood types are based on genetic differences in cell membrane structure. These structural differences are important in clinical medicine because they can induce antibodies that may cause clinical disease. Two examples are hemolytic transfusion reactions and hemolytic disease of the fetus and newborn. A blood group system is a family of related antigens determined by alleles at a gene locus or a cluster of linked genetic loci. There are more than 20 systems of red cell antigens. The systems vary considerably in clinical importance. The goal of this chapter is to describe the red cell antigens that are the most important in blood transfusions and to explain why the systems vary in importance.

Red Cell Antigen Systems

The ABO System

The ABO blood cell antigen group of red cell antigens was discovered in a simple experiment in 1901 by Karl Landsteiner, who took blood samples from himself and five of his colleagues, separated the serum from the red cells, and mixed each serum with a sample of each of the six red cells. In some of these serum-cell mixtures, he noted visible agglutination or aggregation of the red cells; in others, he saw no change in the red cell suspension. From the patterns of agglutination, Landsteiner proposed the ABO and blood cell antigen system.

GENETICS AND BIOCHEMISTRY

By 1910, it was proved that a person's ABO group is inherited. The ABO locus is on chromosome 9. In addition to the original three alleles (A, B, and O), there is a fourth allele that produces a weaker A antigen. The two A alleles are called A_1 and A_2. A weak antigen (H) was found on group O cells. **Table 9-1** gives the antigen and antibody complement in the six phenotypes and the possible genotypes for each phenotype.

The ABO antibodies are usually IgM, but may be IgA or IgG. The reason for sustained IgM production is not known. These antibodies typically react well at room temperature or below (cold-reacting) and do not need additional reagents to enhance agglutination (saline-reacting; complete). IgG anti-A and anti-B usually are found only in group O persons. Anti-A and anti-B antibodies are easy to detect in the laboratory. Regardless of their immunoglobulin type, these antibodies produce visible agglutination of A and B red cells, respectively (Table 9-1).

TABLE 9-1. ABO Phenotypes, Genotypes, Antigens, and Antibodies

Phenotype	% Frequency	Genotypes	Antigens on Red Cell	Antibody in Serum
O	44	O/O	H	Anti-A, -B, -
AB				
A_1	42	A_1/A_1 A_1/A_2 A_1/O	A_1, A_2, small amount of H	Anti-B
A_2		A_2/A_2 A_2/O	A_2, moderate amount of H	Anti-B
B	10	$B/B, B/O$	B, small amount of H	Anti-A
A_1B	4	A_1/B	A_1, B, small amount of H	None
A_2B		A_2/B	A_2, B, small amount of H	None

The ABH antigens have been demonstrated on almost all body cells and are important in organ transplantation as well as in blood transfusion. Eighty percent of normal people ("secretors") have ABH antigens in saliva, sweat, tears, urine, bile, milk, and other body secretions. The ability to form the water-soluble antigens requires an additional secretor gene (*Se*).

In classical genetic terminology, the *O* gene is recessive to the A and B genes, and the O gene phenotype can be detected only when the *O* gene is present in double dose, that is, in group O. The *A* and *B* genes are both dominant over *O*. Thus, the heterozygotes, A/O and B/O, cannot be distinguished from the corresponding homozygotes, A/A and B/B, by typing of the red cells. The *A* and *B* genes are codominant to each other, so the A/B heterozygote has both A and B antigens on each cell. The A_2 gene is recessive to the A_1 gene.

The A, B, and H antigens are located on glycosphingolipid molecules. The carbohydrate chains are synthesized by the sequential action of transferase enzymes. Each transferase adds a specific sugar to a substrate. The H chain ends with a terminal fucose, a required substrate for enzymes produced by the *A* and *B* genes. A, B, and O are alleles of the same gene encoding a sugar transferase. Enzymes encoded by different alleles differ in several amino acids critical for enzyme specificity. The *A* gene produces an enzyme that adds *N*-acetyl-galactosamine to the H chain. The product is called an **A chain**. The *B* gene produces an enzyme that adds the galactose, converting H chains to B chains. The *O* gene is alleleic to the *A* and *B* genes but encodes a truncated protein without transferase activity. Group O chains are unaltered H chains (Fig. 9-1).

ANTIBODIES

Anti-A and anti-B antibodies are called "naturally occurring" and "regularly occurring," because they are always found in the blood of normal persons who lack the corresponding antigen. The carbohydrate chains carrying the ABH antigens are present on cell membranes of the fetus and newborn, but the child does not begin to make A and B antibodies until 3 to 6 months of age. Once antibody production begins, it continues for life, with declining antibody titers over the decades.

Why do these antibodies appear? The current view is that they are a product of an immune response to similar antigens in the environment. Carbohydrate chains similar to the A, B, and H chains are found on the cell membranes of bacteria, plants, and other animal species. An infant comes in contact with these carbohydrate chains in food or via the bacterial flora of the gastrointestinal tract. Those chains that are not present on infants' own cells induce an antibody

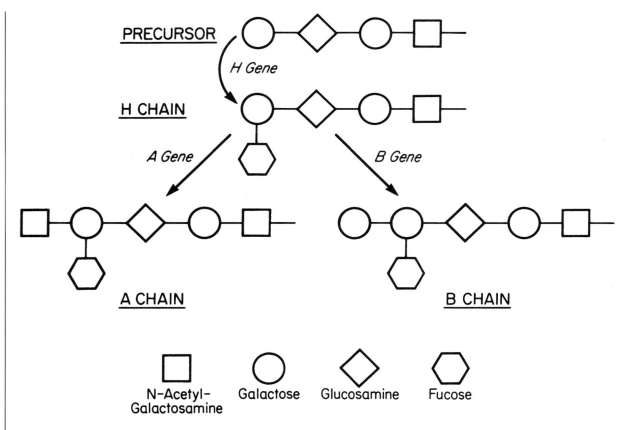

FIGURE 9-1.

Biochemistry of the ABO blood group. The *H* gene adds a fucose to the end of the glycosphingolipid chain. Under *A* gene influence, an *N*-acetyl-galactosamine is added. The *B* gene adds a galactose at the same site. If the *O* gene is dominant, the transferase is not functional.

response. For example, the group O infant makes antibodies against both the A and B antigens. The group A child makes only anti-B, and the group B child, anti-A. Why are no anti-H (anti-O) antibodies formed? The enzymatic conversion of H to A to B chains is not total. A few uncovered H chains remain on the cells of A, B, and AB individuals, presumably rendering them tolerant to H chains.

CLINICAL IMPORTANCE

The ABO system is the most important of all blood group systems because of the naturally and regularly occurring antibodies. Anti-A or anti-B antibodies or both are found in 95% of normal persons—all but those who are of group AB! If the ABO groups of patient and donor are not considered before blood is selected for transfusion, the patient's anti-A or anti-B antibodies may destroy the transfused red cells, sometimes leading to the death of the patient. The risk of ABO mismatch from a random donation of blood is about 30%.

Therefore, the first step in pretransfusion testing is to determine the patient's ABO group. Donor blood of the same ABO group is selected for transfusion. The donor red cells must not carry antigens that can be attacked by naturally and regularly occurring antibodies in the patient's plasma. Such blood is said to be ABO-compatible. In an emergency when there is insufficient time to type the patient's blood, we may transfuse group O red cells. We remove the plasma from the donor blood and give only the red cells, since the red cells of recipient, who is not group O, may be damaged by the anti-A and anti-B antibodies of the donor plasma.

The Rh System

From 1900 to 1940, blood transfusions were sometimes followed by hemolysis of the donor blood even though the patient and donor were of the same ABO group. No unusual red cell antibodies could be found in the sera of patients who had suffered such reactions. In 1939, Levine and Stetson discovered an antibody that was related to clinical transfusion reactions. The patient was a woman who had just given birth to a stillborn infant who had died from hemolytic anemia (hydrops fetalis). This was her second pregnancy. Because of bleeding during delivery, she was transfused with blood from her husband. A severe hemolytic reaction occurred in spite of the fact that she and her husband were of the same ABO group.

When Levine retested the woman's serum, he found an antibody that reacted with her husband's red cells as well as the cells of 80 of 104 ABO-compatible donors. He called the antibody **anti-Rh**, because it reacted to the same red cells as did an antibody to human red cells that had been raised in Rhesus monkeys. He postulated that the woman had been immunized to this new blood group antigen by her baby through the following sequence of events:

- The fetus inherited the antigen from the father.
- A few fetal red cells crossed the placenta into the mother's circulation.
- The mother made antibody against the foreign antigen.
- The antibody crossed the placenta and attacked the fetus's red cells, producing a severe hemolytic anemia.
- The fetus died from severe hemolytic anemia.

After delivery, when the woman was transfused with her husband's blood, this same antibody destroyed the transfused red cells, causing a second "disease," a hemolytic transfusion reaction.

Anti-Rh antibodies were found in the sera of some patients who had had hemolytic transfusion reactions and in the sera of some mothers of babies with hemolytic disease of the newborn. Rh antibodies were probably present in more of these patients, but were too weak to be detected in the laboratory. Rh antibodies are usually IgG, and, unlike the ABO antibodies, they do not readily agglutinate red cells suspended in saline solution. During the next few years, four other antibodies and their corresponding antigens were identified, which were categorized as part of the Rh antigen group: C, E, c, and e. C and E appeared to be related to D because C and E almost never were found in people who lacked D. Since c was always present when C was absent, it seemed to be a product of a gene allelic to C. E and e also behaved as products of allelic genes. A weaker form of D was found (Du) later, as was another type of C antigen (Cw). When methods were developed to detect IgG antibodies, many other rare Rh antigens were discovered.

GENETICS AND BIOCHEMISTRY

The *Rh* gene or genes are located on the short arm of chromosome 1. There are two closely linked genes, one for the D protein, the other for Cc/Ee. The *Cc/Ee* gene encodes the polypeptide carrying the Ee antigens, whereas, by alternative splicing, shorter polypeptides are produced that carry the Cc antigens. An individual who is Rh(D)-negative may have a homozygous deletion of the *D* gene or an active suppressor gene. The *D* and *Cc/Ee* genes have 96% homology and are

TABLE 9-2. The Rh System—Antigens

D	C	E
Du	c	e
(d)	C^W	E^W
	C^X	E^T
	ce*	e^S
	cE*	
	Ce*	

Compound antigens are produced when the corresponding genes are located on the same chromosome (cis position).

subject to crossing-over, gene deletion and mutation, or suppressor genes, explaining variant antigens (Table 9-2). In rare individuals, both the *D* and the *Cc/Ee* genes are nonfunctional (Rh null) and a chronic hemolytic anemia results. This suggests that the Rh proteins serve a function on the red cell membrane other than causing trouble for the blood bank.

The Rh system is the most complex of the human blood group systems. There are now more than 30 antigens, including compound antigens produced only when the required C and E alleles are present in *cis* position (i.e., on the same chromosome; see below). Rarities such as weak or absent antigens also occur. Tables 9-2 and 9-3 list the more common antigens and genotypes. In routine pretransfusion testing, only the original Rh antigen Rho(D) is tested for. The terms Rh-positive and Rh-negative refer only to the presence or absence of the immune-dominant Rho(D) antigen. Approximately 85% of whites are Rh-positive, and 15% are Rh-negative. Among American blacks, about 92% are Rh-positive and 8% are Rh-negative.

ANTIBODIES

Antibodies against the Rh antigens are uncommon (irregular). This is the opposite of the situation in the ABO system. Anti-Rho(D) antibodies appear in less than 5% of Rho(D)-negative persons. Antibodies against the C and E antigens are even more uncommon. When Rh antibodies are found, they are almost always "immune"—alloimmune; that is, they are the result of an identifiable not-self antigenic stimulus. Therefore, Rho(D) antibodies are found only in Rho(D)-negative persons who have been immunized by previous blood transfusions or by pregnancy.

Approximately 50% of Rho(D)-negative persons are immunized by a single exposure to the antigen through red cell transfusion (Table 9-4). Another 20%

TABLE 9-3. More Common Rh Genotypes

Genotype	Wisconsin Whites 3% Frequency	Rh Type
DCe/dce	32	+
DCe/DCe	7	+
dce/dce	16	−
DCe/DcE	14	+
DcE/dce	13	+
DcE/DcE	2	+

make antibody after a second antigenic stimulus. The remaining 30%, called "nonresponders," cannot be immunized. Rh antibody appears in the serum 2 to 6 weeks after antigenic stimulation. Often the first antibody to be detected is IgG (warm-reacting). Because the antibody is IgG, it is also incomplete; that is, it needs special methods for detection. Significant amounts of IgM antibody are found in only a minority of patients.

The Rho(D) antigen is approximately 20 or more times more effective as an antigenic stimulus than the other Rh antigens. This explains the differences in the prevalence of the non-ABO antibodies generally (Table 9-4).

CLINICAL ASPECTS

In all blood group systems, clinical importance is directly proportional to the incidence of blood group antibodies. Because an Rho(D)-negative person is very likely to be immunized by a transfusion of Rho(D)-positive blood, the second step in pretransfusion testing is to determine the patient's Rh type—positive or negative—for the Rho(D) antigen. Testing for the weak D antigen, Du, and for the C/c and E/e antigens is not routinely done. Once the Rh type is known, then donor blood of this Rh type is selected. Such blood is called "type specific." This means that the ABO group and Rh type of the patient and donor are the same.

In summary, ABO matching is done to prevent an immediate hemolytic transfusion reaction. If the patient and donor Rh types are different, usually no immediate hemolytic consequences occur. Rh matching of patient and donor is done to prevent such immunization, not to prevent a hemolytic transfusion reaction. The rationale for preventing immunization applies primarily to women of childbearing age: an Rh-negative woman who has Rh antibodies may be unable to bear children because, the Rh-positive child may die in utero from hemolytic disease of the newborn.

Hemolytic transfusion reactions due to anti-D occur infrequently because of the standard practice of transfusing only Rh-negative blood to Rh-negative patients. Clinical problems due to antibodies against the various C and E antigens are even less common because these antigens are only weakly immunogenic. When problems do occur, they take the form of hemolytic disease of the newborn or hemolytic transfusion reactions.

Other Red Cell Antigen Systems

Some of the other known systems of red cell antigens are listed in Tables 9-4 and 9-5. The M, N, and S antigens were discovered through deliberate experiments in which animals were immunized with human red cells. The others were almost all discovered as a consequence of clinical problems with transfusion reactions or hemolytic disease of the newborn.

TABLE 9-4. Relative Antigenic Potency

Antigen	% Potency*
D(Rho)	50–70
Kell	10
c(hr')	3
E(rh")	3
Duffy(Fyᵃ)	0.4–1
Kidd(Jkᵃ)	<0.2

*Percentage of persons who lack the antigen who would produce antibody after one exposure to the antigen (i.e., one transfusion).

TABLE 9-5. Other Red Cell Antigen Systems

System	Major Antigens	Comments
Kell	K(ell), k(Cellano)	Anti-K (Kell) is the most commonly occurring red cell antibod after anti-Rho(D). Among whites, 10% are Kell-positive, and 0% are Kell-negative.
Duffy	Fy^a, Fy^b, Fy–	Null gene (Fy–) very common in blacks (70%); has greater resistance to malaria.
Kidd	Jk^a, Jk^b	Antibodies to Jk^a may cause delayed hemolytic reaction.
MNSs	M, N, S, s	Spontaneously occurring antibodies to M are occasionally found.*
Lewis	Le^a, Le^b	Antigens are located on same chain as ABO antigens; antibodies usually IgM.*
I	I, i	Antigens are located on same chain as ABO. The common "cold agglutinin" found in cold agglutinin disease in an anti-I with increased thermal amplitude.*

IgM antibodies occur sporadically. They usually react with red cells only at temperatures below 37° C, and so do not cause clinical disease but cause problems in laboratory testing.

BIOCHEMISTRY

In most of the systems, there are two codominant alleles. Only in the last several years have researchers begun to decipher the structures and genetic basis of these "minor" red cell antigens. Antibodies against the minor red cell antigens are very uncommon. They are a result of direct immunization by blood transfusion or pregnancy.

CLINICAL ASPECTS

In the course of routine pretransfusion testing, no attempt is made to determine the patient's complete Rh phenotype or Kell, Duffy, Kidd, or MNSs type, and no attempt is made to match patient and donor for their complements of these various antigens. We know that a transfusion of red cells exposes the patients to antigens that are foreign to them. The risk of immunization is small because of the weak antigenicity of these antigens (Table 9-4). "Unexpected" blood group antibodies, that is, antibodies other than anti-A and anti-B, are found in only 1% to 2% of all patients; many of these are anti-Rho(D) (Table 9-6). When transfusions must be given to one of these immunized

TABLE 9-6. Incidence of Unexpected* Blood Group Antibodies

Antibodies	Incidence (%)
Anti-D(Rho)	0.5 (= 3% of Rh-negatives)
Other Rh (E, c, e, Ce)	0.5
Kell	0.3
Fy^a	0.1
All others	0.1
Total in all patients	1.5

Unexpected in the sense that they are found only occasionally in people who lack the antigen, in people who have been transfused, or in multiparous women. The antibodies are usually IgG immunoglobulins and are detected only by using special laboratory methods, including Coombs' (antiglobulin) test.

patients, the antibody must be detected and identified and donor blood selected that lacks the specific antigen. In other words, to prevent a hemolytic transfusion reaction, the donor red cells should lack the antigen corresponding to the specificity of the antibody in the patient's serum. Antibody screening and cross-matching accomplish this.

Other Blood Group Antigens

Human Leukocyte Antigens

The HLAs are transmembrane glycoproteins involved in self-recognition. Class I antigens (HLA-A, -B, -C) are found on all nucleated cells except spermatozoa and the trophoblast. Red cells carry insignificant amounts of HLA, but platelets probably adsorb HLA from the plasma. Class I antigens have some homology with immunoglobulin molecules. They are recognized by cytotoxic T cells and are the primary targets in graft rejection. These antigens are classified for clinical purposes using alloantibodies in a complement-dependent lymphocytotoxicity assay.

Class II antigens (HLA-DP, -DQ, -DR) are generated by immune response genes limited to hematopoietic progenitors, endothelial cells, monocytes, macrophages, B cells, and some T cells. These antigens are involved in antigen processing and the generation of effector T cells. Structurally, the class II antigens also have some homology with immunoglobulin molecules. Class I and II antigens are inherited as haplotypes—half from each parent—so that one of four siblings is likely to be identical. HLAs are extremely diverse: more than 40 antigens have been defined in the HLA-B region alone. These antigens are very important in organ transplantation. Blood and platelet transfusions may result in immunization to HLAs, mainly from contaminating leukocytes. These antibodies can jeopardize the success of organ transplantations or platelet transfusions. However, grafts fail even without prior sensitization. The fact that a transplant from an HLA-identical sibling to an unsensitized recipient may still result in graft rejection or graft-versus-host disease indicates that other phenomena are not yet accounted for in the present scheme.

Granulocyte Antigens

Several unique granulocyte antigens have been described (e.g., NA1, NA2.). Antibodies against these antigens occasionally cause neonatal granulocytopenia secondary to maternal antibodies, a syndrome analogous to hemolytic anemia of the fetus and newborn. They also cause autoimmune neutropenia. Febrile reactions and pulmonary infiltrates after transfusion are usually due to antibodies against leukocytes. Tests for these antibodies are not generally available. The febrile reactions can sometimes be reduced or avoided by removing leukocytes by filtering the blood.

Platelet Antigens

Four systems of platelet-specific antigens are known: Pl^A, Pl^E, Ko, and DUZO. Antibodies against one of these antigens may cause neonatal alloimmune thrombocytopenia due to antibody produced by the mother. A rare syndrome of post-transfusion purpura may occur in association with platelet-specific antibodies, usually anti-Pl^{A1}. Antibodies against HLA shorten the life span of transfused platelets so that after a period of 5 weeks many chronically transfused patients do not benefit from random-donor platelets. In this situation, HLA-matched platelets are given, usually with good results.

Antigens on Plasma Proteins

Variations in the structure of complement proteins and immunoglobulins, both IgG and IgA, occur. Antibodies against IgA may cause serious transfusion reactions including urticaria, wheezing, and rarely anaphylaxis, especially in IgA-deficient patients. Other transfusion problems are rare.

STANDARD PRETRANSFUSION TESTING

The tests that are ordinarily done before elective transfusion of red cells are listed in Table 9-7.

ABO Typing and Matching

ABO typing and matching of patient and donor ABO groups is the first and most important step. If this were not done, the donor or patient red cells (or both) would be destroyed by the normally occurring anti-A and anti-B antibodies.

Typing for the Rho(D) Antigen

Typing for the Rho(D) antigen, and transfusion of Rh-negative donor blood to Rh-negative patients is standard practice. The Coombs' test (see next section) is used to screen for the RhD antigen.

TABLE 9-7. Standard Pretransfusion Tests for Nonemergency Transfusions of Red Cells and Whole Blood

---

Donor Blood
1. ABO group
2. Rho(D) type (positive or negative); Rh-negatives also tested for weak D (Du)
3. Serum tested for unexpected antibodies to red cells
4. Tests for infectious agents and evidence of infection
   - Hepatitis B (antibodies to core antigens, presence of surface antigen in serum)
   - Hepatitis C (antibodies)
   - Hepatitis—general (alanine transaminse [ALT])
   - HIV-1 (antibodies, presence of P24 antigens in serum)
   - HIV-2 (antibodies)
   - Human T-cell lymphotrophic virus (HTLV)-1 (antibodies)
   - HTLV-2 (antibodies)
   - Syphilis (antibodies)

Patient's Blood
1. ABO group
2. Rho(D) type (positive or negative, no test for Du)
3. Select donor blood of same ABO/Rh as patient (type-specific)
4. Cross-match with patient serum versus donor red cells; blood usable only if cross-match–compatible, i.e., serum contains no antibody that can react with donor cells
5. Antibody screening with patient serum versus reagent red cells; negative (no antibodies) in 99% of patients

---

Antibody Screening

Antibody screening identifies the 1% to 2% of patients who have an unusual, unexpected antibody but not the specificity of the antibody. A sample of the patient's serum is tested against a series of red cell reagents. These reagent cells (group O) have been typed for about 30 antigens—the ones that are the most important in clinical practice—and a sufficient number of different reagents are used in the test to ensure that each of the antigens is present on at least one of the test cells. If the patient's serum does not react with these cells, it is concluded that no "unexpected" antibodies are present. Thus, the patient can be safely transfused with blood that is type-specific, that is, of the correct ABO and Rh type, without regard for any of the other known red cell antigen systems. (But additional testing, the cross-match, is done to ensure that this judgment is correct. See next section.)

In about 1% of patients, positive reactions are observed in the antibody screening. In such patients, the next step is to test the serum against additional reagent red cells to identify the specificity of the antibody, a procedure called "antibody identification." Donor blood is then specifically typed, and donor units are selected that lack the antigen to which the patient has antibody.

Cross-Matching

Cross-matching, the mixing of a sample of the patient's serum with a sample of the donor red cells, is done to double-check the results of the antibody screening and to eliminate the very rare possibility that the patient is immunized to an antigen not represented on the reagent red cells used in the antibody screening test. A sample of the patient's serum is tested against an aliquot of the donor red cells that are to be transfused. This is done in all cases, regardless of the results of the antibody screening. If the patient's serum reacts in the test tube with the donor red cells, then an unexpected antibody is present in the patient's serum, and the corresponding antigen is present on the red cells of this particular blood donor. This blood is incompatible for this patient and must not be transfused. The cross-match is repeated with additional donor units until a sufficient number of cells that do not react with the patient's antibody are found. If the donor red cells are not agglutinated by the patient's serum, they are said to be "compatible," meaning that post-transfusion survival of these cells probably will not be shortened by antibody in the patient's plasma.

METHODS USED IN THE ANTIBODY SCREENING AND CROSS-MATCH PROCEDURES

The Phenomenon of Agglutination

All test methods used today depend on agglutination reactions. Antibody is mixed with red cells in the test tube, and a positive reaction is indicated by agglutination of the test cells. All antibody molecules have at least two combining sites. Agglutination is the visible consequence of the attachment of two combining sites on one antibody molecule to two different red cells, forming a protein bridge that binds them together {#42}. When sufficient antibody cross-linkages form, agglutination can be observed with the naked eye. But agglutination occurs only if the cells can approach each other closely enough for one antibody molecule to attach to two different red cells. We have little control over the distance between combining sites on an immunoglobulin molecule; this is an intrinsic property of the molecule. The laboratory manipulations then consist of changing the distance between red cells.

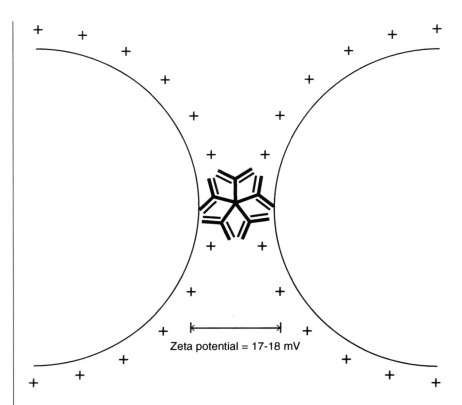

FIGURE 9-2.
The large IgM pentamer is able to agglutinate saline-suspended red cells. The positive charges represent Na⁺ attracted to negatively charged sialic acid groups. (Redrawn from Ortho Diagnostic Systems, Inc, Raritan, NJ. Bulletins: "Ortho Broad Spectrum Anti-Human Serum" (1970) and "Ortho Bovine Albumin.")

Red cells repel each other because of charged amino acid side groups and ionized sialic acid groups on the membrane. The distance between the red cells is partly determined by the ability of the suspending medium to dissipate this electrical repulsion, the **zeta potential** or dielectric constant. Steric hindrance, resulting from water of hydration bound to the cell membrane, is also important in maintaining separation between red cells.

With red cells suspended in 0.85% saline, IgM can bridge the intercellular gap and produce visible agglutination at room temperature (Fig. 9-2). IgG antibodies other than anti-A and anti-B can bind to red cell membrane antigen, but a second red cell does not ordinarily approach closely enough for visible agglutination to occur (Fig. 9-3). This antibody reaction is called "incomplete."

Several methods are used to reduce the intercell distance and allow agglutination of red cells by IgG antibody:

- Suspend the cells in a medium with a greater charge-dissipating capacity (LISS, low ionic strength solution), such as bovine albumin (Fig. 9-4) or synthetic polymers such as dextran, PVP (polyvinylpyrrolidone), or Ficoll.
- Modify the red cell membrane with sialidase, reducing the electrical charge and the water of hydration.
- Link the antibody molecules with an anti-antibody (Figs. 9-5 and 9-6).

The first and third methods are routinely used in blood banking.

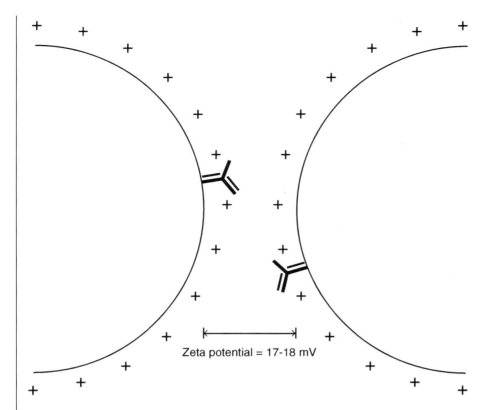

FIGURE 9-3.

The effective length (distance between combining sites) of IgG molecule is too short to produce visible agglutination of saline-suspended red cells. (Redrawn from Ortho Diagnostic Systems, Inc, Raritan, NJ. Bulletins: "Ortho Broad Spectrum Anti-Human Serum" (1970) and "Ortho Bovine Albumin.")

Coombs' or Antiglobulin Technique

The rationale of the Coombs' technique is to link two antibodies or complement molecules together by an anti-antibody to bridge between red cells and produce visible agglutination. A rabbit is immunized against human IgG and complement proteins. The serum from such an animal can be used as a reagent to detect IgG or complement bound to the surface of red cells. The technical name of this reagent is an "antiglobulin," that is, an antibody against immunoglobulin.

Test red cells are first allowed to react with the serum at 37° C to allow maximal binding of blood group antibody to red cell membrane antigen (warm-reacting antibody). The cells are washed with saline to remove unbound antibody. Then Coombs' antiglobulin serum is added. If IgG or complement was bound to the red cells, the antibody will attach to this protein, forming a three-piece bridge between adjacent red cells (red cell antibody, rabbit antibody, red cell antibody; Figs. 9-5 and 9-6). When used in this way, this test is often called the indirect Coombs' test.

A complete cross-match/antibody screening procedure must detect both IgM and IgG antibodies. The techniques always include a saline phase for IgM antibody and a Coombs' (or antiglobulin) phase for IgG.

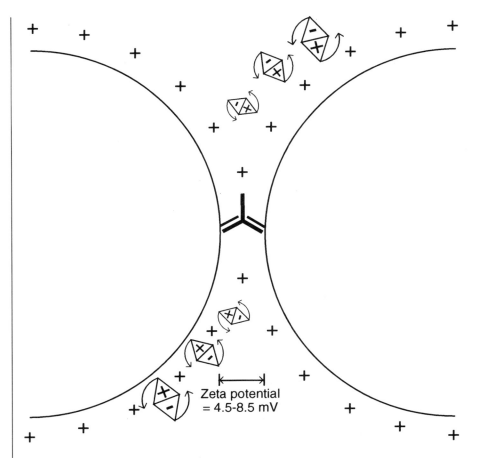

FIGURE 9-4.
Addition of a polar molecule such as bovine albumin in the suspending medium increases its ability to dissipate the repulsive force between red cells. The cells approach each other closely enough for an IgG molecule to span the intercell gap. (Redrawn from Ortho Diagnostic Systems, Inc, Raritan, NJ. Bulletins: "Ortho Broad Spectrum Anti-Human Serum" (1970) and "Ortho Bovine Albumin.")

In the figure: Zeta potential = 4.5-8.5 mV

Direct Coombs' Test

One can use the Coombs' technique to detect an antibody-red cell antigen reaction that is occurring in the patient's circulation. Examples are autoimmune hemolytic anemia; hemolytic disease of the newborn, in which antibody from the mother crosses the placenta and attacks the child's red cells; and a hemolytic transfusion reaction, in which the donor red cells are attacked by antibody from the patient's plasma.

A blood sample is drawn, and the red cells are washed several times with saline to remove all nonattached immunoglobulins. Then the Coombs' or antiglobulin reagent is added. If agglutination occurs, IgG or complement proteins are present. This test is called the "direct" Coombs' test because the antibody was attached in vivo. The indirect Coombs' test is the procedure used in blood banking for detecting antibodies that are attached to the red cell in vitro.

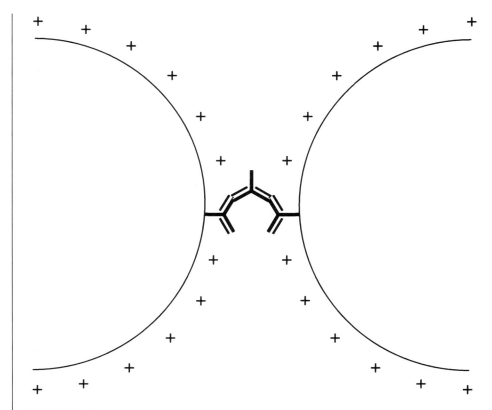

FIGURE 9-5.
Coombs' or antiglobulin reaction. The IgG molecules that have bound to red cell membrane antigen are linked by adding a heterologous antibody, which attaches to the heavy chains of the human immunoglobulin. The red cells are now cross-linked by a three-way immunoglobulin bridge. (Redrawn from Ortho Diagnostic Systems, Inc, Raritan, NJ. Bulletins: "Ortho Broad Spectrum Anti-Human Serum" (1970) and "Ortho Bovine Albumin.")

TRANSFUSION REACTIONS

Infections

The highest risk of infection is from hepatitis B and C viruses. About 1% of patients per unit of blood develop abnormal liver functions. Some patients infected with hepatitis B, especially with hepatitis C, develop chronic liver disease culminating with cirrhosis and hepatoma. HIV infection is more uniformly dangerous, but the risk is much less, less than 0.001%. Other infections rarely transmitted by blood include cytomegalovirus, toxoplasmosis, malaria, and syphilis. A potentially lethal infection can develop from transfusion of bacterially contaminated blood.

Traditionally, patients with chronic anemia were transfused below Hb 10 g/dL. The threshold for giving blood in cases of chronic anemia has changed from Hb of 10 g/dL to 7 g/dL. The reason for the previous threshold was the observation that the cardiac output begins to increase at hemoglobins below 10 g/dL. The emergence of HIV and recognition of the potential viciousness of hepatitis C, however, forced the medical community to reexamine this criterion. The public also reacted to the fear of HIV by demanding autologous transfusion for elective procedures. The risks listed below are being diminished by screening, but more subtle problems such as immune impairment and increased risk of cancer are also being described. Table 9-8 outlines some transfusion risks.

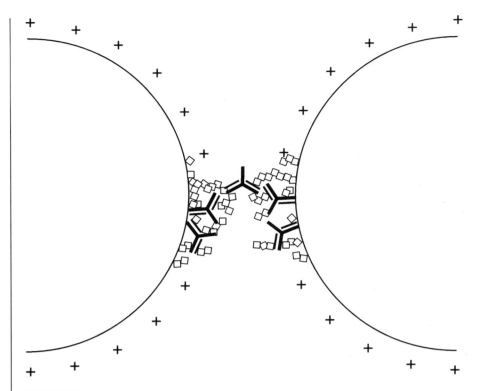

FIGURE 9-6.
Broad-spectrum Coombs' serum also contains antibody against complement proteins (C3 and C4), so it will cross-link red cells that have complement (*open boxes*) bound to their surfaces. (Redrawn from Ortho Diagnostic Systems, Inc, Raritan, NJ. Bulletins: "Ortho Broad Spectrum Anti-Human Serum" (1970) and "Ortho Bovine Albumin.")

One recent development to increase the safety of transfusion is the use of autologous transfusion for elective surgical procedures. Patients donate their own blood for their use two or three times before having coronary bypass, hip surgery, or prostate resection. This process bypasses the risks of reaction; however, only a small percentage of the patients who need blood are candidates for autologous transfusion.

Immune Transfusion Reactions

Transfusion reactions are classified according to their cause. Immunologic reactions are due to interaction between antibody and antigen. Usually, the antibody is present in the patient's plasma before the transfusion, and it reacts with some cellular or protein component of the donor blood. The offending antigen may be located on the cell membrane of red cells, platelets, or leukocytes, or on plasma protein molecules.

Immune Hemolysis

Two to five percent of patients experience a transfusion reaction when they receive blood transfusions. Transfusion reactions vary in severity from trivial problems, such as one or two hives, to death. Of 70 fatalities associated with

TABLE 9-8. Risks of Red Blood Cell Transfusion

Risk	Frequency per Transfusion
Infection	
Cytomegalovirus	Common
Non-A, non-B hepatitis*	1/3000–5,000
Hepatitis B	1/60,000–65,000
HIV	1/500,000
Immune reactions	
Fever, chills, urticaria	1/50–1/100
Hemolysis	1/25,000
Hemolysis with death	1/500,000
Graft-versus-host phenomena	Unknown but real

*Mostly hepatitis C.

blood transfusion, 56% were due to hemolytic reactions and *half of those were due to clerical error in preparing or administering blood.* Fortunately such events are rare (Table 9-8). Studies by blood banks have shown that the tendency to human error is such that there always is a chance of mixup, no matter how well-trained and well-meaning the personnel.

Intravascular Hemolysis

THE FATE OF TRANSFUSED RED CELLS

Intravascular hemolysis usually occurs because the patient is inadvertently given donor blood of the wrong ABO group. The most common mismatch is the transfusion of group A blood to a group O patient. The group A donor red cells are attacked immediately in the patient's plasma by the circulating anti-A antibodies, which are almost always complement-binding. Activation of the complement system produces holes in the membrane of the donor red cells, and the sequence of intravascular hemolysis described in Chapter 6.

THE FATE OF THE PATIENT

Mismatched transfusions are accompanied by immediate and severe symptoms, usually beginning with shaking chills and fever. The patient may complain of headache or pain in the chest, back, or extremities. Shortness of breath (dyspnea), nausea, vomiting, and diarrhea are common. One of the most serious changes is hypotension, which may be severe enough to constitute outright shock. Hypotension is accompanied by compensatory tachycardia. Peripheral vasodilation results from the release of vasoactive compounds, such as serotonin and histamine from platelets and mast cells, and complement fragments (C3a and C5a). Norepinephrine released from the adrenal medulla constricts the renal arterioles and causes renal cortical ischemia. Necrosis of the cells lining the renal proximal convoluted tubules may occur. The renal ischemia results in a period of oliguria or anuria of varying duration (Fig. 9-7).

The ischemic damage to the kidney may be aggravated by disseminated intravascular coagulation. The clotting system is activated by the direct effect of antigen-antibody complexes on factor XII and is accelerated by phospholipids released from platelets, leukocytes, and the stroma of the lysed red cells. The small fibrin clots that are produced tend to localize in those organs in which the circulation is the slowest in this clinical situation, the kidneys (Fig. 9-8).

The adverse effects of hemolysis are dose-related: the more incompatible blood the patient receives, the worse the consequences. Review of the clinical course of adult patients who have received 200 to 500 mL of ABO-incompatible blood showed that 85% to 90% experienced an immediate episode of shock and anuria lasting 1 to 2 hours. The symptoms were self-limited and disappeared as the vasoactive compounds are removed from the circulation and the fibrin clots are lysed. Of the remaining patients, some died of irreversible shock within a few hours. In others, prolonged renal vasoconstriction and extensive intravascular coagulation resulted in ischemic necrosis of the cells lining the convoluted tubules. The overall mortality rate from acute hemolytic transfusion reactions has been estimated at 10%.

Immediate Extravascular Hemolysis

Extravascular removal of red cells from the circulation occurs when antibody is bound to red cell membrane antigen without complete activation of complement. The IgG coated red cells are phagocytized by macrophages. Extra-

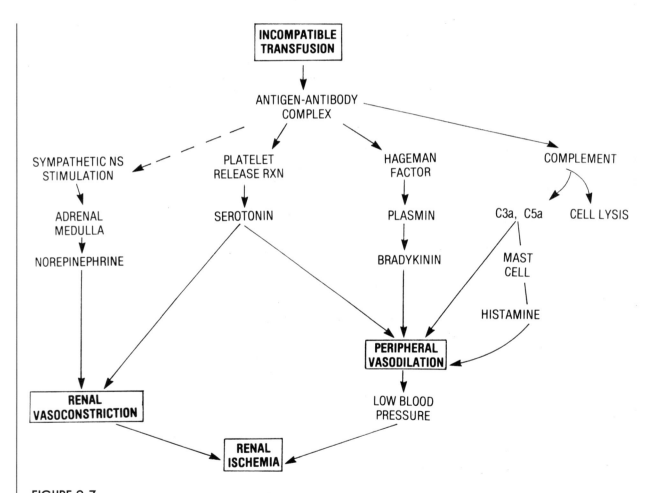

FIGURE 9-7.

Pathophysiology of vascular complications of incompatible red cell transfusion. The kidney is the target organ. NS, nervous system; RXN, reaction. (Adapted from Goldfinger D. "Complications of Hemolytic Transfusion Reactions: Pathogenesis and Therapy in New Approaches to Transfusion Reactions," Arlington, VA: American Association of Blood Banks.)

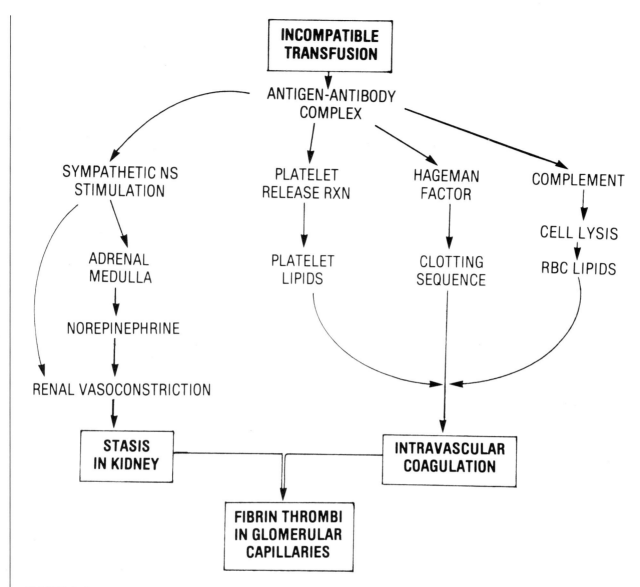

FIGURE 9-8.
Initiation of coagulation by incompatible red cell transfusion. Effects are concentrated on the kidney. NS, nervous system; RXN, reaction. (Adapted from Goldfinger D: "Complications of Hemolytic Transfusion Reactions: Pathogenesis and Therapy in New Approaches to Transfusion Reactions," Arlington, VA: American Association of Blood Banks.)

vascular hemolytic reactions are rarely fatal. The immediate symptoms are usually limited to chills and fever. If phagocytosis is rapid, bilirubin excretion by the liver may not keep pace with production, and jaundice may begin after a few hours. Mismatches in the Rh, Duffy, Kell, or Kidd system usually fit this description.

Delayed Hemolysis

Since the patient and blood donor are ordinarily matched only for their ABO and Rho(D) type, immunization to other red cell antigens is always a possibility. If antibody begins to appear in the circulation before all of the donor red cells have lived out their expected life spans, the remaining cells will be destroyed by the newly formed antibody. This clinical situation is called a "delayed hemolytic transfusion reaction." The patient is usually asymptomatic, and the condition is diagnosed when a recently transfused patient exhibits a falling hemoglobin in the absence of blood loss. The direct Coombs' test is positive as long as donor cells remain in the circulation. Delayed hemolytic reactions are rare, occurring only once for every 20,000 to 30,000 units of blood transfused, but more commonly in frequently transfused patients.

Other Transfusion Reactions not Involving Red Cells

Fever not due to red cell antigen-antibody reactions is the most common transfusion reaction (3% to 5% of transfused units) and may be stimulated by foreign leukocytes, platelets, or plasma components. **Urticaria** may be caused by reactions to allergens that the donor ingested; hence, donors are asked to come to the blood center fasting. Rarely, a white cell agglutination reaction is accompanied by dyspnea and pulmonary infiltrates. **Anaphylaxis** may be caused by anti-IgA antibodies in a patient deficient in IgA. The anaphylactic reaction caused by IgA in transfused blood can be avoided by giving washed red cells.

Volume-Related Transfusion Reactions

Finally, patients whose entire blood volume is replaced with donor blood within a period of 12 to 24 hours may develop special problems, generally related to changes that occur in the donor blood during storage. Such complications may include:

- Hypocalcemia due to citrate overload (citrate binds free Ca^{2+})
- Hyperkalemia (potassium leaked from stored red cells)
- Acidosis (hydrogen ions in storage solution plus glycolytic products)
- Alterations in oxygen transport (2,3-BPG is depleted in stored blood)
- Bleeding from dilution of clotting factors
- Respiratory insufficiency due to fluid overload

SUMMARY POINTS

Transfusion of the components of blood—red cells, platelets, whole plasma, and purified plasma proteins—is important for treatment of a wide variety of diseases. Risks of transfusions fall into two major categories—immunologic reactions with alloantigens and transmission of infection. A working knowledge of the relative importance of various red cell antigens and of transfusion-transmitted diseases is required for the practice of medicine.

CASE DEVELOPMENT PROBLEM: CHAPTER 9

History: Mrs. D.R., a 66-year-old woman, was admitted on March 2, for treatment of a bleeding duodenal ulcer. On admission, she was vomiting blood. Her blood pressure was 110/60 lying and 80/50 standing; pulse rate was 130/minute standing. Her history revealed a cholecystectomy 28 years before and hysterectomy 14 years before. She had been transfused both times. She had never been pregnant.

Laboratory values on admission: HCT 21%, Hb 7 g/dL, bilirubin 0.4 mg/dL. The patient was grouped B, Rh-negative. No unexpected antibodies were present in the serum. Because of the urgency of the situation and the unavailability of B, Rh-negative blood, she was given 4 units of B, Rh-positive packed red blood cells. All 4 units were compatible on cross-match.

1. What is the incidence in the population of B, Rh-negative blood?
2. Why was the patient given packed red cells instead of whole blood?
3. How could the units be compatible on cross-match if the patient was Rh-negative and the blood given was Rh-positive?
4. What is the likelihood that these Rh-positive transfusions will immunize the patient to the D antigen? In how many days do you expect this new antibody to first be detectable?
5. Assuming no further bleeding, what do you expect the hemoglobin and hematocrit to be after 4 units of blood?

   Subsequent hospital course: Hematocrit values on subsequent days were as follows:

   > 32% on March 4
   > 31% on March 7
   > 29% on March 9
   > 27% on March 11
   > 24% on March 14

6. What are the possible explanations for the fall in hematocrit?

   On March 14, the patient's stool guaiacs and gastric aspirate guaiacs were negative for occult blood. She was noted to be jaundiced with a bilirubin of 8.2 mg/dL, of which 6.6 mg/dL was indirect.

7. What is the likely explanation for the jaundice in this patient?
8. What further laboratory studies would confirm your diagnosis?

   The patient's pretransfusion cross-matches were rechecked and reconfirmed as negative. A direct Coombs' test on the patient's blood on March 14 was 2+ positive, and an irregular antibody was found in her serum. This was characterized as anti-D.

9. How do you explain these findings?
10. When did the initial antigenic stimulus probably occur?
11. Why were the cross-matches compatible on admission?
12. What kind of transfusion reaction is this? How could it have been prevented?
13. Where was the hemolysis probably taking place in this patient?
14. (a) Define "extravascular transfusion reaction." (b) What complications are associated with it? (c) In what Ag-Ab system are extravascular transfusion reactions likely to occur?
15. (a) In what Ag-Ab systems are intravascular transfusion reactions likely to occur? Why? (b) What are the symptoms? (c) What are the complications? What is the pathophysiology of each complication? (d) How do you confirm that an intravascular transfusion reaction has occurred? (e) What do you do for the patient if you suspect that an intravascular transfusion reaction is occurring?
16. List the other transfusion complications and their causes.
17. The patient, now 94, is in good health but obsessed with the fear that she contacted AIDS from prior blood transfusions. Can you reassure her?

CASE DEVELOPMENT ANSWERS

1. Incidence of B, Rh-negative: 11% × 15% = 1.7%. Because of the rarity of B, Rh-negative blood, the patient was given B, Rh-positive blood.
2. The patient shows evidence of acute loss of 25% to 30% of her blood volume (blood pressure changes, tachycardia). She also has had chronic blood loss

because her hematocrit is about half normal. She has an immediate need for plasma to replace blood volume losses and red cells to replace oxygen carrying capacity. Logistics favor the use of separated plasma and packed red cells.

3. The patient does not have preformed anti-D antibody. Rh antibodies are found in people who have been immunized by previous contact with human red cells, but not all such people become immunized, in part because immunologic tolerance is induced by the large volume of antigen given in the usual transfusion.

4. The likelihood of immunization to the Rho(D) antigen by a transfusion of 1 unit of blood is 50% to 100%. Antibody usually is detected in the serum after several weeks. Antibody production probably starts in 2 to 3 days, but synthesis is slow at first and all of the antibody is "mopped up" by the transfused RH-positive donor cells.

5. A simple rule of thumb is that in adults, each unit of blood increases the hematocrit by 3%. Therefore, 4 units increase the hematocrit by 12 percentage points, to 33%.

6. Falling hematocrit is most likely due to continued bleeding. If this is ruled out, then hemolysis due to newly formed antibody should be looked for. Immune hemolysis probably occurs after less than 5% of clinical transfusions. It is more likely in this patient because of the history of previous transfusions.

7. Hemolysis by antibody is most likely.

8. Indicated laboratory tests: Coombs' test, antibody screening, re–cross-match sample from the 4 donor units (if still available), with a new blood sample from the patient.

9. Immunization has occurred; probably it is a secondary or anamnestic response.

10. First immunization to Rho(D) antigen probably occurred with transfusions given 28 years before. At this time, the Rh system had been only recently discovered and Rh typing was not widely done because of the unavailability of IgM anti-D reagents and lack of knowledge of methods for detecting IgG antibodies in the test tube.

11. Antibody level was below the threshold for in vitro tests.

12. Hemolysis is extravascular. It could have been prevented by transfusing Rh-negative red cells. In this case, there was no B, Rh-negative blood available, but group O, Rh-negative packed red cells could have been given. (Group AB plasma might be given also to provide greater increase in blood volume. We do not give O, Rh-negative whole blood because the anti-B antibodies in group O plasma may destroy the patient's red cells.)

13. Red cells are destroyed in the spleen and other monocyte-macrophage organs.

14. (a) Extravascular hemolysis is characterized by destruction of red cells with IgG antibodies by splenic trapping and phagocytosis. (b) If antibody had been present in high titer at the time of transfusion, the patient would have had chills and fever, and jaundice after 5 to 6 hours. In this case, hemolysis is slower and symptoms are therefore unlikely. Hemolysis is evident only from falling hemoglobin, jaundice, and late-developing positive direct Coombs' test. (c) Antigen systems usually involved are Rh, Kell, Duffy, Kidd, S, and so on.

15. (a) Intravascular hemolysis is almost exclusively seen with ABO incompatibility because of regularly occurring high-titer IgM antibodies that bind complement. (b) Symptoms: chill, fever, hives, dyspnea, fall in blood pressure and tachycardia, nausea and vomiting, pain in extremities and back, and other locations. (c) Complications are shock, renal failure, and bleeding diathesis. Pathophysiology is discussed in the text. (d) Hemolysis is confirmed by free hemoglobin in plasma and urine. (e) Stop the transfusion;

hydrate; give diuretics (furosemide); give heparin if disseminated intravascular coagulation is present.

16. Febrile reactions, allergic reactions, and volume-related reactions.
17. Yes. Transmission of AIDS is most likely from transfusions received between 1979, when AIDS was first recognized, and 1985, when rigorous donor selection and screening of donated units for anti-HIV antibodies became mandatory in this country.

CHAPTER 10

Immune Hemolysis

Robert E. Exten

OUTLINE

OBJECTIVES

- Know the major sites of extravascular hemolysis and how red cells are targeted to those sites.
- Know causes of hemolytic disease of the newborn (HDN) not mediated by antibodies and mediated by antibodies.
- Know how HDN is prevented and treated.
- Understand the thermal range, characteristics, and specificity of warm and cold antibodies, site of hemolysis, and clinical manifestations.
- Know diseases associated with warm and cold antibodies.
- Understand why splenectomy works in warm autoimmune hemolyic anemia and not in cold autoimmune hemolytic anemia.
- Describe the pathophysiology of Raynaud's phenomenon.
- Understand mechanisms of different types of drug-induced immune hemolysis and the prototypic drugs.

Immune hemolysis is antibody-mediated destruction of circulating red cells. It can be classified broadly into isoimmune, autoimmune, and drug-induced immune reactions. This chapter discusses all three.

INTERPRETATION OF COOMBS' TEST

An essential requirement for classifying a hemolytic anemia as immune is the demonstration of an antibody or complement on the erythrocyte membrane. Antibody or complement on the erythrocyte can be detected by the direct antiglobulin (Coombs') test. As described in Chapter 9, the antiglobulin reagent agglutinates red cells by attaching simultaneously to antibody or complement molecules on two or more erythrocytes.

False-Negative Results

Most patients with antibody-mediated hemolysis have a positive result from the direct Coombs' test. However, false-negative test results do occur. Broad-spectrum antiglobulin serum cannot detect fewer than 100 to 500 molecules of antibody or C3 per erythrocyte. A lower density of antibody or C3 molecules can at times produce hemolysis but a false-negative Coombs' test. (For reference, fewer than 35 molecules of IgG can be found on the normal erythrocyte.). Two percent to 5% of patients with immune hemolytic anemias have a false-negative direct antiglobulin reaction, and special methods are required to detect the antibody. The addition of polyvinylpyrrolidone or other low-ionic-strength solutions, decreases the zeta potential and enhances weak reactions. Immune hemolytic anemia with a truly negative direct antiglobulin test result is rare.

False-Positive Results

A positive result from the Coombs' test is not proof of immune hemolysis. A false-positive direct antiglobulin test may occur in the presence of coexisting autoimmune disease or drug therapy or in the absence of known causes. False-positive results occur as a rare coincidental finding in patients with nonimmune hemolytic anemia.

The IgG subclass is an important determinant in autoimmune hemolytic disease. IgG3 antibodies are associated with marked shortening of the erythrocyte life span. IgG1 antibodies are occasionally associated with premature erythrocyte destruction. IgG2 and IgG4 antibodies are rarely associated with shortening of erythrocyte survival. Thus, the presence of IgG2 or IgG4 on the erythrocyte is one explanation for a positive direct antiglobulin reaction in the absence of overt hemolysis.

GENERAL MECHANISMS

Extravascular Hemolysis

Extravascular autoimmune hemolysis is much more common than intravascular autoimmune disease. It is caused primarily by IgG autoantibodies and occasionally by IgM antibodies with incomplete complement activation. The antibody class and the presence or absence of the complement component C3b determine the predominant site of extravascular hemolysis. The spleen is an efficient filter of IgG-coated erythrocytes. Splenic macrophages have receptors for the Fc fragment of IgG with specificity for IgG1 and IgG3. Some of these macrophages also have receptors for the activated third component of complement, C3b. These receptors act synergistically in binding IgG and C3b, and erythrocytes coated with both IgG and C3 are cleared more efficiently than those coated with IgG alone.

The liver has a relatively small concentration of macrophages with IgG receptors compared with the spleen, although the hepatic macrophages have a larger number of receptors for C3b. Clearance of IgM-coated erythrocytes occurs through partial activation of the complement sequence, attachment of C3b to the erythrocyte membrane, and detection of erythrocyte C3b by the hepatic macrophage receptor. As a result, the liver is the predominant site of extravascular hemolysis of IgM-coated erythrocytes. If phagocytosis does not occur in the hepatic macrophages, however, C3b inactivator cleaves C3b to C3d. Since the hepatic macrophages have no receptor for C3d, these erythrocytes are released from the hepatic macrophages. Erythrocytes coated with C3d survive normally in the circulation.

Red cell survival is proportional to the number of either IgG or IgM antibody molecules per cell. Since the liver receives 30% of the cardiac output (whereas the spleen receives 5%), the liver becomes the major site of hemolysis when large numbers of IgG molecules are present on the cell. Hepatic clearance of IgG-coated erythrocytes is enhanced by high plasma concentration of specific IgG antibody and high concentration of specific antigenic binding sites on the erythrocyte membrane.

Intravascular Hemolysis

Intravascular hemolysis in immune hemolytic anemia requires fixation and complete activation of complement. Although IgM isoantibodies (ABO incompatibility) predictably cause intravascular hemolysis, IgM autoantibodies usually do not. They most often bind complement only through C3b, and the red cells are removed by liver macrophages. Several factors are involved in whether hemolysis will be intravascular or extravascular, such as the nature and subclass of the antibody and the frequency and proximity of the antigenic sites.

- IgM autoantibodies are more likely than IgG antibodies to activate complement to C9, but occasionally IgG can also do so. One molecule of IgM or two molecules of IgG are necessary to completely activate one molecule of complement. In intravascular hemolysis due to IgG, complement activation occurs when two IgG molecules, a "doublet," are within 250 to 400 angstroms on the erythrocyte membrane.
- A second determinant of complement activation by IgG is the antibody subclass. IgG4 does not activate complement. The IgG1 and IgG3 subclasses are strong activators of complement, whereas IgG2 is a weak activator of complement.
- A third determinant of complement activation by IgG consists in the proximity and number of antigen-binding sites on the erythrocyte membrane. There are 10,000 to 20,000 Rho(D) antigens per red cell, but about 800,000 A and B antigens per red cell. This is another reason why intravascular hemolysis is typical of ABO mismatches, whereas Rh mismatches usually result in extravascular hemolysis.

HEMOLYTIC DISEASE OF THE NEWBORN

There are at least five causes of hemolytic disease of the newborn (HDN): hereditary elliptocytosis, hereditary spherocytosis, glucose-6-phosphate dehydrogenase deficiency, α-thalassemia, and maternal antibody. In this chapter, discussion of HDN is limited to maternal antibody. Maternal IgG antibody may be naturally occurring or due to sensitization by transplacental hemorrhage or previous transfusion. Ninety-eight percent of cases of HDN are due to ABO or Rho(D) incompatibility between mother and fetus.

Pathogenesis

HDN is caused by passage of an IgG antibody from the mother across the placenta and attachment of the IgG to a fetal erythrocytic antigen. Hemolysis occurs extravascularly in the spleen, resulting in anemia and the production of unconjugated bilirubin. Unconjugated bilirubin is not dangerous to the fetus because it is cleared by the placenta and metabolized in maternal liver. When hemolysis is severe, normoblasts proliferate in the liver and spleen, and normoblasts appear in the blood (erythroblastosis fetalis). The liver becomes obstructed and injured by this normoblastic hyperplasia, leading to massive hepatosplenomegaly, edema, and ascites (hydrops fetalis). Babies are born dead or with a high neonatal mortality.

Two normal changes in the newborn may aggravate the severe hemolytic disease. The first is the diminished stimulus to erythropoiesis owing to the increased concentration of oxygen in the blood after birth. The second event is the delayed appearance of glucuronyl transferase. Jaundice occurring during this early postpartum period in normal infants is called "physiologic jaundice of the newborn" and is due to the inability of the immature liver to conjugate bilirubin. In the infant born with significant hemolytic disease, extremely high levels of unconjugated bilirubin may accumulate. Indirect bilirubin levels greater than 20 mg/dL are associated with neurologic damage resulting from deposition of unconjugated bilirubin in the basal ganglia (kernicterus).

The clinical expression of HDN depends on the following variables:

- Concentration of IgG antibodies that cross the placenta into the fetal circulation
- Capacity of the fetal monocyte-macrophage system to destroy antibody-coated erythrocytes
- Ability of the fetal bone marrow to increase red cell production
- Rate at which the newborn resumes erythropoiesis after the normal physiologic increase in oxygen
- Ability of the neonatal liver to synthesize glucuronyl transferase (i.e., hepatic maturity)

Hemolytic Disease of the Newborn Due to ABO Incompatibility

Maternal-fetal ABO group incompatibility is the most common cause of HDN. Most episodes of hemolytic disease due to ABO incompatibility are asymptomatic or mild; only 10% of severe hemolytic disease is due to ABO incompatibility. The disease is mild because (1) most anti-A is IgM and does not cross the placenta; (2) 80% of the population are ABH antigen secretors and are called "secretors"), so that the antibody has many more soluble antigen combining sites besides the red cell; and (3) the ABO blood group antigens are not well developed at birth. ABO incompatibility is almost always seen in infants born to type O mothers, since naturally occurring IgG anti-A and anti-B antibodies occur in the sera of group O individuals. Since the offending antibodies are usually naturally occurring, no primary immunization is necessary, and HDN may occur with the first pregnancy that is ABO-incompatible. Unlike Rho(D) hemolytic disease, the development of ABO-incompatible HDN with one pregnancy is of no prognostic value in predicting the incidence or severity of ABO-incompatible hemolytic disease with subsequent pregnancies.

Hemolytic Disease of the Newborn Due to Rho(D) Incompatibility

In contrast to ABO hemolytic disease, Rho(D) incompatibility requires prior sensitization and is likely to cause severe hemolysis. Although small volumes (0.1 mL) of fetal erythrocytes may cross the placenta during pregnancy, such quantities are usually not sufficient to immunize the mother. Hemolytic disease, therefore, does not usually occur with the first pregnancy. However, significant transplacental hemorrhage may occur at labor and delivery, so that immunization can occur and subsequent pregnancies with Rho(D)-positive fetuses are at risk for hemolytic anemia. Primary immunization can also occur when an Rho(D)-negative woman aborts an Rho(D)-positive fetus. Since immunization is more likely to occur with large numbers of Rho(D)-positive erythrocytes, transfusion of Rho(D)-positive erythrocytes is more likely to immunize an Rho(D) recipient than is a pregnancy with an Rho(D)-positive fetus. About 15% of Rh-negative mothers with Rh-positive babies become immunized to the Rho(D) antigen during labor and delivery.

After primary immunization, the small numbers of erythrocytes that cross the placenta during a subsequent pregnancy are sufficient to induce a secondary immune response. The secondary immune response results in an increase of the maternal Rho(D) antibody titer. The appearance of Rho(D) antibody in the maternal circulation is an important prognostic sign: all future pregnancies with Rho(D)-positive fetuses will be affected, and the severity of the disease tends to be progressive with each Rho(D) pregnancy.

ABO antigens have an important effect on Rho(D) HDN. When pregnancy occurs with an ABO-compatible, Rho(D)-positive fetus, the incidence of immunization is about 15% per pregnancy. However, when pregnancy occurs with an ABO-incompatible, Rho(D)-positive fetus, immunization occurs in about 3% per pregnancy. This protective effect of ABO incompatibility occurs because ABO-incompatible fetal erythrocytes entering the maternal circulation are rapidly destroyed intravascularly by complement-fixing anti-A or anti-B alloantibodies before they reach the monocyte-macrophage system, where primary immunization against Rh antigens could occur.

Treatment

Treatment for HDN is intended to prevent complications caused by anemia and hyperbilirubinemia. In mild HDN, as is often seen with ABO incompatibility, delivery effectively interrupts the source of maternal antibody. No specific therapy is necessary, since the residual antibody-sensitized erythrocytes are cleared by macrophages, and the infant's bone marrow and liver are able to compensate for the mild degree of hemolysis.

Simple transfusions may be used in infants with only mild anemia and mild hyperbilirubinemia. However, severe HDN (cord blood Hb <12 g/dL and cord bilirubin >20 mg/dL) is treated with exchange transfusions of group O, Rho(D)-negative erythrocytes resuspended in group AB plasma. Exchange transfusions correct the newborn's anemia and prevent kernicterus by removing indirect (unconjugated) bilirubin. In addition, maternal antibody is removed from the newborn's circulation, decreasing hemolysis. Also, the Rh-negative cells transfused are not subject to destruction by any residual maternal antibody.

Phototherapy is used as adjunctive therapy for hyperbilirubinemia. Blue-violet and yellow-green light slowly oxidizes bilirubin pigments in the skin to water-soluble compounds that are excreted in the urine.

Erythroblastosis fetalis should be suspected in pregnant women with a history of neonatal hemolytic disease or hydrops fetalis after a previous pregnancy or with sensitization to the Rho(D) antigen. Amniocentesis should be performed when rising antibody titers are found on serial antibody screens (indirect Coombs' test). In a sensitized mother, the level of bilirubin in the amniotic fluid is directly related to the severity of erythroblastosis in the fetus. Intrauterine transfusion may prevent hydrops fetalis in a fetus with erythroblastosis (<34 weeks' gestation). Beyond 34 weeks' gestation, when pulmonary maturity is suggested by amniocentesis, early delivery may be necessary to interrupt severe erythroblastosis fetalis.

Prevention

Rho(D) sensitization is preventable. Rho(D)-negative women of child-bearing age should not be transfused with Rho(D)-positive erythrocytes except in life-threatening circumstances. Routine prenatal screening of pregnant women should include ABO and Rho(D) typing. An antibody screening of the mother's serum should be done at both 2 to 3 months' and 7 to 8 months' gestation. The Rh type of the fetus should be determined at birth. Rho(D)-positive pregnancies in unsensitized Rho(D)-negative women should be treated with Rh immuno-globulin within 72 hours of delivery. Any Rho(D)-negative woman who becomes pregnant should receive Rh immunoglobulin if she has previously received a transfusion of erythrocytes, platelets, or granulocytes from an Rho(D)-positive donor. Rh immunoglobulin (Rhogram) should be given to all Rh-negative women after an abortion.

Rh immune globulin is fractionated from the plasma of human volunteers containing anti-Rho(D) antibody. The mechanism of action of Rh immune globu-lin is not known. Simple antigen blockade explains only some of the effect; there is also evidence that a central inhibition of the immune system by IgG immune complexes inhibits the primary immune response.

Administration of Rh immune globulin is effective; it prevents immunization in 90% of the women at risk. The remaining 10% of women who are therapeutic failures probably have had significant transplacental hemorrhages in the third trimester. A controversy presently exists as to whether Rh immune globulin should be given at 28 or 34 weeks' gestation in addition to the currently recommended postpartum dose. But measures described have resulted in reduced fetal death due to antibody-mediated hemolytic disease by 90% in recent years.

AUTOIMMUNE HEMOLYTIC ANEMIA

Incidence

The annual incidence of autoimmune hemolysis is approximately 1 in 80,000. Although autoimmune hemolysis does not always appear to have a genetic basis, there are patients with autoimmune hemolytic anemia who have family histories of other autoimmune diseases.

Etiologic Classification of Autoimmune Hemolytic Anemia

The autoimmune hemolytic anemias are classified according to the presence or absence of an underlying disease process and according to the thermal optimum of the autoantibody (Table 10-1). In approximately one third of all autoimmune hemolytic anemias, no underlying disease is identified. Secondary autoimmune hemolytic anemias usually are seen with malignancies (especially lymphomas), infections, rheumatologic disorders, and drugs. Warm auto-antibodies are predominantly IgG, with optimum antibody activity at 37° C. Cold autoantibodies, usually IgM, are more active at 0° to 4° C or at room temperature than at 37° C.

TABLE 10-1. Etiologic Classification of Immune Hemolysis

I.   Neoplastic processes
     A. Malignant:
        1. Lymphoproliferative disorders C,W
        2. Breast cancer W
        3. Colon cancer W
     B. Benign: ovarian teratoma W

II. Infections
     A. *Mycoplasma* pneumonia (anti-I) C
     B. Infectious mononucleosis (anti-i) C
     C. Viral hepatitis C,W
     D. Syphilis (anti-P) C
     E. Measles W

III. Immune disorders
     A. Granulomatous disease (rare)
        1. Sarcoidosis W
        2. Ulcerative colitis W
     B. Immunoglobulin disorders
        1. Hypogammaglobulinemias W
        2. Dysglobulinemias W
     C. Rheumatologic disorders
        1. Rheumatoid arthritis C,W
        2. Lupus erythematosus C,W
        3. Scleroderma C,W
        4. Vasculitis C,W

IV. Drugs
     A. Quinidine C
     B. Penicillin W
     C. α-Methyldopa W
     D. Cephalosporins W
     E. Procainamide W
     F. Hydralazine W

C, cold autoantibodies; W, warm autoantibodies.
Note: One third of cases of autoimmune hemolysis have no known cause.

Pathogenesis and Clinical Description of Warm Autoimmune Hemolysis

IgG autoimmune hemolytic anemia is characterized by a positive direct anti-globulin test and extravascular hemolysis. The antibody is active in a thermal range of 25° to 37° C. Complement is not usually activated, or only partial complement activation through C3 occurs. The antibody may show general affinity for the Rh group of antigens. IgG antibody has no effect on the red cell in vitro. Damage comes from contact with macrophages in vivo. Hemolysis occurs predominantly in the spleen.

The clinical manifestations of warm-type autoimmune hemolytic anemia vary according to the severity of the anemia and according to the presence of an underlying disease. Weakness, malaise, dyspnea on exertion, and light-headedness are usually attributable to anemia. Congestive heart failure, or angina pectoris, may be seen in patients with underlying cardiovascular disease. The blood smear shows polychromatophilic macrocytes and, in many cases, spherocytes

{#44, 45}. Spherocytes are the result of membrane injury from contact with macrophages. Agglutination on the blood smear is not seen in warm autoimmune hemolysis.

Pathogenesis and Clinical Description of Cold Autoimmune Hemolysis

The clinical manifestations of cold autoimmune hemolytic anemia depend on the amount of antibody coating the erythrocytes, the thermal amplitude of the antibody, and the ability of the antibody to fix complement. A minimum antibody concentration of 20 IgM molecules per cell is required to cause increased erythrocyte clearance in humans. If the upper thermal limit of antibody activity is less than 28° C, then obvious hemolysis is unlikely. Clinically significant hemolysis and erythrocyte agglutination occur when the thermal limit is above 28° C. Hemolysis may be either intravascular or extravascular. Most of the cold autoantibodies are of the IgM class, and their efficiency in binding complement determines whether intravascular hemolysis will occur or whether enough C3b will be bound to cause the cell to be attached to the C3b receptors of the hepatic macrophages. Table 10-2 compares warm and cold red cell antibodies.

The Cold Agglutinin Syndrome

The cold agglutinin syndrome is an autoimmune hemolytic anemia due to an IgM antibody. Most IgM cold agglutinins adhere to erythrocyte membranes at less than 25° C, and clinical hemolysis is unusual because temperatures in the extremities do not usually fall below 30° C. However, some cold agglutinins are active up to body temperature and cause hemolysis even at low antibody density. In such cases, agglutination is apparent on the blood smear {#42}. When complement is completely activated, intravascular hemolysis occurs. In most instances, however, incomplete complement activation through C3b occurs, with extravascular hemolysis occurring predominantly in the liver.

Raynaud's phenomenon is occasionally seen in association with the cold agglutinin syndrome. When the thermal range of a cold antibody extends about 28° to 32° C, the skin temperature of the extremities may fall to within the active range of the antibody, and agglutination of erythrocytes occurs within the capillaries. Vascular sludging results, so that impaired circulation to the affected extremities occurs. Signs and symptoms include pain, paresthesias, and cyanosis of the extremities.

TABLE 10-2. Warm versus Cold Antibodies

Type	Warm	Cold
Immunoglobulin	IgG	IgM
Temperature at which antibody is usually active	37° C	<32° C
Complement activation	None or partial	Partial, rarely complete
Antibody specificity	Broad specificity Rh system	I, i
Predominant site of erythrocyte destruction	Spleen	Liver or intravascular
Common underlying causes (if any)	Drugs, B-lymphocyte malignancies, collagen vascular disease	Infections, B lymphocyte malignancies

The cold agglutinin syndrome may be idiopathic but is seen after infectious disease (*Mycoplasma* pneumonia and infectious mononucleosis) and in association with malignant lymphomas. Most idiopathic cold agglutinins, including those associated with mycoplasma infections, are directed against the I antigen on the erythrocyte membrane. Cold agglutinins seen with infectious mononucleosis and some malignant lymphomas are directed against the i antigen. Hemolysis is rarely associated with anti-i, since the i antigen is not well expressed on adult erythrocytes.

Paroxysmal Cold Hemoglobinuria

Paroxysmal cold hemoglobinuria is a rare cold autoimmune hemolytic anemia characterized by an IgG antibody. IgG becomes attached to the erythrocyte in the cold and fixes complement. Upon rewarming to 37° C, the IgG elutes off the erythrocyte, complement is completely activated, and intravascular hemolysis occurs. This pattern of thermal activity results in a biphasic direct antiglobulin reaction. The anti-IgG antiglobulin test is negative at 37° C, but positive at 4° C, whereas the anti-complement antiglobulin test is positive at 37° and 4° C. When the IgG antibody has specificity for the "P" erythrocyte antigen, it is known as the Donath-Landsteiner antibody. Paroxysmal cold hemoglobinuria is usually idiopathic, but in the past was an occasional complication of syphilis.

Note. Paroxysmal cold hemoglobinuria is *not* the same as paroxysmal nocturnal hemoglobinuria (PNH), described in Chapter 6. In PNH, red cells lack several glycolipid-linked membrane proteins that protect the cell from buildup of complete complement complexes. Thus, the red cells are so sensitive to complement-induced lysis that lysis occurs without specific anti–red cell antibodies.

Drug-Induced Hemolytic Anemia

Drugs cause 16% to 18% of all acquired immune hemolytic anemia. The essential features of drug-induced immune hemolysis are a positive direct antiglobulin test, with evidence of increased erythrocyte destruction in association with current or recent drug therapy.

Drug-induced positive Coombs' tests are subclassified according to four underlying mechanisms: immune complex adsorption to erythrocytes ("innocent bystander"), drug adsorption onto erythrocytes (hapten), membrane modification, and true autoimmunity (suppressor cell). Membrane modification is not associated with hemolysis. These four mechanisms are outlined in Table 10-3, and a list of drugs that cause a direct Coombs' test and hemolysis is given (Table 10-4).

Immune Complex Adsorption to Erythrocytes

In the immune-complex type of hemolytic anemia, drug and antidrug antibody combine and are absorbed onto the erythrocyte membrane, which is an innocent bystander (**Fig. 10-1**). The prototypic drugs are quinidine, stibophen, and phenacetin. The antidrug antibody in the serum usually is of the IgM class and fixes complement through C9, causing lysis. The direct antiglobulin test is positive with anticomplement serum. Hemolysis can occur after ingestion of a small quantity of drug. A similar mechanism occurs in drug-induced thrombocytopenia.

Drug Adsorption onto Erythrocytes

Immune hemolysis due to drug adsorption onto erythrocytes occurs in approximately 1% of patients receiving massive doses of intravenous penicillin; 3% will

TABLE 10-3. Mechanisms of Drug-Induced Positive Coombs' Test

Mechanism	Prototype Drugs	Clinical Findings	Antibody Class	Antiglobulin
Immune adsorption	Quinidine	Acute IV hemolysis Hemoglobinemia, hemoglobinuria; thrombocytopenia may occur; recovery with withdrawal of drug	IgM fixes complement completely the erythrocyte	Drug and antibody in a patient's serum form a complex attached to
Drug adsorption onto erythrocytes	Penicillins, cephalosporins	Extravascular hemolysis occurs in 1% of patients receiving >10 million units IV penicillin	IgG. May rarely I incompletely fix complement	Requires drug-coated erythrocytes and patient's serum as a source of antibody
Membrane modification	Cephalosporins	Hemolysis is not known to occur	IgG and other nonspecific proteins	Requires drug-coated erythrocytes and patient's serum as a source of antibody
True autoimmunity	α-Methyldopa	Extravascular hemolysis in 0.8%	IgG. May rarely incompletely fix complement; antibody commonly has Rh specificity	Presence of drug not necessary; requires normal erythrocytes and patient's serum as source of antibody

Adapted from Garratty G, Petz L. Drug-induced hemolytic anemia. Am J Med 1975;58:398–407.

develop a positive direct antiglobulin test (Fig. 10-2). Penicillin readily reacts with tissue proteins to form haptenic groups and can be detected on the erythrocyte membranes of all patients receiving large intravenous doses. The major haptenic determinant is the benzyl penicilloyl group. Penicillin-induced hemolytic anemia is characterized by an IgG antibody, extravascular hemolysis, and complete recovery after cessation of penicillin therapy. Because of continuous exposure to penicillin in our environment, over 80% of unselected normal sera contain IgM penicillin antibodies. Hemolysis does not occur in these individuals because not enough penicillin is present in their serum to form haptenic groups with their erythrocytes. There is no correlation between penicillin-induced immune hemolysis and other manifestations of penicillin allergy.

TABLE 10-4. A Partial List of Drugs Reported to Cause a Direct Antiglobulin Test and Hemolysis

Analgesics
  Phenacetin
  Acetaminophen
  Ibuprofen
Antibiotics
  Cephalosporins
  Sulfonamides
  Tetracycline
  Stretptomycin
  Isoniazid

Cardiovascular drugs
  Procainamide
  Hydralazine
  Methyldopa
  Hydrochlorothiazide
Miscellaneous
  Chlorinated hydrocarbons
  Chlorpromazine
  Sulfonylureas

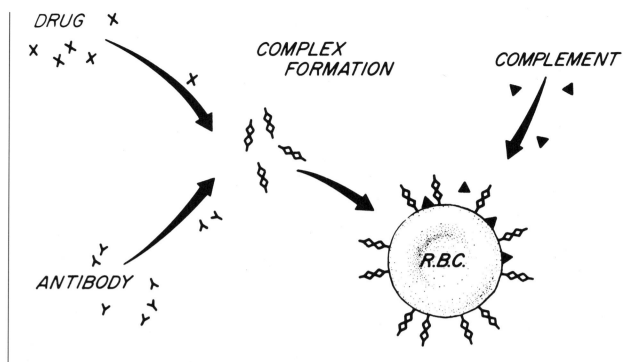

FIGURE 10-1.

Immune complex–type of drug-induced hemolysis. The antibody is usually IgM and fixes complement, leading to intravascular hemolysis. (From Garratty G, Petz L. Drug-induced immune hemolytic anemia. *Am J Med* 58:398.)

Membrane Modification

A positive Coombs' test may develop, but hemolysis does not occur when erythrocyte membranes are modified by cephalosporins (Fig. 10-3). This leads to nonimmunologic (nonspecific) absorption of proteins by the erythrocyte, and the cells become coated with various plasma proteins (albumin, IgG, IgA, and fibrinogen) in a nonspecific fashion. Results from the direct antiglobulin test are positive when antisera to various serum proteins are used.

True Autoimmunity

True drug-induced autoimmune hemolytic anemia occurs with the antihypertensive drug α-methyldopa (Aldomet). α-Methyldopa induces the production of an IgG antibody, which commonly has Rh antigen specificity. After discontinuation of α-methyldopa, the direct antiglobulin test becomes negative in 1 month to 2 years. Recent investigations suggest that α-methyldopa alters the immune system by inhibiting suppressor T-cell function, which results in unregulated autoantibody production by B cells in affected patients.

A further question is to what extent these models of drug–antibody–cell interaction have been found for platelets and granulocytes. In most cases, the innocent-bystander mechanism has been found for both platelets and granulocytes, but the penicillins can also induce the haptenic form of immune destruction of granulocytes. Heparin-induced platelet antibodies are relatively common and particularly troublesome because they induce platelet aggregation, leading to the risk of serious thrombotic complications. This is frustrating, since heparin was used to prevent thrombosis in the first place. Drug antibody-mediated injury to granulocyte stem cells has also been described.

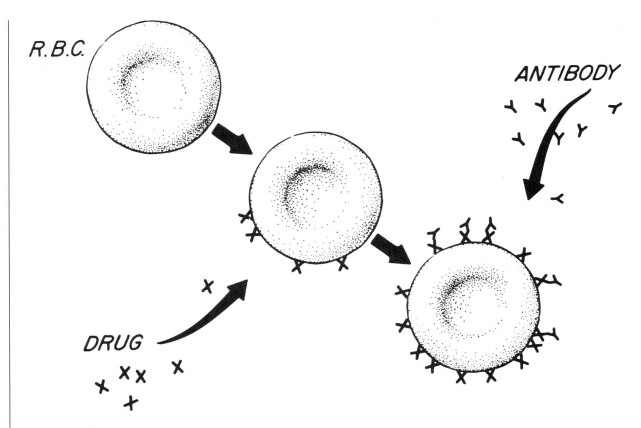

FIGURE 10-2.
Haptenic type of drug-induced hemolysis. The antibody attaches to the drug bound to the red cell membrane. (From Garratty G, Petz L. Drug-induced hemolytic anemia. *Am J Med* 58:398.)

Treatment of Autoimmune Hemolytic Anemia

If hemolysis is mild and compensated, no therapy is necessary. In most secondary autoimmune hemolytic anemias, successful treatment of the underlying disease controls the hemolytic anemia. Patients with drug-induced immune hemolysis usually respond to withdrawal of the offending medication.

Patients with warm-type IgG immune hemolysis usually respond to corticosteroid therapy. Corticosteroids act by two mechanisms: an immediate decrease in macrophage Fc-γ-receptors and a slower decrease in the production of the abnormal IgG antibody. Intravenous γ-globulin is also effective in temporarily interfering with antibody-mediated hemolysis, as well as immune thrombopenia and neutropenia. Its action is multifactorial, but blocking the Fc-γ-receptor is at least part of the mechanism.

Splenectomy is also effective in IgG immune hemolysis, because it removes both a site of red cell destruction and a major site of antibody production. Splenectomy is reserved for patients who fail to respond to corticosteroids and for patients who require prolonged therapy with corticosteroids to maintain an adequate hematocrit. Immunosuppressive therapy with alkylating agents is used in patients resistant to corticosteroids and splenectomy.

Corticosteroids are less effective in cold-type IgM immune hemolysis, especially when the hemolysis is intravascular. Splenectomy is of little benefit because clearance of IgM-coated erythrocytes also occurs in the liver. Immunosuppressive therapy is occasionally effective in decreasing antibody production. Plasmapheresis may provide temporary improvement in IgM immune hemolysis until more effective medical therapy can be initiated.

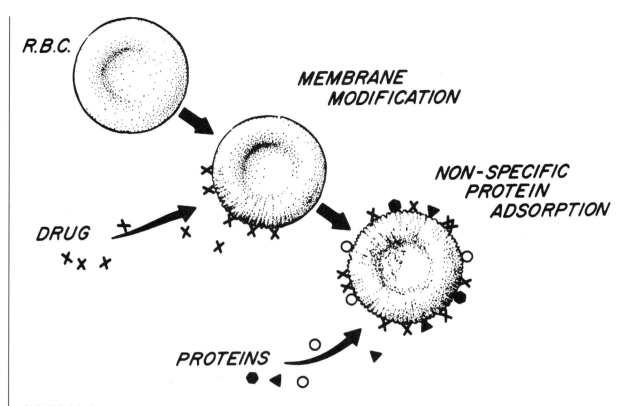

FIGURE 10-3.
Membrane modification type of drug-induced immunoglobulin adherence reaction. Hemolysis does not occur in this nonspecific reaction. (From Garratty G, Petz L. Drug-induced hemolytic anemia. *Am J Med* 58:398.)

Transfusions should be given when serious anemia is present. This usually requires administering blood despite the cross-match indicating incompatibility. The major risk of transfusion in this group is, therefore, that clinically significant alloantibodies may not be detected because of autoantibodies. When compatible donor erythrocytes are transfused, however, the transfused cells usually have a survival rate comparable to that of the patient's own cells. Patients with cold autoantibodies should be transfused with blood that has been run through a warming coil to raise the temperature above 30° C.

SUMMARY POINTS

Immune hemolysis is mediated by the presence of antibody or complement, or both, on the erythrocyte membrane. Antibody production may occur with no identifiable causes (idiopathic) or may be secondary to an underlying disease or to the use of specific medications. Factors that determine whether an antibody causes hemolysis as well as the severity of any hemolysis include the immunoglobulin class and subclass of the antibody, the ability of the antibody to attach complement to erythrocytes and activate the complement cascade, the antigenic specificity of the antibody, the concentration of the antibody, and the number of macrophages that recognize specific antigen-antibody complexes or components of complement on the erythrocyte membrane.

CASE DEVELOPMENT PROBLEM: CHAPTER 10

History: A 62-year-old porcelain factory foreman was first seen 8 years ago with the following diagnoses: diabetes mellitus, peptic ulcer disease, and asthmatic bronchitis. Six months later, he was admitted to the hospital after having passed a massive black stool and fainting. An upper endoscopy showed a duodenal ulcer. Gastrointestinal bleeding stopped after 4 days, and the stool became guaiac-negative, but the reticulocyte count, which had been 12.8%, on admission rose to 23.6%. The hematocrit remained in the mid 30s. The serum bilirubin was 2.5 mg/dL; direct bilirubin 0.2. On discharge, the patient's hematocrit was 39%, the reticulocyte count 9%. He was not treated with iron supplements.

1. What is the significance of a steady-state reticulocytosis greater than 5%?
2. What advice would you give the patient on discharge from the hospital?
   The patient was followed up in the hematology clinic for the next 2 years, demonstrating hematocrits in the high 20s and reticulocyte counts of 25% to 30%. The Coombs' test was positive on several occasions. After 2 years, the patient was admitted with weakness and dyspnea. Hematocrit was 22%, reticulocyte count 48.5%, total bilirubin 7.6 mg/dL, direct antiglobulin 1.0 mg/dL. A ^{51}Cr survival study was performed, and the half-life was 2 days (normal, 30 days). His serum iron concentration was 178 mg/dL, the total iron binding capacity 225 mg/dL.
3. Assuming a red blood cell count of $2.2 \times 10^6/\mu L$, calculate the reticulocyte index.
4. By what factor can the marrow multiply its output?
5. How many times more than normal would the patient's bone marrow output have to be to match this degree of reticulocytosis?
6. List the possible causes of hemolytic anemia in this patient.
7. What are the possible treatments for this patient's disease?
   The patient was given treatment. His hematocrit rose from 22% to 37%, and his reticulocyte count dropped from 48% to 11.5%.
8. How do corticosteroids work in this disease?
   The corticosteroids were tapered to 20 mg every other day, and the Coombs' test 6 months later was negative, although the reticulocyte count was still 14% and the hematocrit 32%.
9. How do you account for the negative Coombs' test?
   The patient was resistant to treatment of his diabetes. He did not follow a diet and refused oral hypoglycemia agents ("I don't like to take pills!"). Two months before he died, the patient was admitted to the hospital for 3 weeks with urinary frequency and urgency. On examination, the foreskin and glans were inflamed and edematous (balanitis). The hematocrit was 22%, the reticulocyte count 9.6%. The urine culture was positive for β-hemolytic streptococci. The blood sugar was 665 mg/dL.
10. Calculate the reticulocyte index assuming a red cell count of 2.2 million/μL.
11. Outline a series of pathophysiologic events leading to the exacerbation of the patient's anemia.
12. Is this an aplastic crisis?

CASE DEVELOPMENT ANSWERS

1. Reticulocytosis, which is associated with bleeding or the response to a specific hematinic such as iron or vitamin B_{12}, reaches a peak in 7 to 10 days after the beginning of drug administration and then subsides. A steady-state reticulocytosis is highly suggestive of hemolysis.

2. Return to the clinic in 2 weeks. Patients with hemolytic anemia need to be observed closely.

3. $\dfrac{2.2 \times 10^6 \times 48.5 \times 10^{-2}}{5 \times 10^4} \times \dfrac{1}{2} = 10.67$

4. The output of the bone marrow is estimated to be 10 times normal. Although this value is much larger than the maximum of fivefold quoted in Chapter 1 (the kinetic analysis of anemia), similar numbers are commonly encountered in brisk hemolytic anemia.

5. The patient's maximum output yielded only half the normal hematocrit. We estimate that a 16-fold increase in production would be required to produce a normal hematocrit. Note also that the ^{51}Cr survival is 2 days rather than 30, an estimated 15-fold reduction.

6. (a) Drug. In a patient with so many diseases (the problem list eventually reached 23), the possible list of drugs is long. However, in this case the patient took only a proprietary mixture of aminophylline, ephedrine, and amobarbital for asthma. Consult the list of drugs in your text to see whether any of these three is implicated in acquired hemolytic anemia. (b) Lymphoma. Observation over 2 years makes this possibility unlikely. (c) Idiopathic. Most patients fall into this category, and no cause was uncovered over 10 years of observation.

7. (a) Corticosteroid use was delayed 2 years because of the patient's diabetes and his peptic ulcer disease. (b) Splenectomy; the patient refused this procedure many times. (c) Immunosuppressive drugs such as azathioprine or cyclophosphamide. These drugs are currently reserved for patients who fail to improve after splenectomy.

8. Corticosteroids interfere with the attachment of the antibody molecule to monocytes or macrophages and decrease the affinity of the antibody for red cells.

9. Corticosteroids also decrease the rate of antibody synthesis.

10. 2.2 million × .096 = 211,000

$\dfrac{211,000}{2.0} = 105,000$

$\dfrac{105,000}{50,000} = 2.1$

11. (a) Diabetes mellitus. (b) Poor control of diabetes plus the use of corticosteroids. (c) Glycosuria (an excellent bacterial culture medium). (d) Superficial infection (balanitis). (e) Urinary tract obstruction and infection. (f) Suppression of marrow production by inflammation.

12. No. Aplastic crisis implies a disappearance of red blood cell precursors in the marrow and absence of reticulocytes in the peripheral blood. It is virus-mediated. The patient's anemia with depressed reticulocytosis (2.5 instead of the expected eightfold) is due to the effect of chronic inflammation: decreased erythropoietin production, increased macrophage avidity for iron, and interleukin suppression of erythropoiesis.

PART III
WHITE BLOOD
CELLS

Granulocytes

CHAPTER 11

Archie A. MacKinney, Jr., Naveen Manchanda

OUTLINE

OBJECTIVES

- Learn the maturation steps and morphology of granulocytes.
- Appreciate the role of granulocytes as the primary form of defense against many foreign invaders.
- Acquire insight into clinical disorders that involve granulocytes.
- Know the mechanisms of neutropenia.
- Recognize morphologic signs of inflammation in neutrophils.

NEUTROPHIL ORIGIN AND FUNCTION

Granulocytes are the white blood cells primarily responsible for killing foreign invaders and scavenging injured tissue. There are three very different types of granulocytes—neutrophils, eosinophils, and basophils). Their names derived from the light-microscopic appearance of the granules on Wright's-stained smears of blood and bone marrow.

Definitions and Morphology

Neutrophils constitute 60% of the normal adult's total white blood cell count. They have neutral staining and salmon-pink granules interspersed with indistinct lilac-colored granules. The nucleus has three or four segments, and its highly condensed chromatin stains blue-black {#6}. **Eosinophils** represent 2% to 5% of peripheral white blood cells. They are easily recognized by their large orange-pink refractile granules and a dense bilobed nucleus {#8}. **Basophils** are the rarest (0.5%) of all circulating white blood cells. They have large irregular basophilic blue granules, which tend to obscure the large single-lobed or bilobed nucleus {#7}.

Granulocytes share with monocytes the ability to respond to chemotactic stimuli by migrating into tissues. Once in tissues, the three types of granulocytes have specialized functions according to the constituents in the specific granules. For instance, the myeloperoxidase in the primary granule of neutrophilic granulocytes causes formation of hypochlorous acid (bleach) whereas lactoferrin in the secondary granules binds iron needed for bacterial growth.

Origin and Maturation

Granulocytes originate in the bone marrow. They are generated from the granulocyte-monocyte stem cell (CFU [colony-forming unit]-GM) under the control of a variety of growth factors. There are specific factors for each cell type as well as overlapping cytokines with broader ranges of action (Fig. 11-1; see also Chapter 2). One system for inducing G-CSF (colony-stimulating factor) and GM-CSF comes from inflammation. The T lymphocyte signals the monocyte to release interleukin-1 (IL-1), which in turn induces endothelial cells and fibroblasts to make a series of growth factors (Fig. 11-2). In addition, cytokines cause the marrow to release its stored granulocytes. Thus, the bone marrow is tuned to the immune system to respond to antigenic challenge with a rapid response to IL-1, then a more sustained output of granulocytes and monocytes in response to GM-CSF.

The earliest recognizable precursor is the myeloblast. The **myeloblast** is a rare (1% of marrow cells) undifferentiated cell with a prominent nucleolus and no cytoplasmic granules {#1}. During its life, it divides about four times and gives rise to about 16 daughter cells that differentiate into granulocytes. The time from initiation of differentiation to release of the finished cell is 10 days with a minimum of 5 and a maximum of 14. After the myeloblast, five additional stages in granulocyte development are recognized: the promyelocyte, myelocyte, metamyelocyte, band, and segmented cell. The proportion of these cells in the blood and marrow has been shown to have clinical significance (Fig. 11-3).

The **promyelocyte** (4% of marrow cells) is easily identified by its larger size and its population of conspicuous dark-red primary ("azurophilic") granules {#2}. These granules contain myeloperoxidase and acid hydrolases, defensins (small antimicrobial peptides), as well as lysozyme and other cationic antibacterial proteins. Since production of the primary granules stops at this stage, their number decreases with the two subsequent cell divisions.

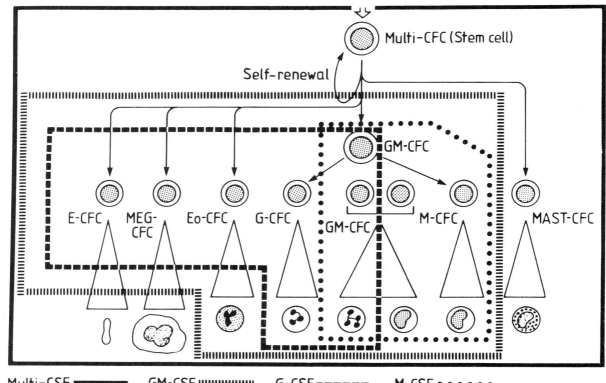

FIGURE 11-1.

Biologic specificity of different hematopoietic growth factors. Each of the colony-stimulating factors (CSFs) stimulates a distinct set of progenitor, blast and immature cells of the hematopoietic system. The cells responsive to each CSFs are included within the boundaries marked. E-CSF is erythropoietin. CFC, colony-forming cell; CFU, colony-forming unit. E-CFC, erythroid CFC; Eo-CFC, eosinophil CFC; G-CFC, granulocyte CFC; GM-CFC, granulocyte-monocyte CFC; M-CFC, monocyte CFC; Mast-CFC, mast cell CFC. (From Walker F. Hierarchical down-modulation of hematopoietic growth factor receptors. *Cell* 43:269.)

During its maturation from a myeloblast to the finished granulocyte, the cell decreases its surface charge and its resistance to deformation and increases its adhesiveness and its ability to spread and form pseudopods. These changes explain in part why the myeloblast stays in the marrow and the segmented neutrophil is able to leave and carry out its mission (Fig. 11-4).

The myelocyte stage (12% of marrow cells) is characterized by the appearance of a secondary population of granules, "specific" granules {#3}. These become more numerous than the primary granules and give the cell its characteristic appearance and name. The secondary granules of the neutrophil are small and faint pink (neutrophilic) and contain lysozyme as well as lactoferrin (which exerts a negative feedback on granulocyte production) and vitamin B_{12}-binding proteins. Tertiary granules and a novel granule containing leukocyte alkaline phosphatase have been identified. The secondary granules that characterize the eosinophil and basophil myelocyte differ from those of the neutrophil and confer on each cell type its distinct name and role. After the myelocyte stage, cell division stops and maturation is parallel in the three types of granulocytes. During the metamyelocyte stage (16% of marrow cells), the nucleus indents {#4}; at the band stage, it is a thin strip {#5}. The final stage is the segmented ("seg") or polymorphonuclear ("poly," neutrophil) nucleus {#6}. The marrow retains a storage pool of 20% segs and bands for emergencies.

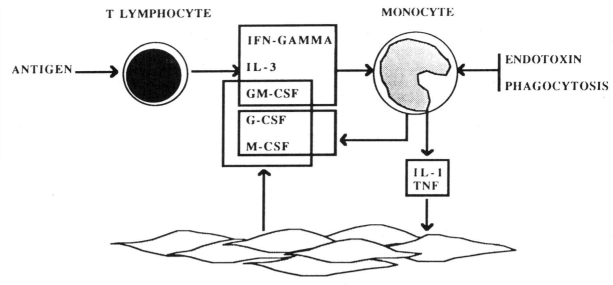

FIGURE 11-2.
Cellular sources and regulation of colony-stimulating factor (CSF) secretion. IL-3, interleukin-3; GM-CSF, granulocyte-monocyte CSF; G-CSF, granulocyte CSF; M-CSF, monocyte CSF; IFN-GAMMA, interferon-γ; IL-1, interleukin-1; TNF, tumor necrosis factor. (From Cannistra SA, Griffin JD. Regulation of the production and function of granulocytes and monocytes. *Semin Hematol* 25:173.)

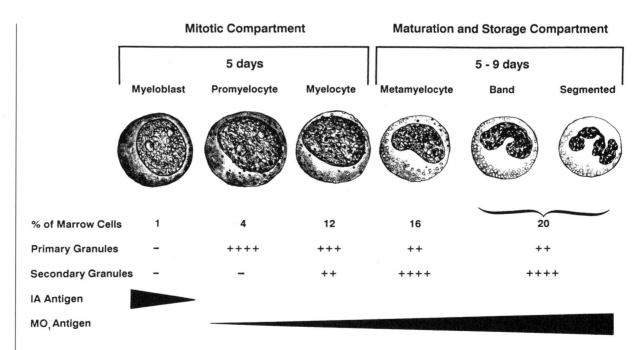

FIGURE 11-3.
The flow of granulocytes through the bone marrow compartment. The compartment is divided into two parts; the myelocyte is the last dividing cell. Primary granules are diluted by division. Appearance of secondary granules is a critical part of differentiation. $M0_1$[CD11b] is an adhesion protein that permits neutrophils to stick to endothelium. IA antigens are major histocompatibility antigens.

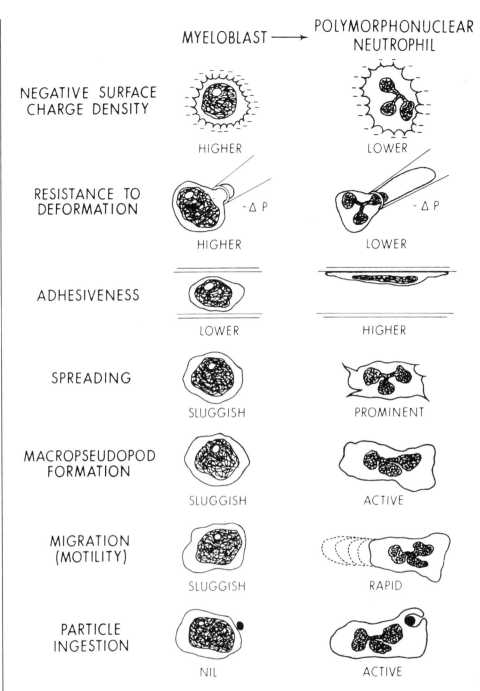

MYELOBLAST ⟶ POLYMORPHONUCLEAR NEUTROPHIL

NEGATIVE SURFACE CHARGE DENSITY
HIGHER — LOWER

RESISTANCE TO DEFORMATION
$-\Delta P$ HIGHER — $-\Delta P$ LOWER

ADHESIVENESS
LOWER — HIGHER

SPREADING
SLUGGISH — PROMINENT

MACROPSEUDOPOD FORMATION
SLUGGISH — ACTIVE

MIGRATION (MOTILITY)
SLUGGISH — RAPID

PARTICLE INGESTION
NIL — ACTIVE

FIGURE 11-4.
A summary of the differences between the myeloblast and the polymorphonucelar neutrophil. The changes in charge, deformability, adhesiveness, and motility in part explain the ability of the neutrophil to leave the marrow and perform its functions. (From Lichtman MA, Weed RI. Alteration of the cell periphery during granulocyte maturation: relationship to cell function. *Blood* 39:301.)

Compartment Kinetics

Neutrophils circulate for an average of 10 hours. In the circulation, half of the neutrophils are in the axial stream and half are rolling along the endothelial surface where they would not be counted in a blood sample. Figure 11-5 shows

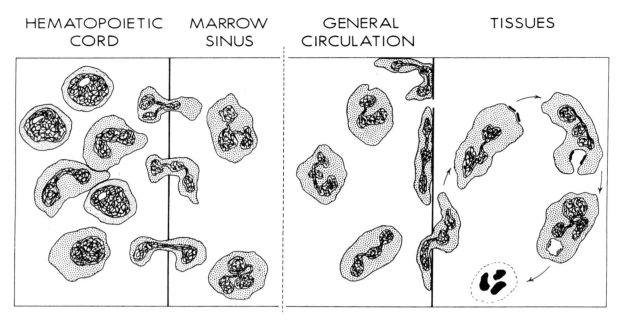

HEMATOPOIETIC CORD   MARROW SINUS   GENERAL CIRCULATION   TISSUES

FIGURE 11-5.

Major compartments involved in granulocyte kinetics. The restrictive barrier separating marrow hematopoietic cord from marrow sinus is depicted. 1:1 distribution of neutrophils free and marginated in the circulation is depicted. Adhesion of bacteria and pseudopod formation required for engulfment are shown in the tissue compartment. (From Lichtman MA, Weed RI. Alteration of the cell periphery during granulocyte maturation: relationship to cell function. *Blood* 39:301.)

the two compartments of the peripheral blood neutrophils in equilibrium. Hence, the white cell count measures only half of the neutrophils present in the blood. The neutrophils then migrate into the tissues to phagocytize and die. Monocytes, in contrast to the fully differentiated, short-lived granulocytes, can adapt to the organs to which they migrate and become long-lived, specialized macrophages. For more on monocytes, see Chapter 13.

A series of adhesion reactions governs the neutrophil movement to and through the endothelium. When neutrophils are activated, they roll along the endothelial surface of the vein in response to adhesion molecule(s) called selectins and then pass through the endothelium in response to integrins. The five steps are illustrated in Figure 11-6.

Phagocytosis

Neutrophils defend against microorganisms that cause acute infections (e.g., pneumococci and staphylococci) by engulfing, oxidizing, and digesting them. Having fought, these neutrophils die and disintegrate into the cell debris we call pus. Monocytes can digest bacteria and live to fight another day. Eosinophils are phagocytic for IgE-antigen complexes and parasites, and they modulate the inflammatory activity of basophils.

Steps in Inflammation

Once skin or mucous membranes are breached by bacteria or fungi, neutrophils are the first cells in the immune system to respond {#55–58}. As the first line of defense, neutrophils have a highly refined system for detecting invasion, are able

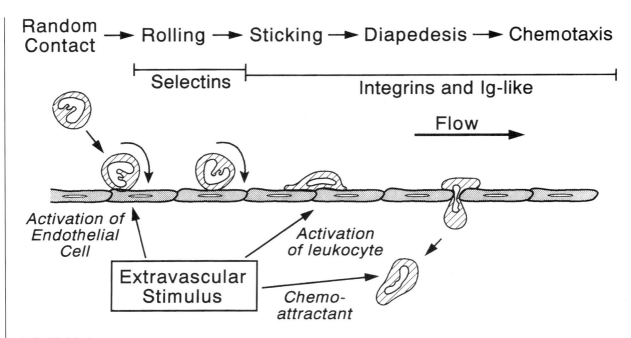

FIGURE 11-6.

Adhesive reactions during leukocyte migration. Five steps are outlined, dependent on selectins, integrins, and Ig-like molecules. (From Carlos TM, Harlan JM. Leukocyte-endothelial adhesion molecules. *Blood* 84:2068.)

to respond rapidly, are able to recognize foreign material and have potent systems for killing a wide variety of microorganisms. The 10 steps are outlined and elaborated in the following text.

1. **Mobilization**. Interactions between macrophages and endotoxin lead to the release of *interleukins (IL-1, IL-6), interferons (IFN), and tumor necrosis factor-α* (TNF-α). IL-1 induces fever by raising the hypothalamic temperature set point. It also releases the marrow granulocyte storage pool. (IL-1 has numerous other functions that do not involve granulocytes.) Epinephrine and glucocorticoids release marginated granulocytes from the vessel walls.

2. **Expanded production**. CSF-GM induces the marrow to increase granulocyte production.

3. **Activation**. C5a, G-CSF, GM-CSF, and leukotrienes prime or activate the circulating granulocytes to their new task.

4. **Adherence to endothelium**. The local inflammatory mediators allow neutrophils to adhere to the normally nonsticky endothelial cells. The key molecular event is up-regulation of two classes of endothelial cell surface proteins: selectins, which mediate neutrophil rolling by transient interactions with carbohydrates on the neutrophil surface and various cell adhesion molecules, which act as counterreceptors for heterodimeric cell surface leukocyte receptors of the integrin class (e.g., CDIIa/18).

5. **Diapedesis**. Neutrophils pass between endothelial cells without causing disruption of the vessel wall (this feat involves recognition of a cell surface molecule called CD31 that lines the potential space between endothelial cells) and move up a chemotactic gradient to the site of invasion.

6. **Chemotaxis**. The chemotactic factors are peptide fragments from bacterial protein metabolism (formyl-methionyl-leucyl-phenylalanine [FMLP]),

products of clotting (fibrinopeptide), arachadonic acid products from platelets or neutrophils (prostaglandins, leukotriene B4 [LTB$_4$]), complement components (C5a), neutrophil granule products (fibronectin, lactoferrin), and chemokines (especially IL-8).

7. **Attachment**. Bacterial capsules are negatively charged and hydrophilic, representing a barrier to the negatively charged lipid membrane of the neutrophil. Opsonization with antibody and complement overcomes these barriers.

8. **Ingestion**. Phagocytosis does not occur with complement alone unless fibronectin and FMLP are present. When the plasma membrane surrounds the bacterium, it forms a phagosome. Lysosomal granules fuse with the phagosome and deliver their enzymes. The internalized membrane is activated, and degranulation starts in a few seconds. The specific (or secondary) granules fuse first, and in 30 seconds the internal pH of the vacuole begins to fall from 7.0 toward 4.0, dropping as low as 3.5 in a matter of minutes. At that time, the primary (or azurophilic) granules fuse with the phagosome and release their contents, all of which have acid pH optima. These events depend on intact cytoskeletal and cytomuscular elements and are energy-dependent. If the particle is too big to be ingested, granule release occurs externally. Even with small particles, secretion of granules into the medium is a normal event. Corticosteroids and antimalarial drugs impede degranulation.

9. **Killing**. Bacterial killing involves both enzymatic digestion and oxidation by potent oxygen radicals. Within 90 seconds of attachment, neutrophils develop a "respiratory burst," oxygen uptake, glucose consumption, and superoxide ($O^2\bullet^-$) generation. Early investigators were surprised by the oxygen uptake because mature neutrophils have very few mitochondria. This led to the discovery of the nicotinamide adenine dinucleotide phosphate (NADPH) oxidase complex, which shuttles electrons from glucose in an electron transport chain located in the plasma membrane surrounding the phagocytized particle. The oxidase complex becomes functional when NADPH oxidase is linked to cytochrome b, which is in the specific granules. The reactive oxygen species are:

$$O_2 + e^- \rightarrow O_2\bullet^- \text{ (superoxide)}$$

$$2O_2\bullet^- + 2H^+ \xrightarrow{\text{SOD}} H_2O_2 + O_2$$

$$H_2O_2 + Cl^- + H^+ \xrightarrow{\text{MPO}} HOCl + H_2O$$

where SOD I = superoxide dismutase and MPO = myeloperoxidase.

Superoxide is formed by the univalent reduction of molecular oxygen. Superoxide dismutes to hydrogen peroxide slowly or enzymatically by superoxide dismutase. Myeloperoxidase, an azurophilic granule enzyme, combines peroxide with chloride to make hypochlorous acid (HOCl). HOCl, H_2O_2, and $O_2\bullet^-$ are all potent oxidants capable of killing microorganisms. If these oxidants leak back into the cell, ascorbic acid and glutathione peroxidase can inactivate them.

Other killing systems include cationic proteins in primary (azurophilic) granules, which can punch holes in the membranes of gram-negative rods. Lysozyme digests the peptidoglycan layer of bacteria. Lactoferrin complexes iron to prevent bacterial growth and virulence.

10. **Secretion**. During phagocytosis, enzymes and oxygen radicals leak or are secreted from the neutrophil. This leads to digestion of nearby tissue and proteins. Degraded fibronectin is a potent monocyte chemoattractant. Thus, the neutrophil sends out signals to the monocyte to initiate the second phase of inflammation.

Since we know that activation may begin in the circulation, the neutrophil may do harm if the activator concentration is too high. Activation of complement by exposure of blood to foreign material (e.g., renal dialysis membrane) induces neutrophils to aggregate in the lung and cause dyspnea and chest pain. Adult respiratory distress syndrome, which occurs after operations or sepsis, may be the result of neutrophils adhering to pulmonary vascular endothelium. Neutrophils appear to be an important cause of injury to ischemic, reperfused myocardium.

PATHOLOGY OF NEUTROPHILS

Kinetics

Normally, about 50% of circulating neutrophils "marginate" or adhere reversibly to vascular endothelium (Fig. 11-5). Epinephrine release causes rapid demargination. Corticosteroids and exercise have a similar effect. (If a patient comes into your office late, running to her appointment, expect the white cells to be elevated.) Corticosteroids inhibit the motility of neutrophils and keep them from moving out of the blood. Under physiologic regulation, corticosteroids may aid the mobilization so that neutrophils can congregate at sites of inflammation. At pharmacologic concentrations, corticosteroids inhibit granulocyte function. Certain viruses shown to infect endothelial cells in vitro increase the adherence of neutrophils; this may explain vascular injury by viruses (e.g., measles).

In infection, the initial event is increased margination and egress of neutrophils from the circulation. This is followed by inflow of mature cells from the marrow stores. The usual increase in circulating neutrophils in infection occurs because this inflow persists and exceeds outflow (Fig. 11-7). When the infection is severe or the marrow is incompetent, peripheral demand for neutrophils may outstrip the supply, the peripheral neutrophil count may become subnormal, and the store of marrow neutrophils may become depleted. An alcoholic with pneumonia and a low white cell count has a bad prognosis.

Thus, during acute infection, the blood counts are often low in the early hours as neutrophils rapidly leave the circulation. These cells are restored by the storage pool so that an overshoot in granulocytes is expected. Younger cells (bands and metamyelocytes) appear. The azurophilic granules are more prominent than normal ("toxic granulation"). Traces of RNA ("Döhle's bodies) and vacuoles may be seen {#50}. Pseudopods indicate activation. Bacteria are almost never seen in the blood and, if present, are indicative of overwhelming infection. For *Ehrlichia*, which is a tick-borne infection of woodsmen, gardeners, and golfers who drive into the rough, detection of the organism in neutrophils is the major diagnostic clue.

Quantitative Abnormalities

Neutropenia

Neutropenia is the term used to identify an absolute neutrophil count of fewer than 1800/μL in whites and fewer than 1400/μL in African Americans. When neutrophils are lower than 1000/μL, the patient is prone to overwhelming infection and must be evaluated promptly and thoroughly for any fever. Neutrophil counts below 500 are a danger to life and require isolation of patients from crowds, barns, cut flowers, and so on. **Agranulocytosis** means no circulating neutrophils. Death is the expected outcome. Patients can survive agranulocytosis up to 40 days in the hospital on modern antibiotic support. After 40 days, resistant bacteria and fungi emerge. Based on the cost of this antibiotic support, the worth of neutrophils is approximately $5 per neutrophil per μL per day!

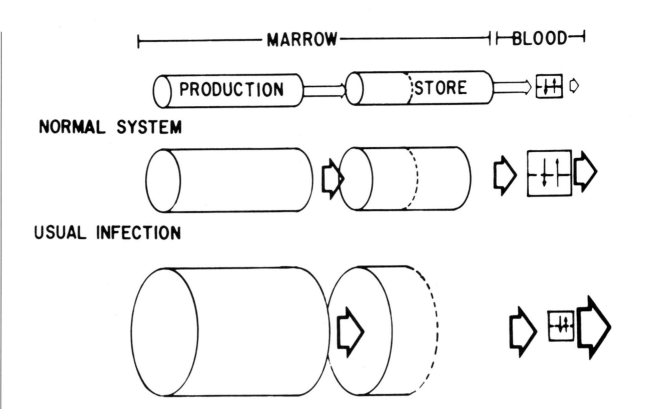

MARROW ⊢————————————————————⊣⊢**BLOOD**⊣

PRODUCTION ⟶ STORE ⟶

NORMAL SYSTEM

USUAL INFECTION

INFECTION WITH NEUTROPENIA AND STORAGE EXHAUSTED

FIGURE 11-7.
Neutrophil kinetics in acute infection. The normal system has a small flux of neutrophils into the tissues from blood. The usual infection expands the marrow and peripheral blood compartments with a large flux into the tissues (*large arrows*). In infection with neutropenia and with storage exhausted, the flux into the tissues leads to a decrease in the blood pool as well as a disappearance of the marrow metamyelocytes, segmented neutrophils, and bands. (From Boggs DR, Winkelstein A. *White Cell Manual*. Philadelphia: FA Davis.)

Table 11-1. Neutropenia Due to Common Drugs

Drug Treated	Incidence per 1000	Dose-Related	Antibody-Mediated
Ticlopidine	24	?	Probably
Clozapine	10	Yes	No
Phenylbutazone	10	Probably	Yes
Aminopyrine/dipyrone*	8		Yes
Antithyroid drugs	4	Yes	Yes
Phenindione*	2	?	No
Sulfonamides	1	Yes	Yes
Phenothiazines	0.8	Yes	No
Chloramphenicol	<0.01	?	No

Discontinued drug.

Neutropenia can be divided into four pathophysiologic groups:

- Decreased production due to hypoproliferative or ineffective myelopoiesis.
- Increased destruction due to drug-dependent or autoimmune antibodies.
- Increased utilization (or loss). In overwhelming infections, neutrophils may be destroyed faster than the marrow can supply them.
- Sequestration. Neutropenia may occur when the spleen is enlarged and no antibody is demonstrated, as in cirrhosis of the liver. How the enlarged spleen affects neutrophil kinetics is not clear.

DECREASED PRODUCTION

Decreased bone marrow production of neutrophils is most often due to primary hematologic malignancies (e.g., acute leukemias, myeloma), carcinomas that metastasize to the marrow (lung, breast cancers), drug toxicity, hereditary factors, or a combination of factors. The drugs most commonly associated with absolute neutropenia (<1800/μL) are listed in Table 11-1. Predictable drug toxicity to the bone marrow from chemotherapeutic drugs is the most common form of neutropenia in hospitalized patients. Damage to the stem cell (from radiation or chloramphenicol), antimetabolite-induced interruption of DNA synthesis (from methotrexate), inhibition of mitosis (from vinca alkaloids or colchicine), damage by alkylating agents (e.g. cyclophosphamide), and interference of protein synthesis (from antibiotics) are some therapy-related mechanisms that induce hypoproliferation.

Hereditary neutropenias may be severe (as in infantile agranulocytosis) and may be associated with other constitutional defects (cartilage-hair hypoplasia) as well as with immunologic defects (hypogammaglobulinemia). Cyclic neutropenia is characterized by a low normal neutrophil count alternating with neutropenia and may be associated with significant infections. Treatment with corticosteroids has proved helpful. Some ethnic groups have significantly lower neutrophil counts than whites: people of African extraction, West Indians living in Britain, and Yemenite Jews in Israel. No disease is associated with this benign neutropenia.

INCREASED DESTRUCTION

Drugs can interact with neutrophils as they do with red cells and cause immune neutropenia much as they cause hemolytic anemia. Aminopyrine, an analgesic no longer used (Table 11-1), is a well-known inducer of antibody-mediated neutropenia. Clozapine is used to treat psychiatric disorders and must be monitored frequently with white blood counts. Felty's syndrome is an example of autoimmune neutropenia, in which patients with rheumatoid arthritis develop splenomegaly and neutropenia. In Felty's syndrome, IgG is bound to the neutrophil membranes, and the neutrophils are destroyed in the spleen. The study of immune neutropenia has been hampered by the lack of a reliable Coombs' test for granulocytes, so the mechanisms of neutropenia in many cases have not been clarified.

Neutrophilia

When the number of white blood cells exceeds 12,000/μL, the term "leukocytosis" is used. "Granulocytosis" and "neutrophilia" refer to an increase in neutrophils to more than 8000/μL. "Leukemoid reaction" describes a peripheral white blood cell count high enough to resemble leukemia but actually due to other causes (e.g., infection, nonhematopoietic infiltrative malignancy of the marrow). The white blood cell count rarely exceeds 100,000/μL in non-leukemic conditions. A variety of conditions cause neutrophilic leukocytosis (Table 11-2).

Qualitative Abnormalities

Abnormal Morphology

Morphologic abnormalities of neutrophils in the peripheral blood occasionally may be the only sign of an underlying disorder. Normally, there are up to 5% five-lobed neutrophils. Neutrophils with six lobes and macrocytic red blood cells should lead to suspicion of a megaloblastic process, such as B_{12} or folate deficiency. Chemotherapeutic drugs that block DNA synthesis produce the same neutrophil morphology.

The Pelger-Huët anomaly refers to a bilobed nucleus resembling glasses that fasten on the bridge of the nose (pince-nez) {#52}. This is usually a benign, heterozygous autosomal dominant variant (1 in 6000 individuals) but can sometimes be seen as an acquired abnormality in patients who have an abnormal clone of hematopoietic stem cells and are felt to be preleukemic. Döhle's bodies, associated with acute infections, are light-blue cytoplasmic inclusions (rough endoplasmic reticulum) attached to the inner surface of the plasma membrane of a neutrophil {#50}. In the May-Hegglin anomaly, another benign disease, the hereditary presence of Döhle's bodies is also associated with large platelets with decreased granules {#53}.

Abnormal Chemotaxis or Motility

Both extrinsic and intrinsic factors have been found to affect the ability of neutrophils to move in an appropriate directed fashion toward their prey. Deficiencies of opsonins (antibody) can be congenital (agammaglobulinemia) or acquired (chronic lymphocytic leukemia, plasma cell myeloma), and affected patients have an increased risk for bacterial infections. Recently, an anaerobic bacterium (*Capnocytophagia*) associated with gum infections was found to impair the ability of neutrophils to respond to a chemotactic stimulus, although they

---

Table 11-2. Some Conditions Associated With Neutrophilia Greater Than 8000/μL

Immune
  Infection
  Rehumatoid arthritis, acute
Hormones and drugs
  Pregnancy
  Thyrotoxicosis
  Hypercorticism
  Lithium treatment of bipolar disorders
Redistribution
  Splenectomy
Rebound
  After marrow-suppressive chemotherapy
  After treatment of megaloblastosis
Malignancy
  Chronic myelogenous leukemia
  Polycythemia vera

---

still moved in a random fashion. Deficiencies in almost all components of the complement cascade have been described, and most are associated with recurrent infections in affected persons. A large family in which C5 was absent had no chemotactic activity but surprisingly few infections, whereas lack of C3 caused life-threatening infections in another kindred. Systemic illnesses such as diabetes mellitus and uremia lead to neutrophil dysfunction and a susceptibility to infections.

Disorders intrinsic to neutrophils and causing clinical problems due to abnormal mobility include inability of neutrophils to adhere (shown to be due to lack of CDIIa/18 membrane cell adhesion receptors), a defect in polymerization of the intracellular actin so that the cells cannot move (the lazy leukocyte syndrome), and lack of adenine triphosphate due to hypophosphatemia.

Abnormal Granules

Inherited absence of the enzyme myeloperoxidase came to the attention of scientists when the enzyme was used to mark neutrophils in automatic differential counters. One of 2000 people were found to lack the enzyme. Infections are not significantly increased except in the presence of diabetes. Perhaps the higher hydrogen peroxide levels compensate for the deficiency. Acquired absence of myeloperoxidase has been found in leukemic and dysplastic cells.

Chédiak-Higashi syndrome is a rare recessive disorder in which lysosomes fuse abnormally, producing functionless giant granules in numerous organs {#102}. This is associated with albinism, neuropathy, decreased numbers of leukocytes and platelets, and a greatly increased susceptibility to infection, because, although neutrophils ingest particles normally and have a normal respiratory burst, bacteria are not killed effectively owing to poor fusion of the giant granules with phagosomes.

Enzyme Deficiencies

Chronic granulomatous disease (CGD) of childhood is a rare (1 of 1 million) X-linked or autosomal disorder characterized by recurrent infections with catalase-positive organisms (*Staphylococcus aureus*, most gram-negatives, *Candida albicans*, *Aspergillus*). The defect is due to the genetic lack of one of the components of the NADPH oxidase system, resulting in a failure of the respiratory burst in response to phagocytosis or membrane stimulation. Therefore, these organisms are ingested but cannot be killed. Most commonly, the defect is in cytochrome b. CGD neutrophils can kill pneumococci or streptococci, which contain no catalase, because these organisms also generate H_2O_2, and, when combined with the myeloperoxidase in the primary granules, these organisms kill themselves in the phagosomes. Severe deficiency of glucose-6-phosphate dehydrogenase, which is rare, has been associated with neutrophil dysfunction. Any person with a history of unexplained recurrent infections should be evaluated for CGD. Clinical testing involves assessing patients' leukocytes for their ability to generate $O_2 \bullet^-$ and change nitroblue tetrazolium (NBT test) from yellow to blue.

EOSINOPHILS

Like neutrophils, eosinophils respond to chemotactic stimuli, have an array of lysosomal enzymes, phagocytize microorganisms, and develop a respiratory burst to membrane stimuli. Unlike neutrophils, however, eosinophils decrease rapidly in the blood with acute inflammation or corticosteroid administration. Corticosteroids cause increased margination of eosinophils on the vascular epithelium (the reverse of their effect on neutrophils) so that they disappear from the circulation temporarily. The finding of eosinopenia is a useful diagnostic test for recognizing high levels of adrenal cortical hormones, as in Cushing's syndrome. Eosinophilia (an increase in eosinophils), on the other hand, results from a deficiency of corticosteroids (Addison's disease) or is induced by IL-5 released by stimulated T lymphocytes.

Eosinophils are involved in seemingly unrelated diseases such as allergies, parasitic infestations, malignancies, skin diseases, and certain chronic infections. Recent studies provide a unifying hypothesis: eosinophils participate in repeated or persistent tissue inflammatory responses by playing two contrasting roles. They are phagocytic cells, similar to neutrophils, but they are also immunomodulatory. They are able to kill invaders, especially large organisms such as helminths, by extracellular release of enzymes. Eosinophils have been shown to surround large schistosomes and suddenly destroy them. The peroxidase of eosinophils has less oxidizing power than myeloperoxidase and is thought to mediate oxidation of key parasitic enzymes rather than to oxidize macromolecules indiscriminately. The major basic protein in eosinophils has poorly understood toxic properties. Eosinophils seem to work best, even in parasitic infections, in concert with other cells (mast cells, macrophages, T lymphocytes) rather than alone, strengthening the hypothesis of their complex role in inflammation.

Eosinophils are also anti-inflammatory, immunomodulatory cells, which restrain and localize immune inflammation. Their role as homeostatic immune modulators in intimate cooperation with basophils is good evidence for such a hypothesis. Eosinophils are present during the late stages of almost all inflammatory reactions (infectious, traumatic, or neoplastic) and are most often found at the periphery of the inflammatory process. They also are ubiquitous in hypersensitivity reactions in which antigens fix to mast cells or basophils via IgE. This attachment causes the basophils to release the tetrapeptide eosinophilic chemotactic factor of anaphylaxis, and histamine. Eosinophils then approach and secrete prostaglandins E_1 and E_2 (which suppress mast cell degranulation), histaminase, and arylsulfatase, which inactivates mast cell slow-reacting substances of anaphylaxis (slow-reacting substance of anaphylazis [SRS-A], leukotriene B_4 [LTB$_4$], leukotriene C_4 [LTC$_4$]).

Eosinophilia

Increased numbers of eosinophils ($>450/\mu$L) {#8} occur in a wide variety of conditions. Most important are the common allergic diseases, such as allergic rhinitis, asthma, and atopic dermatititis. Parasitic infestations constitute another worldwide cause of eosinophilia. Unlike neutrophils, disorders of eosinophils do not appear to be accompanied by morphologic abnormalities.

BASOPHILS

Basophils {#7} have been the scientific orphans of the blood, largely because they are few and therefore difficult to isolate and study. But their role in acute hypersensitivity reactions and their interaction with eosinophils have stimulated great interest. The relation between basophils and tissue mast cells has not been firmly established. Despite similarities of morphology, contents, and function, basophils and mast cells may not have a common origin. Little is known about production of basophils. Recent investigation shows that T lymphocytes and their secretory products are important in the differentiation of basophils (and eosinophils) from their marrow precursors.

The release of mast cell contents results when specific antigen becomes bound to IgE fixed to their surfaces. The response of basophils to corticosteroids is similar to that of eosinophils. Agents that increase intracellular cAMP (cyclic adenosine monophosphate), such as adrenergic compounds, prostaglandin E, and methylxanthines (e.g.,theophylline) inhibit the histamine release of tissue mast cells, a mechanism by which these drugs control bronchial asthma.

Basophilia (>50 cells/μL) is a nonspecific finding, seen in a wide variety of hypersensitivity reactions, chronic lung disease, and other inflammation. Basophilia also has been noted with hypothyroidism, suggesting that these cells may be controlled by thyroid hormones.

SUMMARY POINTS

Neutrophils constitute the linchpin of the body's defenses against infection. Quantitative defects are much more common than qualitative. During the chemotherapy of malignancy, neutrophils are frequently decimated and the patient is sustained by multiple antibiotics. A knowledge of granulocyte kinetics enables the clinician to predict the return of the white cells. Transfusions of white cells are logistically useless except for very narrow indications.

SUGGESTED READINGS

Butcher EC. Leukocyte-endothelial recognition: three (or more) steps to specificity and diversity. *Cell* 1991;67:1033–1036.

Gallin JI, Goldstein IM, Snyderman R. *Inflammation: Basic Principles and Clinical Correlates*. New York: Raven Press, 1988.

Julia A, Olona M, Bueno J, et al. Drug induced agranulocytosis: prognostic factors in a series of 168 episodes. *Br J Hematol* 1991;79:366.

Logue GL, Shastri KA, Laughlin M, et al. Idiopathic neutropenia: antineutrophil antibodies and clinical correlations. *Am J Med* 1991;90:211.

Metcalf D. Control of granulocytes and macrophages: molecular, cellular and clinical aspects. *Science* 1991;254:529.

Rotrosen D, Gallin JL. Disorders of phagocyte function. *Ann Rev Immunol* 1987;5:127.

CASE DEVELOPMENT PROBLEMS: CHAPTER 11

Problem I

History: A 57-year-old man was hospitalized with a myocardial infarction. The infarction was complicated by congestive heart failure and frequent premature ventricular contractions. Subsequently, he developed runs of ventricular tachycardia and had to be resuscitated. He was eventually able to return to normal activity on captopril to reduce his systolic pressure and procainamide to control his arrhythmia. Three months later, the patient was seen by a dentist with the complaint of a sore on his lip. The dentist called in a consultant, and the patient was admitted to the hospital. Shortly after admission, the patient had a shaking chill.

Physical examination: The patient's lower lip had an odd-looking 1-cm painless mass with a black surface and no surrounding erythema. The rest of the examination was negative except for a 1 × 3 cm perirectal ulcer that the patient had not noticed. There was no pain or drainage.

Laboratory data: WBC 3600/μL, with 66% lymphocytes, 34% monocytes; platelets were 421,000/μL, HCT 34%.

1. Calculate the absolute neutrophil count.
2. Ulcers without pain are unusual. Why is infected tissue normally tender?
3. What is your impression in this case? Why did the perirectal ulcer not show any drainage?
4. What should be done now?
5. The specimen was hypocellular. The differential was 2% myeloblasts, 6% promyelocytes, 16% eosinophils, 46% normoblasts, 16% small lymphocytes, amd 16% monocytes. What is your interpretation?
6. Shortly after admission, the patient had fever of 101° F. He was given antibiotics and the fever resolved. What should be done now?
7. Did the marrow behave as you would have expected

Problem II

History: A 65-year-old man with recent coronary artery bypass was admitted with fever, anorexia, and drainage from his sternotomy wound of 2 weeks' duration. His medical history included diabetes, and he has been taking oral hypoglycemic agents for 2 years. He had had an amebic hepatic abscess in the 1940s. In 1950, he had a colon resection with a large postoperative abscess. A thalamic abscess was drained in 1973. He had a dental abscess in 1983. There was no family history of infection.

Physical examination: The patient had a 10-cm open sternotomy wound with a small amount of purulent drainage.

Laboratory data: White count 11,000/μL with 73% segs. No abnormal forms were seen. Blood glucose >200 mg/dL; wound culture positive for *Candida tropicalis*.

In the hospital: in spite of good control of his diabetes, the patient developed a purulent meningitis due to group B streptococcus. He eventually died from this infection.

1. The history of this patient indicates more frequent infections than would be expected. The thalamic abscess stands out as a very unusual event. *Candida tropicalis* is not ordinarily a pathogen. What possibilities come to mind?

CASE DEVELOPMENT ANSWERS

Problem I

1. 3600 white cells/μL) × (0 neutrophils/100 white cells) = 0 neutrophils.
2. The lack of pain, swelling, and tenderness suggests that neutrophil kinins have not been released locally. The absence of pus also indicates that neutrophils are not present.
3. Life-threatening agranulocytosis.
4. Culture the blood. He is in grave danger of overwhelming sepsis. Examine the bone marrow to learn why neutrophils have disappeared.
5. There is less than expected neutrophil production. Growth of other cell lines appeared intact.
6. Search the drug literature to see whether any of the patient' s drugs causes neutropenia.
   It was found that captopril induces a significant risk of neutropenia. In more than 75% of patients with neutropenia, procainamide had also been administered. (Incidentally, the patient also had an antinuclear antibody titer of 1:160, probably related to the use of procainamide.)
   Impression: captopril neutropenia. The drug should be stopped.

7. Ten days later, the first neutrophils emerged into the blood. In 14 days after stopping the captopril the absolute neutrophil count was >3000/μL and the patient was discharged from the hospital.

Problem II

1. A thalamic abscess and the development of a *Candida tropicalis* infection suggest a defect in immunity. Common variable immunoglobulin deficiency is a possibility, but these patients have predominantly sinopulmonary infections. The complement deficiencies would be expected to be seen in the family. The defect is much milder than chronic granulomatous disease of childhood. It is compatible with myeloperoxidase deficiency. Note that the patient had hyperglycemia. Diabetes makes myeloperoxidase deficiency much more likely to become symptomatic.

   In this case, the infectious disease consultant recognized the probable diagnosis and requested a peroxidase stain of the granulocytes. The stain was negative and the diagnosis confirmed. There is no accepted treatment, although granulocyte transfusions were tried.

Disorders of Marrow Production

Archie A. MacKinney, Jr., Deane F. Mosher

CHAPTER 12

OUTLINE

Aplastic Anemias
Myelodysplasia
Acute Leukemia and Myeloproliferative Syndromes
   Chronic Myeloproliferative Disorders
   Acute Leukemias

Summary Points
Case Development Problem
Case Development Answers

OBJECTIVES

- Understand how aplastic anemia is different from anemia, neutropenia, and thrombocytopenia.
- Survey the diseases grouped under the myelodysplastic and myeloproliferative syndromes.
- Learn about chronic myelogenous leukemia as a model neoplastic condition.
- Understand the log-kill theory.
- Distinguish remission from cure when applied to acute myelocytic and lymphocytic leukemias.

Disorders of bone marrow production can be grouped into three classes: aplasias, in which few or no cells are seen; myelodysplasias, in which defective cells are seen; and hyperplasias in which one or more cell types overgrow the others. All the hyperplasias listed are considered malignancies; the dysplasias have a significant risk of malignancy, and the aplasias are benign disorders with malignant potential. Many of the aplasias and most of the hyperplasias are treatable; the dysplasias are quite refractory.

APLASTIC ANEMIAS

When the marrow appears empty of red cell, white cell, and platelet precursors, it is by definition aplastic {#87}. The aplastic anemias are rare devastating diseases with symptoms and mortality rates closely resembling acute leukemia. In both aplastic anemia and acute leukemia, the failure to make differentiated cells—red cells, granulocytes, and platelets—leads to anemia, infection, and bleeding. Most patients die of infection.

Although differentiated cells are absent in the aplastic bone marrow, in most cases stem cells lurking among the few residual lymphocytes can be demonstrated by tissue culture techniques. Aplastic anemia is a syndrome, that is, a collection of similar diseases with different causes, rather than a single disease. In clinical reports, several causes have been described:

- Loss of stem cells. The bone marrow does not grow under any experimental conditions. Bone marrow transplantation should be effective in replenishing the stem cell pool.
- Suppression by macrophages. Suppression of macrophage function or related prostaglandins may be helpful treatment.
- Suppression by lymphocytes. Immunosuppression should be effective treatment.
- Failure of stromal elements. No treatment is likely to benefit. The soil will not accept the seed.

In practice, the first order of business is to stop agents that may cause aplastic anemia (Table 12-1). If no such agents are implicated, then empiric therapy is given. Most patients with aplastic anemia who are not candidates for bone marrow transplantation are tried on a course of immunosuppressive treatment with antithymocyte globulin and/or cyclosporine and glucocorticoids. About 40% of patients have a remission on this treatment, suggesting that immune mechanisms are important in almost 50% of patients. Most hematologists consider allogeneic (from a human leukocyte antigen (HLA)–matched sibling or unrelated donor) bone marrow transplantation to be the treatment of choice. Bone marrow transplantation is effective in about 40% of patients who are eligible for such a procedure. A few patients respond to androgens and corticosteroids.

Ethanol is the most common cause of chemical marrow injury. In ethanol poisoning, there is usually a mild pancytopenia (decrease in all three major cell types), which in itself is not life-threatening. The marrow is rarely severely hypocellular. The morphologic evidence of ethanol toxicity consists of vacuoles in the normoblasts and, in some cases, ringed sideroblasts. When combined with nutritional deficiency (folate and ascorbic acid) and compounded by the other complications of alcohol abuse, however, the marrow injury may be the final straw. Fortunately, ethanol marrow injury is reversible. Patients almost always improve with abstinence and good diet.

Benzene is the most important industrial marrow toxin. Benzene is an important solvent in the rubber industry, printing business, and shoe repair business. It is ubiquitous in the oil-refining, gasoline-dispensing industry. Gasoline is 2% to 8% benzene. Workers who are chronically exposed to more than 100 ppm (parts per

TABLE 12-1. Agents Associated With Aplastic Anemia

Agents Regularly Producing Marrow Hypoplasia If Dose Is Sufficient:
  Ionizing radiation
  Benzene and derivatives (toluene, etc.)
  Chemotherapy drugs (6-mercaptopurine, cyclophosphamide, methotrexate,
  daunorubicin, etc.)
  Other poisons (inorganic arsenic)

Agents Occasionally Associated With Marrow Hypoplasia:

Class	Infrequently	Rare
Antianxiety		Chlorpromazine
		Chlordiazepoxide
Anticonvulsant	Mephenytoin	
	Phenytoin	
Anti-inflammatory	Phenylbutazone	
Antimicrobial	Chloramphenicol	Amphotericin B
	Organic arsenicals	Sulfonamides
	Sulfasoxazole	
Antithyroid	Carbimazole	
	Tapazole	
Hypoglycemic	Tolbutamide	
Insecticide	DDT	
	Parathion	
Miscellaneous	Colchicine	
	Acetazolamide	
	Hair dyes	
	Gold salts	

million) benzene in inspired air have a 50% chance of showing a decrease in one or another cell type. Aplastic anemia is usually not reversed by stopping the exposure. Acute leukemia or myelodysplasia may develop. Benzene exposure also increases the risk of lymphoma. Chloramphenicol, an antibiotic used to treat serious infections, has been the prototypic drug causing aplastic anemia on an unpredictable basis (Table 12-1).

MYELODYSPLASIA

The five myelodysplastic syndromes are stem cell disorders, particularly seen in the elderly, and associated with a high risk of evolving into acute leukemia (Table 12-2). Defects in cell production occur in spite of normal or hypercellular marrow. That is, the marrow demonstrates ineffective hematopoiesis. Production defects are accompanied by visible evidence of poor development (dysplasia). The red cell series commonly shows ringed sideroblasts {#19} or megaloblastic changes. Granulocytes may lose peroxidase or primary granules or may show a pseudo–Pelger-Huët nuclear anomaly. Micromegakaryocytes ($\sim 15\ \mu$) are seen in the marrow. Platelets are often large and hypogranular.

The visible dysplastic features are associated with poor cell function. Patients are anemic, even though the marrow may show plentiful normoblasts; they have poor response to infection and easy bleeding often in spite of adequate blood cell counts. Autoimmune disorders appear to be increased, suggesting that the lymphoid system is also involved. Patients with myelodysplastic diseases, in contrast to those with acute leukemia, respond poorly to chemotherapy. One may infer that the totipotent stem cells are subverted and no normal stem cells are available to regenerate.

TABLE 12-2. The Myelodysplastic Syndromes

Name	Description	Marrow (%) Blasts	Risk of Acute Leukemia
Refractory anemia	Anemia unresponsive to all nutritional agents	<5	15
Refractory anemia	Ringed sideroblasts	<5	15
Refractory anemia, excess blasts (RAEB)	Pancytopenia, dysplasia of all cell lines	5–20	30
RAEB in transition	Marrow suggesting acute leukemia	20–30	100
Chronic myelomonocytic	>1000 monocytes/μL	5–20	40

The approach to patients with myelodysplastic disorders is usually aimed at providing transfusion and antibiotic support. Younger patients should be considered for allogeneic bone marrow transplantation. Vitamin B_6, B_{12}, or folate deficiency must be ruled out.

ACUTE LEUKEMIA AND MYELOPROLIFERATIVE SYNDROMES

One or more of the bone marrow cell populations may proliferate without any apparent physiologic stimulus or beneficial effect. This group of disorders is called "myeloproliferative" and has two main features: the uncontrolled growth of one or more of the marrow elements and an interrelationship among the disorders. The myeloproliferative disorders are divided into chronic and acute forms. The acute disorders are all acute leukemias. The chronic disorders have individual descriptive names.

Chronic Myeloproliferative Disorders

Erythrocytosis

When only the red cell count is elevated, there are four issues to consider:

- An increase in the red cell mass or a decrease in the plasma volume
- Hypoxia
- A nonhypoxic increase in erythropoietin due to cysts or tumors
- Autonomous red cell production, that is, a myeloproliferative disorder

A rigorous approach to these questions would entail a measure of the red cell mass by radioisotope labeling, estimate of blood gases, and scanning of organs for masses. In practice, the patient's history and physical examination and screening laboratory studies usually make these tests unnecessary.

For example, when the hematocrit is above 52%, the red cell mass is almost always elevated. If the hematocrit is marginally elevated (52%), the erythrocytosis may be a combination of slightly increased red cell mass and decreased plasma volume, a condition labeled stress erythrocytosis, spurious polycythemia, or Gaisböck's syndrome. This syndrome is seen in obese adults who smoke, have mild hypoxia, decreased plasma volumes, and increased probability of hypertension and cardiovascular disorders.

It is important to exclude tissue hypoxia as a cause of erythrocytosis. Hypoxia may be due to cardiopulmonary disease, high blood levels of carbon monoxide (>5%), or rarely abnormal hemoglobin with high oxygen affinity. If the patient is not hypoxic, the erythropoietin level may be useful. Some endocrine tumors (androgenic) should be kept in mind because they also raise the hematocrit.

In about half the patients with erythrocytosis, no explanation can be found for the elevated red cells, and the erythropoietin level is normal or low. These patients are presumed to have autonomous erythropoiesis. Most of this group goes on to develop elevated platelet and white cell counts and eventually the disorder is labeled polycythemia vera (see section that follows).

Regardless of the cause of erythrocytosis, high viscosity of whole blood leads to an increased risk of clotting—stroke, deep vein thrombosis, and myocardial infarction. Regular phlebotomy is used to control the hematocrit to reduce the whole blood viscosity and decrease the risk of thrombosis.

Thrombocythemia (Idiopathic Thrombocytosis)

When the platelet count is greater than $1 \times 10^6/\mu L$ {#104} and no iron deficiency, infection, or other malignancy is found, the patient is said to have idiopathic thrombocythemia. This is a clonal disorder of the stem cell in which only the platelet production is increased. The patient may have either thromboses or a bleeding tendency. Drug suppression of the high platelet counts with hydroxyurea or anegrelide decreases the risk of either problem.

Polycythemia Vera

When the hematocrit, platelet count, and white cell count are elevated, with emphasis on the hematocrit, the disorder is called polycythemia vera. The criteria for polycythemia vera are an elevated red blood cell mass and any two of the following: white blood cell count greater than $12,000/\mu L$ or platelet count greater than $400,000/\mu L$, an increased leukocyte alkaline phosphatase, or an increased serum B_{12} or B_{12} binding capacity. (B_{12} binding capacity refers to transcobalamins or R binders, which are synthesized by granulocytes in proportion to their numbers.)

Polycythemia vera is a clonal stem cell disorder involving all three major cell lines. Bone marrow cultures have uncovered the interesting observation that polycythemia vera red cell precursors do not require added erythropoietin for growth. Precursors presumably respond to the traces of erythropoietin on their membranes and are able to grow exuberantly at the expense of the normal clones. A small change in receptors makes the polycythemia vera red cell clone independent of normal regulation and gives it a competitive advantage over the normal cells.

Polycythemia vera is a disease of the fifth and sixth decade of life. Most patients are diagnosed incidentally. Patients often are ruddy or "plethoric"; they look healthier than normal people. If untreated, patients may be troubled by venous thrombosis (increased blood viscosity) and pulmonary embolus, gastrointestinal bleeding (peptic ulcer plus poor platelet function), itching (histamine release from increased basophils), inability to eat a full meal (large spleen compressing stomach), or gout (increased uric acid production from increased hematopoiesis). They have enlarged spleens and hypercellular bone marrow with increased megakaryocytes. Examination of the marrow is often unnecessary, however, because the hyperplasia is typically predictable from the appearance of the peripheral blood.

Phlebotomy (bleeding) to hematocrit 45% increases the median survival time from 18 months to over 10 years but does not totally prevent thrombotic complications. Phlebotomy induces iron deficiency, which restrains red cell production by hypoproliferation (see Chapter 5). Most patients need a myelosuppressive drug such as hydroxyurea in addition. Some patients develop acute leukemia, others gradually develop a fibrotic marrow (myelofibrosis), but most progress to a burned-out phase in which anemia develops and transfusions must be given.

Chronic Myelogenous Leukemia

Chronic myelogenous leukemia (CML) is a model malignancy. Like polycythemia vera, it is a clonal disorder involving all three major cell lines, with emphasis on the granulocytic series. CML was the first neoplastic disease defined by a specific chromosomal abnormality: the Philadelphia (Ph1) chromosome is found in more than 95% of the patients and now defines the disease. The Ph1 chromosome has been found in erythrocytic, myelocytic, megakaryocytic, and monocytic cells and occasionally in B lymphocytes. The implication is that the colony-forming unit–granulocytic-erythrocytic-monocytic-megakaryocytic (CFU-GEMM; see Chapter 2) or its precursor, CFU–lymphoid-myeloid (CFU-LM) is affected. Leukocyte alkaline phosphatase is another, less expensive, screening test for patients with unexplained leukocytosis; it is virtually absent in patients with CML.

The cause of CML remains unclear, but ionizing radiation (from exposure at Hiroshima or Nagasaki), radiation therapy for ankylosing spondylitis or heavy benzene exposure clearly increase the incidence of both acute and chronic myeloid leukemias in humans (Fig. 12-1). CML affects a younger age group (25 to 60 years old) than the other myeloproliferative diseases, thrombocythemia, polycythemia vera, and myelofibrosis).

The Ph1 chromosome is due to the reciprocal translocation of chromosome 9 to chromosome 22, t(9;22) (Fig. 12-2). This translocation leads to the apposition of the c-abl oncogene from chromosome 9 to the break-cluster region (bcr) of chromosome 22. Abl is a cytoplasmic and nuclear tyrosine kinase, and the c-abl oncogene when fused with the bcr makes a new protein kinase, named p210. The new kinase has different substrate specificity, which is similar to that of the v-abl gene in mouse leukemias induced by the Abelson leukemia virus. Although the Ph1 chromosome has been used to define CML, bcr-abl gene fusion is also easily detected and can be found in patients who have a balanced translocation and therefore do not appear to have the Ph1 chromosome by cytogenetic analysis. Other chromosomal abnormalities, such as second Ph1 chromosome or additional group C chromosomes, may appear in the abnormal clone as the disease progresses. Thus, CML is an excellent example of a malignancy in which a genetic change allows establishment of a clone, which then acquires further genetic changes.

The peripheral blood is a showcase of granulocytic precursor cells of all kinds, with a differential rather like the normal bone marrow differential {#80}. Eosinophils and basophils are numerous. The white cell abnormality overshadows the red cell and platelet changes: white cell counts as high as 300,000/μL are found in untreated patients, whereas the platelet count and hematocrit are often close to normal.

CML is an almost uniformly fatal disease without allogeneic bone marrow transplantation. Initially, treatment with mild chemotherapy such as hydroxyurea may alleviate symptoms and decrease the white blood cell count. However, the risk of developing acute leukemia (blast crisis) is about 10% per year (or 90% overall). Interferon treatment has been reported to cause disappearance of the t(9;22) translocation. Patients who achieve this kind of remission have a longer life span than those with conventional treatment. Nevertheless, treatment strategy is dominated by studies showing that patients with an HLA-matched sibling or an unrelated donor may be cured by receiving a bone marrow transplant during the chronic phase. Recently, a specific inhibitor of kinase activity of the p210 bcr-abl fusion protein has shown great promise on clinical trials and may change treatment strategies in the future.

CML is an inherently unstable disease. The patient may develop erythrocytosis, thrombocytosis, or marrow fibrosis during the course of treatment (Fig. 12-3).

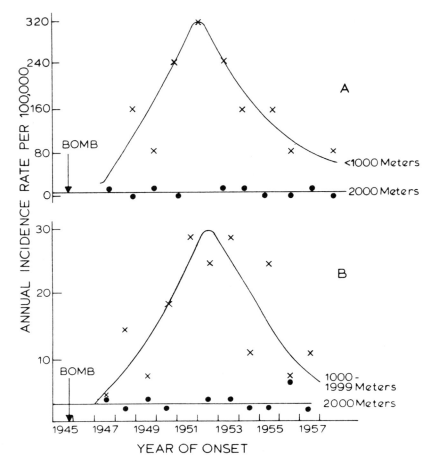

FIGURE 12-1.
Annual incidence rate of leukemia after the atomic bomb explosion among survivors who were residents of Hiroshima at the time of diagnosis. (A) Persons less than 1000 meters from the hypocenter compared with persons 2000 meters or more from the hypocenter at the time of explosion. (B) Person 1000 to 1999 meters from the hypocenter compared with persons 2000 meters from the hypocenter at the time of explosion. (From Lilienfeld AM. *Foundations of Epidemiology.* New York: Oxford University Press, 1976:41.)

Early in the course, the stem cell can differentiate to make functional cells, but ultimately differentiation is lost and only blasts are made. The characteristics of the blast can take many forms as suggested by the multiple progeny of the CFU-LM (see stem cell diagram, Fig. 2-1): myeloblastic, erythroblastic, megakaryoblastic, or lymphoblastic cells may be expressed. The blast crisis does not respond well to drugs, and patients die of infection, hemorrhage, and organ infiltration by leukemic cells.

Myelofibrosis

Myelofibrosis is the most complex of the chronic myeloproliferative disorders. In myelofibrosis, fibrous tissue replaces the normal marrow {#91}. The fibroblasts, however, have a normal karyotype. They are not malignant but are stimulated by a myeloproliferative disorder. In many cases, the previous disorder has been obvious: the patient has had polycythemia vera or CML or idiopathic thrombocytosis (Fig. 12-3). Anemia with nucleated red cells and tear-drop forms, and giant platelets with thrombopenia and megakaryocyte fragments appear in the blood, signaling a change in the marrow. But in some cases, myelofibrosis appears with no previous myeloproliferative disorder. Then, insidious weight loss and a

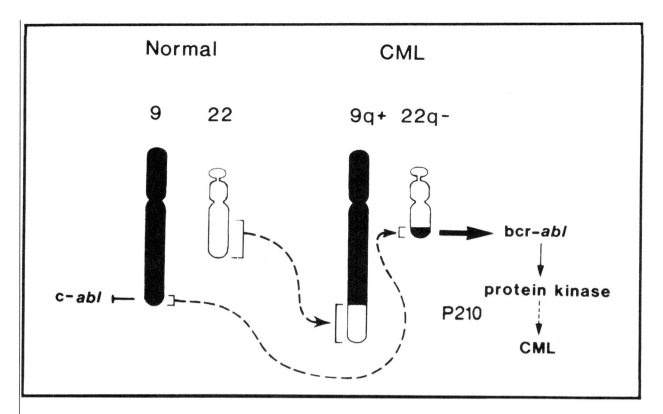

FIGURE 12-2.

Reciprocal translocation between parts of the long arms of chromosome 9 and 22—the Philadelphia chromosome. The region on the long arm of chromosome 9 (9q), which carries the *abl* oncogene, is translocated to the distal end of chromosome 22 (22q). In its new site, the *abl* oncogene is deregulated and produces an overactive protein product, the P210 protein kinase. (From Gordon H. Oncogenes. *May Clin Proc* 60:697.)

grossly enlarged spleen bring the patient to medical attention. The marrow shows dense connective tissue with entrapped megakaryocytes and vanishing erythroid and granulocytic precursors. Usually, hematopoietic islands are found in liver and spleen (myeloid metaplasia).

Growth-promoting factors such as platelet-derived growth factor from platelets and megakaryocytes are probably responsible for the growth of fibroblasts that overrun the marrow in this disease. Special studies using glucose-6-phosphate dehydrogenase heterozygotes or abnormal chromosomes have shown that the hematopoietic cells but not the fibroblasts are derived from one clone and, by inference, are neoplastic. Treatment of this disease is generally unsatisfactory, but reversal of the myelofibrosis does occur occasionally.

The red cell abnormalities seen in myelofibrosis—tear-drop cells and marked poikilocytosis—are more prevalent than in the other myeloproliferative disorders. Anemia rather than erythrocytosis is expected, but up to one third of patients have increased platelets. The bone marrow biopsy serves to distinguish myelofibrosis from thrombocythemia. However, some patients with either myelofibrosis or thrombocythemia have chromosomal translocations, including the t(9;22), or Ph1, which is diagnostic for CML. This serves to emphasize that the myeloproliferative disorders are interrelated through disease in the totipotent stem cell (Fig. 12-3).

Acute Leukemias

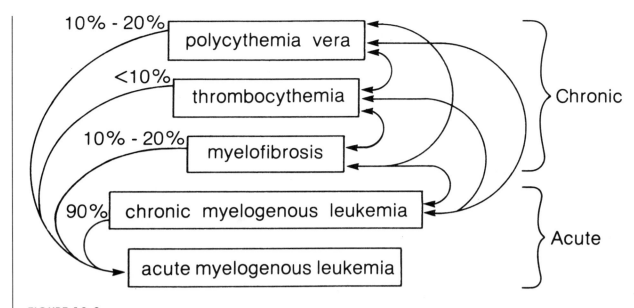

FIGURE 12-3.
Interrelationships among myeloproliferative disorders. The apparent complexity is probably due to the
subversion of the totipotent stem cell, which permits the development of multiple pathways of malignancy.

Acute leukemia is a disease in which undifferentiated cells (blasts) {#65, 76–78}
replace the normal marrow elements, leading to anemia, bleeding, and infection.
Acute leukemia is "acute" because its onset is usually explosive and the duration
of life is less than 1 year without treatment. The incidence of acute leukemia in
the United States and Europe is 3.5 per 100,000 persons per year, a rate comparable to cancer of the esophagus, brain tumors, and malignant melanoma. Eighty
percent of adult acute leukemia is myelogenous; 20% is lymphocytic. Reversed
ratios of acute leukemia are seen in childhood.

The incidence of acute leukemia appears to be increasing. Patients with the
chronic myeloproliferative and myelodysplastic syndrome are being kept alive
longer, allowing acute leukemia to develop. The risk of developing leukemia is
also increased in patients receiving successful long-term chemotherapy for
ovarian carcinoma, polycythemia vera, and multiple myeloma, as well as in
patients treated with both chemotherapy and radiation therapy for Hodgkin's
disease.

Acute Lymphocytic Leukemia

ALL is the most common fatal disease in childhood. It is a malignancy of pre-B
cells, and the chemotherapy is different from that used for patients with AML.
Since the blast cells of ALL are difficult to distinguish from the blasts of AML
{#65}, histochemistry, flow cytometry, and chromosome analysis are needed for
diagnosis. One distinctive but rare microscopic feature is the red cytoplasmic
Auer rod seen in AML but not in ALL.

ALL in childhood is a curable disease. It was the first neoplastic disease to be
successfully treated with combination chemotherapy, and current treatment
leads to a 5-year survival rate of 50% of affected children. Intensive therapy for
childhood ALL includes drug given in the spinal fluid and brain irradiation to
treat or prevent central nervous system leukemia. From studies of childhood
ALL, current principles of combination chemotherapy have been derived
and have led to improved results in adults with ALL or AML. The cure rates in

childhood ALL are good enough so that survivors in the United States are approaching 100,000.

Acute Myelogenous Leukemia

AML has been classified into seven subtypes, based on morphology and the degree of maturation of the leukemic cells {#59, 76–78} (**Table 12-3**).

Acute promyelocytic leukemia (M3) is unusual for two reasons. First, it has a higher risk than the other leukemias for a bleeding disorder that may be fatal. Bleeding is usually most severe during chemotherapy. It is due to release of pro-coagulants and plasminogen activators from granules as the leukemic cells die. Clotting factors are consumed, and fibrinolysis is activated. Acute promyelocytic leukemia is also unique because it responds to a vitamin—retinoic acid! The translocation of chromosome 15 to 17, t(15;17), puts the retinoic acid receptor-α (RARα) on chromosome 17 against a gene (*PML*) on chromosome 15, which may encode a transcription factor. All-*trans* retinoic acid by mouth induces remissions by differentiating leukemic promyelocytes rather than destroying them. This is a new and potentially revolutionary advance in treatment of cancer, which has, until now, focused entirely on cell kill. However, the patients suffer relapse quickly unless treated with standard chemotherapy such as daunamycin and cytosine arabinoside.

Although the pathophysiology of acute leukemia is very difficult to study in humans, a great deal of information has been obtained from studying animal models. Since the basic objective in the management of a rare disease is treatment rather than prevention, much of the following discussion deals with the rationale of treatment. The relentless treatment of malignancies in which there are no physical or clinical signs of residual tumor requires explanation.

From animal studies we know the following:

- A single viable leukemic cell inoculated into the peritoneal cavity of the L1210 mouse can proliferate to a number that is lethal to the host.
- A drug-induced increase in the life span of leukemic mice is largely the result of leukemic cell kill, rather than slowed proliferation or selection of a homogeneous leukemia population with a longer doubling time.
- To cure leukemia, it is necessary to kill leukemic cells faster than they are generated..
- Effective antileukemic drugs kill a larger proportion of malignant cells than normal cells.
- Some antileukemia agents are cell-cycle–specific; others attack cells in the resting phase as well. Most cycle-specific agents attack the cell during DNA synthesis phase, and a few, in mitosis.

TABLE 12-3.   Classification of Acute Myelogenous Leukemia

Code	Description	Characteristics
M1	Acute myeloblastic	No differentiation
M2	Acute myeloblastic	Differentiation toward promyelocyte
M3	Acute promyelocytic	Bleeding syndrome from primary granule enzymes
M4	Acute myelomonocytic	Mixture of monoblasts and myeloblasts
M5	Acute monocytic	Infiltration of mucosa and meninges by monoblasts
M6	Erythroleukemia	Mixture of erythroblasts and myeloblasts
M7	Acute megakaryocytic	Rapidly fatal, with acute myelofibrosis

An estimated 10^9 leukemic blast cells are necessary to kill a mouse (Fig. 12-4). (Approximately 10^{12} blasts are found in advanced adult acute leukemia.) Animals bearing as many as 10^5 cells are cured of leukemia by intense treament with an alkylating agent. This schedule is assumed to destroy all of malignant cells ($0.01\% \times 10^4 = 1$, or hopefully zero cells remaining). When drug was given at longer intervals, malignant cells were allowed to grow and destroy the host. (The effect of different programs for the mouse is diagrammed in Fig. 12-5).

Estimates of Kinetics

From the mouse data, we better understand acute leukemia in humans. The doubling of time of leukemic cells in humans is estimated to be as short as 4 days,

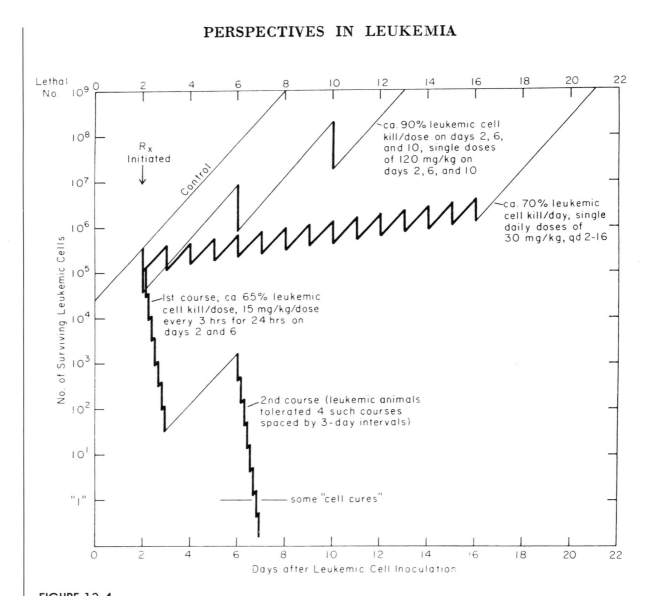

PERSPECTIVES IN LEUKEMIA

FIGURE 12-4.

Schematic results obtained using three chemotherapy schedules of arabinosylcytosine in the L1210 system in the mouse. The effective cell kill that achieves cure is shown by the protocol on the lower left. (From Skipper HE. *Perspectives in Leukemia.* New York: Grune & Stratton, pp. 187–216.)

and the number of cells necessary for the clinical diagnosis approaches 10^{12}, a liter of leukemic cells replacing the marrow. If we assume that doubling continued exponentially without limitation due to crowding or other feedback regulation, then 40 doublings would yield 10^{12} cells, and the patient would be clinically ill 160 days after the first cell had begun to replicate (Table 12-4). It is unlikely that acute leukemia could be recognized by the proportion of blasts in the marrow before the 37th doubling, when there would be 10^{11} blasts ($10^{11}/10^{12}$ = 10% of total marrow cells).

A good treatment schedule could kill 99.99% of the cells, reducing the number of cells by 4 logs and leaving 10^8 cells. If the host were able to tolerate a massive dose of such therapy and recover within 1 or 2 weeks and if another treatment of comparable killing power were available, one could conceivably reduce the population again by 4 logs to 10^4. The difficulty of curing acute leukemia after it reaches the clinical threshold of 10^{12} cells is apparent.

The study of leukokinetics of acute leukemia in humans, however, shows that leukemic cell treatment is more complicated than the mouse leukemia model.

Consider these problems:

1. Blast cells out of mitotic cycle
2. Leukemic sanctuaries
3. Nature of the stem cell—normal or malignant
4. Status of residual leukemic cells
5. Drug resistance
6. Stem cell exhaustion

Blast cells. In the laboratory model, leukemic growth resembles a bacterial population in log phase. The growth rate of human acute leukemia, at least during the time of recognition of the disease, is slower than that of the normal marrow cells. As leukemic blast cells replicate, they become smaller, nondividing blasts, which are preferentially released into the blood. Unlike normal mature granulocytic cells, these smaller blasts may reenter the mitotic cycle and resume mitosis. Since acute leukemia chemotherapy is generally designed for cells that are in the mitotic cycle, it appears likely that some failures of chemotherapy are due to an inability to kill cells that are not in the mitotic cycle.

Leukemic sanctuaries. Another problem of treatment is that drugs do not penetrate all tissues equally, leaving some organs as sanctuaries. The bone marrow may show a remission, whereas the patient has leukemia appearing in the testis, central nervous system, or connective tissue, where drug concentrations were too low to sterilize the tissue. This is the rationale of the use of central nervous system treatment of acute lymphocytic leukemia in children.

Nature of the stem cell. A third problem of treatment is that successful chemotherapy depends on a totipotent stem cell that is normal and can repopulate the marrow after the malignant cells have been killed off. This is probably the case in 80% of patients, but a malignant totipotent stem cell that cannot generate normal cells may account for a the failure of chemotherapy in 10% to 20% of patients. Patients with myelodysplasia who develop acute leukemia are in this category. Patients with acute leukemia who have the Ph1 chromosome, t(9;22), also have a poor prognosis for this reason and are prime candidates for bone marrow transplantation.

Residual leukemic cells. Another difference between humans and the experimental mouse is that residual malignant cells can be found in patients even after prolong remission. Tissue culture of remission bone marrow after treatment of acute leukemia has shown that malignant clones of cells can still be grown. Polymerase chain reaction techniques show that many patients thought to be cured (5-year relapse-free survival) have 10^5 or more malignant cells remaining in the marrow. The more malignant cells that are found, the greater the risk of

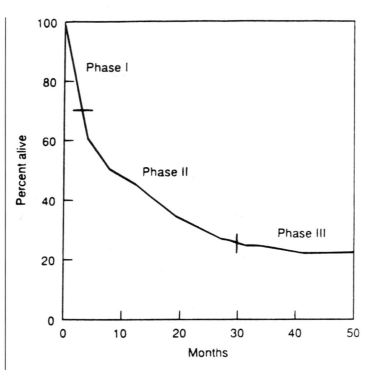

FIGURE 12-5.
Generic Kaplan-Meier curve for patients with acute myelogenous leukemia. The overall survival for patients is divided into three phases. Phase I is induction therapy. The overall survival during this phase reflects the complete remission rate and the ability of the patient to tolerate chemotherapy and prolonged neutropenia and thrombocytopenia. Most patients who fail to respond die of infections or hemorrhage. True resistant disease account for less than 15% of induction failures. The complete response rate is approximately 60% to 80%. Phase II comprises the first 2 years after attainment of complete remission. During the first 2 to 6 months, patients receive consolidation and perhaps intensification and maintenance therapy. Many patients in complete remission suffer relapse and die of their leukemia in these first 2 years. Phase III begins 2 years after complete remission is attained. Patients in remission for more than 2 years have a markedly increased chance for prolonged survival; 75% to 80% of patients in complete remission at 2 years have a prolonged disease-free survival. However, the curve of this phase is not flat, and patients continue to suffer relapse 3 to 10 years after attaining complete remission.

eventual relapse. The mechanism that holds these cells dormant for long periods of time is not yet known.

Drug resistance. This is a complex problem. Suffice it to say that treatment that does not eradicate the malignancy permits the escape of clones that may resist new drugs as well as the ones to which they were previously exposed (multiple-drug resistance).

Stem cell exhaustion. Although most stem cells are out of the mitotic cycle and are relatively insensitive to chemotherapy, the barrage of chemotherapy takes a toll. The inability of the patient to recover after multiple-course chemotherapy is referred to as "burnout" and may be due to injury to the marrow microenvironment as well as to depletion of stem cells.

Treatment Strategies

Use of multiple drugs in adult acute leukemia can induce clinical remissions in up to 80% of patients. A clinical remission reduces the blast population by 2 to 3

TABLE 12-4. A Simple Model of Leukemic Cell Doubling

Patient	Cell Number	Weight Weight	Volume Volume	Time (Days)	Doubling
Subclinical	10^0	1 pg	10^{-12} L	0	0
	10^3	1 μg	10^{-9} L	40	10
	10^6	1 mg	10^{-6} L	80	20
	10^9	1 g	10^{-3} L	120	30
Sick	10^{12}	1 kg	1 L	160	40
Dead	10^{13}	*10 kg*	*10 L*	*200*	*50*

logs, so that blasts are not visibly increased in marrow. Remission is accompanied by an increase in platelets, red cells, and neutrophils to normal or near-normal levels. Remissions that are not pursued with further treatment are short, suggesting that the blast population begins to proliferate promptly and 10^{12} cells are again present within a few months. For this reason, several strategies are applied to the treatment of acute leukemia.

Chemotherapy of acute lymphocytic leukemia is divided into four phases:

- Induction—to reduce leukemic population and induce remission
- Consolidation—given as soon as possible to further reduce the leukemic population and sustain remission
- Intensification—used after a period of rest to attack residual leukemic nests
- Maintenance—low-level chemotherapy used in ALL, controversial in AML

The overall goal of treatment is to achieve cures as outlined in Figure 12-5. If cure is not possible, the goal then is to achieve a long-term remission. The definition of a complete remission is normal blood counts, normal marrow, and absence of any cells with genetic characteristics of the original leukemia. Cure is defined by a flat Kaplan-Meier curve. If the curve becomes flat for 5 years for a sufficiently large number of patients treated in the same way, those patients can be said to be cured of their disease.

The combination of daunamycin or idarubicin and cytosine arabinoside usually eradicates 99% of leukemic cells. All visible leukemic cells are killed, and in the process any normal hematopoiesis is lost and the skin and gut are also temporarily damaged. The process can be described as burning a field of weeds so that good plants can grow. For about 3 weeks, the patient is dependent on red cell and platelet transfusions and broad antibiotic coverage.

Another therapeutic approach is to stimulate immunity, either nonspecifically or specifically, against the leukemic cell. A third approach is to transplant normal bone marrow when the patient has achieved a remission. Best results are obtained in childhood acute leukemia, where an estimated 50% are living more than 5 years. However, cures are achieved probably not because the cytoreduction chemotherapy kills the last remaining leukemic cells but because the engrafted marrow has immunity against the leukemic cells of the host. Evidence for this proposition is (1) that transplantations from identical twins do not result in cures; (2) patients who are cured after allogeneic bone marrow transplantation are those with manifestations of chronic graft-versus-host disease (and graft-versus-leukemia effect).

SUMMARY POINTS

The bone marrow may exhibit four kinds of intrinsic disorders: disappearance of cells (aplastic anemia), production of poorly made cells (myelodysplasia), exuberant production of normal-appearing cells (chronic leukemias), or production of undifferentiated precursors (acute leukemias). Since in most of these cases, the patient suffers from the failure of normally functioning cells, complaints of weakness, fever, weight loss, or bleeding may be expected. Because of the metabolic demands of the myeloproliferative diseases, the patient may present with decreased energy, weight loss in spite of good appetite, or loss of work tolerance. Treatment is difficult and in some cases life-threatening, but rewarding.

CASE DEVELOPMENT PROBLEM: CHAPTER 12

History and Laboratory Data: You are reviewing laboratory data at the end of a clinic day and turn up these values: hematocrit 49%, RBC $6.4 \times 10^6/\mu L$, mean corpuscular volume (MCV) 76 fL, WBC 14,000/μL, platelet count 480,000/μL. The white cell differential is normal. The patient is a middle-aged woman who had come in for a yearly checkup. She did not drink or smoke. She appeared well, and the physical examination was normal.

1. Are these counts normal?
2. (a) Are these separate abnormalities or part of a pattern? (b) If you think of these as separate abnormalities, what possibilities can you think of?
   Actually, you should avoid thinking of data as individual bits. One of the basic rules of medicine is to look for patterns rather than separate abnormalities.
3. If you think of all the data together, what disease comes to mind?
4. What should you do? Do you want to see her again or let the matter go?
5. The patient returned in 2 months and the counts were unchanged. But on your reexamination, you feel the spleen tip. What is your thought now?
   The patient did not return. Two years later, you are consulted by a doctor in another hospital about anticoagulating a patient. It is this same patient. She is in bed with her swollen left leg elevated. Doppler studies confirm that she has a femoral vein thrombus. Her hematocrit is 50%, WBCs 18,000/μL, platelet count 850,000/μL, MCV 72 fL.
6. There are many causes of venous thrombosis. Does any possibility seem obvious from these data?
7. One puzzle remains. (a) Why is the patient's MCV low? (b) Is she iron-deficient? (c) How would you find out?
8. Do you have an explanation for this finding?
9. Should we treat her for this condition?
10. How can you be sure that the patient does not have chronic myelogenous leukemia?
11. What treatment would you offer?

CASE DEVELOPMENT ANSWERS

1. The hematocrit, platelet count, and white cell count are all somewhat above the normal limits. Also, the MCV is low.
2. (a) A high hematocrit may be secondary to hypoxia or erythropoietin (or androgen)-secreting tumors. The patient could have a left-shifted hemoglobin. (b) A slightly elevated white count could be from anxiety, exercise, or an undetected infection, among many other possibilities. An elevated platelet

count occurs in iron deficiency (note that the MCV is low), infection, or malignancy. The low MCV may be due to iron deficiency, but the hematocrit is normal.

3. Elevated white cell count, red cell count, and platelet count indicate polycythemia vera.

4. The patient does not appear ill, and the elevations in her counts are marginal. Let us see her again in 2 months.

5. Polycythemia vera is the first choice. The enlarged spleen is additional evidence for this. See her again in 6 months.

6. The platelet count has doubled and may have caused the thrombosis. She will have further trouble from a high platelet count and a high hematocrit if nothing is done for her.

7. The serum ferritin was 10 μg/L; the serum iron (transferrin-bound iron) was 40 μg/dL; the iron-binding capacity (apotransferrin) was 350 μg/dL. The data support iron deficiency.

8. Polycythemia vera patients are often iron-deficient. They have an increased risk for gastrointestinal bleeding (make a mental note to screen the patient for gastrointestinal blood loss). In these patients, marrow stores are used to make excess numbers of red cells.

9. Iron therapy would be disastrous. It would release her marrow to make more and larger red cells. Her hematocrit might go up to 65%, with greatly increased risk of stroke, myocardial infarction, and deep vein thrombosis. Her iron deficiency should be left alone and a warning left in her chart not to treat her with iron.

10. The white cell differential showed no young cells, and no increase in eosinophils or basophils. Her leukocyte alkaline phosphatase was elevated, and the Ph1 chromosome was not found. Chronic myelogenous leukemia is excluded.

11. For now the patient must be given anticoagulation (heparin followed by warfarin) for her deep vein thrombosis. She needs phlebotomy to bring down her hematocrit quickly. Hydroxyurea is the treatment of choice for the high platelet count and should be started soon.

Monocytes and Macrophages

Archie A. MacKinney, Jr.

OUTLINE

OBJECTIVES

- Compare and contrast the maturation and morphology of monocytes/macrophages and granulocytes.
- Appreciate the varied roles of monocytes/macrophages.
- Acquire insights into clinical disorders that involve monocytes/macrophages.

MONOCYTES

Monocytes are ubiquitous, multifarious, and omnivorous. They are found everywhere from the skin to the brain, they perform many different tasks, and they eat anything. The monocyte/macrophage, and its fraternal twin, the neutrophil, are the principal phagocytes (cell eaters) of the body. They attack bacteria, but also attack crystals, splinters, and dead cells. In addition, the monocyte/macrophage is an antigen-presenting cell. Monocytes are important in defense against malignancies and virus diseases. They are also the basic unit of the granuloma. Malignancies of the monocyte are unusual (e.g., acute and chronic myelomonocytic leukemia, histiocytosis X). Genetic diseases (e.g., Gaucher's disease, Niemann-Pick disease) are rare. This chapter integrates material you have read or will read about in other chapters or other courses.

Origin

The monocyte originates in the bone marrow from the common stem cell for the granulocytic and monocytic series (CFU-GM). Few promonocytes and monocytes are counted in the normal marrow differential; yet the monocyte is the precursor of a large organ—the monocyte-macrophage system (MMS), which hides in interstitial spaces throughout the body. The promonocyte is the only recognized bone marrow precursor, and the transit time of the developing monocyte in the marrow is short—2 to 5 days. Because the marrow transit time of the monocyte is shorter than that of the neutrophil, the appearance of monocytes in the blood after serious marrow injury precedes and predicts the recovery of granulocytes. The monocyte is not stored in the bone marrow."

Circulation

The monocyte is one of the less common cells in the peripheral blood {#9, 72}. It is an immature phagocyte when circulating, and it has a characteristic "horse shoe" nucleus and abundant gray cytoplasm with a few granules and vacuoles. Its normal count in blood is about $400/\mu L$. Monocytes are not a homogeneous population and have been subdivided by their membrane antigens into $CD14^+CD16^+$ and $CD14^+CD16^-$ cells. The major population of $CD14^+CD16^-$ cells produce interleukin-10 (IL-10), which enhances T-cell function. The $CD14^+CD16^+$ cells are a minor population that is expanded in sepsis and produces tumor necrosis factor (TNF). CD14 is a receptor with high affinity for lipopolysaccharide, enhancing the phagocytosis of gram-negative bacteria and subsequently leading to the release of IL-10 ($CD14^+CD16^-$).

Monocyte half-life ($t_{1/2}$) in the circulation is 3 days, about 10 times longer than that of the granulocyte. Monocytes roll along the blood vessel and exit through endothelium in response to chemotactic stimuli. The marginal pool of monocytes is estimated to be three to five times greater than the circulating pool. Data on the monocyte compared with the neutrophil are given in Table 13-1.

Monocytosis ($>1000/\mu L$) occurs in Hodgkin's disease, tuberculosis, and syphilis. Grossly elevated monocyte counts ($>20,000/\mu L$) occur in acute or chronic myelomonocytic leukemia and acute monocytic leukemia. Monocytopenia is not common, but it is a feature of hairy cell leukemia {#79}, AIDS,

TABLE 13-1.   Comparison of Monocyte and Neutrophil

Characteristic	Monocyte	Neutrophil
Marrow transit time	2.5–5 days	8–14 days
% Marrow	1	50
Marrow storage	No	Yes
Daily delivery	0.4×10^9	1×10^{11}
Number in blood/μL	400	4,000
Half-life in blood	70 hours	7 hours
Corticosteroid effect	Decrease in blood	Increase in blood
Marginal/circulating pool	3–5/1	1/1
Destiny	Tissues	Tissues
Life span in tissues	Months to years	Hours
Function	Phagocytosis	Phagocytosis
Division outside marrow	Yes	No
Participation in delayed hypersensitivity	Yes	No
Participation in viral immunity	Yes	No
Consequence of deficiency	?	Septicemia
Histochemistry		
Peroxidase	Weak	Strong
Nonspecific esterase	Strong	Weak

and bone marrow failure. Total absence of monocytes is so rare that one suspects it is incompatible with life.

TISSUE MACROPHAGES

Monocytes migrate into the tissues to become fixed or loose macrophages with a variety of names: Kupffer's cell (liver), littoral cell (spleen), alveolar macrophage (lung), Langerhans' cell (dermis), microglial cell (brain), osteoclast (bone), and others.

Macrophages probably have a life span extending into months in the tissues except in the lung, where sputum losses account for some of the daily turnover. This has been established by slow conversion of tissue macrophages from recipient to donor type after bone marrow transplantation. Macrophages are easily overlooked in histologic sections unless loaded with particles, such as lipid or hemosiderin, or identified by special stains.

The monocyte differs from the neutrophil in its ability to induce enzyme formation during activation. Transition of the monocyte to a macrophage in response to interferon-γ is marked by an increase in the number of mitochondria, increased activity of enzymes, and increased phagocytosis and mobility. Macrophages in various tissues have metabolic characteristics peculiar to that tissue. For example, alveolar macrophages have two to three times the oxygen consumption of peritoneal macrophages. These differences are believed to be due to macrophage adaptation rather than to different sites of macrophage origin.

The number of macrophages in the tissues depends on marrow input, but also, in contrast to the granulocytes, on local proliferation. Growth of monocytes in culture depends on granulocyte-macrophage colony-stimulating factor (GM-CSF), M-CSF, both elaborated by macrophages, and IL-3. Furthermore, IL-1 and TNF, also secreted by macrophages, induce other cells to make GM-CSF and M-CSF. Thus, activated cells of the monocyte series appear to stimulate their own production directly and indirectly. In the tissues, proliferation also depends to the workload of ingested particles. Local increase in spleen DNA synthesis can be observed when splenic macrophages are presented with increased numbers of injured erythrocytes to ingest. Prostaglandins, especially of the E series, may inhibit monocyte growth.

Secretion

The macrophage has been reported to secrete or excrete at least 100 products. The list includes:

- Enzymes (elastase, collagenase)
- Antibacterial oxidants such as superoxide, hydroxyl radicals, and nitric oxide
- Complement components (C1–C5) involved in cell lysis
- Coagulation factors, as well as plasminogen activator and fibronectin
- Mediators, such as prostaglandins, fibroblast growth factor, pyrogen (IL-1), interferon-α and -β, and TNF
- Nutrients (thymidine)

Most of the factors are released during activation or phagocytosis.

SOME MONOCYTE/MACROPHAGE FUNCTIONS

The monocyte-macrophage may be regarded as a cellular mediator in the hematopoietic system, interacting with kinins, complement, and clotting systems and modulating production and destruction of red cells, granulocytes, lymphocytes, and bone. It influences the brain through endotoxin-mediated pyrogens (IL-1, $TNF\alpha_1$). The complexity of its functions approaches that of the hepatocyte.

Erythrophagocytosis

The macrophage is a storage source of iron for the growing normoblast. In the anemia of chronic inflammation, the macrophage plays a central role by withholding iron from reutilization by new red cells. This leads to restricted red cell production on the one hand, but to restricted nutrient iron passing through the plasma on the other. This short-term iron shortage may inhibit bacterial proliferation.

Monocytes have surface receptors for IgG (Fc) and C3. When erythrocytes are coated with either of these, active attachment occurs. This in vitro observation explains a mechanism by which the spleen traps red cells in Coombs'-positive hemolytic anemia. The macrophage also is the sarcophagus of the red cell, efficiently returning degraded globin to the amino acid pool, extracting heme iron for reutilization, and converting the porphyrin to bilirubin.

Clotting

Tissue monocytes produce procoagulants, such as tissue factor and factors, II, V, VII, IX, and X. The monocyte can be stimulated by a process that requires interaction with lymphocytes to cause the elaboration of fibrin. Kupffer's cells (liver macrophages) remove fibrin particles and activated clotting factors as part of the body's defense against disseminated intravascular coagulation.

Granulocytes

Monocytes stimulate production of colony-stimulating factors. On the other hand, myelopoiesis may be inhibited by prostaglandins secreted by monocytes.

Macrophages are the site of destruction of old granulocytes. When the mass of granulocytes to be recycled is very large, as in chronic myelogenous leukemia, macrophages may show bundles of filamentous debris almost identical with those of Gaucher's disease. They are called pseudo-Gaucher's cells and are a graphic illustration of the macrophage working overtime.

Lymphocytes

Monocytes interact with lymphocytes to amplify mitosis stimulating reactions in vitro. IL-1 is the best-known monocyte activator of lymphocytes. Physical binding of lymphocytes to a central monocyte, an "immunologic island," probably is important in immunologic processing of antigen. Macrophages also act as suppressor cells in some immune reactions by secreting prostaglandins. When macrophages and lymphocytes interact, lymphocytes may release chemotoxin or macrophage inhibiting factor or may impart cytocidal properties to macrophages. The orchestration of these complex functions remains to be described.

Bone Formation

Monocytes are the precursors of the osteoclasts and as such are a major factor in bone remodeling. The osteoclast activating factors include IL-1, TNFα and TNFβ. Osteoclast hyperactivity is an important part of the pain and morbidity in multiple myeloma. It is ironic that monocytes and TNF, which may destroy some tumors, are part of the tumor pathophysiology in multiple myeloma.

Atherosclerosis

The foam cells that are the early pathology of atheroma formation are macrophages full of ingested lipid. Monocyte invasion of endothelium may be the first step in atherosclerosis.

Granulomas

When the body cannot destroy a microorganism or foreign body, a granuloma is formed. Granulomas are formed in reaction to indigestible organisms such as *Mycobacterium tuberculosis, Mycobacterium leprae,* and *Leishmania.* This is also true of chronic granulomatous disease of childhood in which ordinarily susceptible bacteria such as staphylococcus cannot be killed by neutrophils. In the granuloma, the monocyte contributes the epithelioid cell and the multinucleated giant cell. B and T cells and fibroblasts are also present.

Fever

The malaise, somnolence, fever, muscle aches, and anorexia that accompany the flu are well known to most adults. Existing data suggest that the monocyte is a major player in all this. In response to viral or bacterial antigen, it produces IL-1 and TNFα (two of six known fever-producing cytokines), which have profound effects on the body. They raise the temperature set point in the hypothalamus, causing vasoconstriction and shivering and other central nervous system effects, such as somnolence and anorexia. Stored neutrophils are mobilized from the marrow, and apoptosis of neutrophils is inhibited.

Although neutrophils are believed to be important in fever, the monocytes are probably more so. When the marrow has been wiped out by chemotherapy and neutrophils have disappeared, fever continues unabated, probably controlled by tissue macrophages that have not been destroyed by the chemotherapy.

TABLE 13-2. Distribution of Particle Clearance in Three Organs

Organ Particles	Cell	% Cardiac Output	% Phagocytosis of
Liver	Kupffer's cell	25	60–95
Spleen	Macrophage	5	5–20
Marrow	Macrophage	?1	5-25

MONOCYTE-MACROPHAGE SYSTEM

The term "monocyte-macrophage system" (MMS) replaces the older reticuloendothelial system because the principal phagocytic capacity of the body originates in the marrow rather than in the connective tissue. Although the three most important MMS organs are believed to have equal numbers of macrophages, they do not show equal phagocytic ability, in part because of differences in blood flow (Table 13-2).

Kinetics

The MMS may be described in terms of particle clearance and its stimulation or inhibition. In particle clearance, the whole MMS appears to act as a unit. Each particle has its own clearance characteristics, depending partly on size. Saturation of the system by one particle does not necessarily prevent phagocytosis of another kind of particle. Kinetics of whole-body clearance can be analyzed by elegant mathematical models.

Inhibition of particle clearance, however, occurs in viral infections, corticosteroid therapy, and alcohol abuse. Patients with these conditions are more prone to disseminated intravascular coagulation because they do not clear activated clotting factors normally. They are also more prone to overwhelming bacterial infections because they do not clear bacteria efficiently.

Liver versus Spleen

Differences in particle clearance by liver and spleen also depend on antibody class and antibody concentration. Elegant studies of the partition of antibody-coated red cells are summarized in Figure 13-1. Red cell clearance becomes more efficient as the concentration of antibody molecules increases on the cell. IgG antibody-coated cells (anti-Rho[D]) are preferentially trapped in the spleen, whereas IgM antibody-coated cells (anti-A) are caught in the liver. At high concentrations of antibody, however, the liver also efficiently traps IgG-coated red cells. Consequently, one must know both the types and the concentration of antibody on the red cell to accurately predict whether splenectomy will stop antibody-mediated hemolysis. If the antibody concentration on the cell is high, splenectomy will be less effective. The same rule probably applies to immune disorders of platelets and granulocytes.

Work Hypertrophy

If the effective liver blood flow is reduced, as in cirrhosis of the liver, the spleen and marrow increase their proportion of the phagocytic work. This can be seen readily by visualization of radioactive particles used in liver and spleen scanning. If the spleen is removed, the liver and bone marrow MMS becomes hyperplastic. When the spleen is presented with a load of injured erythrocytes, its MMS proliferates to

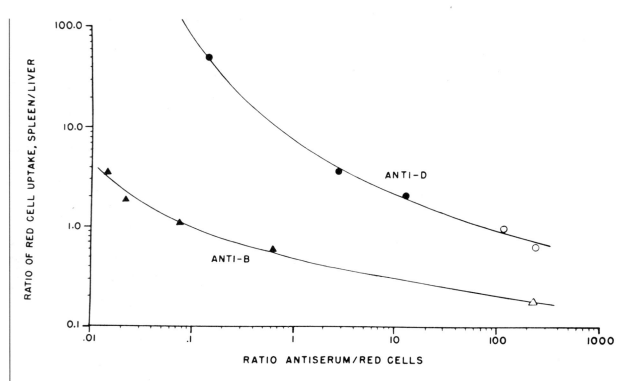

FIGURE 13-1.

Comparison of the trapping of IgG versus IgM antibodies by the liver and spleen in human subjects. The ordinate is the ratio of uptake of radioactive ^{51}Cr-labeled red cells by the spleen/liver. The abscissa is the ratio of antibody to red cells. The upper curve shows IgG antibody (anti-Rh[D]) attached to Rh(D)$^+$ red cells; the lower curve shows IgM antibody (anti-B) attached to B$^+$ red cells. (From Jandl JH, Kaplan MS. The destruction of red cells by antibodies in man. *J Clin Invest* 39:1145).

accommodate. If macrophages are incompetent, work hypertrophy becomes counterproductive (see Lipoidoses and Polysaccharidoses).

THE SPLEEN

Circulation

The spleen, as discussed in Chapter 6, is the body's fine mechanical and immunologic filter. Splenic blood flow is rapid, however, with equilibration of normal red cells occurring at 2 minutes, so that many cells bypass the splenic cords. In some animals, the spleen pools red blood cells at rest and contracts in times of stress, thus abruptly increasing the hematocrit. The spleen in normal humans normally contains only 30 mL of red cells and is not a reservoir of red blood cells.

Platelets also traverse the spleen. Their circulation is different from that of the erythrocytes, because 30% of platelets are normally stored in the spleen. Their transit time also is slower, with a mixing time of approximately 10 minutes. Platelets retained in the spleen can return to the peripheral circulation upon release of epinephrine. When the spleen is very large, up to 90% of the platelets may be stored there. There is little evidence of granulocyte storage in the spleen, but some lymphocytes recirculate through the spleen.

Inclusion bodies, such as Heinz bodies {#40}, Howell-Jolly bodies {#32}, and hemosiderin granules {#18}, are removed by a sieving action that squeezes the straggling particle to the rear of the cell, where it may be pinched off or torn away, leaving the red cell to reseal itself. This process is called "pitting." Deformed or viscous red cells and reticulocytes also are preferentially retained by the spleen, a process called the "culling" function of the spleen.

Splenectomy

When the spleen is removed surgically or is destroyed by infarction as in sickle cell disease, Howell-Jolly bodies (nuclear remnants), target cells, deformed erythrocytes, and increased reticulocytes are seen. The blood smear appears untidy. Leukocyte counts increase to 10,000 to $15,000 \mu/L$, and the platelet count, which is normally 2 to $4 \times 10^5/\mu L$, may temporarily reach 1 to $2 \times 10^6/\mu L$.

The main risk of elective splenectomy is overwhelming bacteremia by grampositive organisms. For this reason, patients undergoing splenectomy should be immunized against encapsulated microorganisms and then given longterm penicillin prophylaxis, if less than 18 years old, and counseled to take antibiotics and seek medical care for infection, if older than 18. Emergency splenectomy for trauma to the spleen is thought to carry less risk of overwhelming infection because of remnants of splenic tissue that may seed the peritoneal cavity.

Workload

Enlargement of the spleen in the presence of a workload is due partly to the volume of cells being destroyed and partly to the hyperplasia of mononuclear cells. Thus, the spleen is not enlarged in idiopathic thrombocytopenic purpura, probably because the platelets have small volumes, whereas the spleen is enlarged and congested in hemolytic anemia because of the volume of retained red cells.

Splenomegaly

The spleen is usually not palpable. Palpation of the spleen tip on physical examination, therefore, requires diagnosis and additional information. Splenomegaly may be due to:

- Workload and work hypertrophy, as in hemolytic anemia
- Infections, notably infectious mononucleosis, typhoid, malaria, histoplasmosis, or leishmaniasis
- Congestion from portal hypertension with cirrhosis of the liver or portal vein thrombosis
- Infiltration in storage diseases such as Gaucher's and Niemann-Pick's disease or amyloidosis
- Tumors such as leukemia, Hodgkin's disease, other lymphoma, or cysts

The list of diseases that lead to a very large spleen is short:

- Chronic myelogenous leukemia
- Myelofibrosis and myeloid metaplasia
- Chronic lymphocytic leukemia
- Leishmaniasis
- Thalassemia major
- Gaucher's disease

The question remains whether a large spleen necessarily leads to splenic dysfunction and harm to the patient. Mild anemia may be due to sequestration and occasionally to destruction of erythrocytes by the large spleen. Mild leukopenia

TABLE 13-3. Macrophage Storage Diseases

Disease	Compound Stored	Clinical Syndrome
Gaucher's disease topenia,	Glucocerebroside	Hepatosplenomegaly, thrombocy-anemia, leukopenia
Sea-blue histiocytosis	Ceroid	Splenomegaly, purpura
Niemann-Pick's disease	Sphingomyelin	Hepatosplenomegaly,cachexia, mental retardation
Fabry's disease	Ceremide trihexoside	Fever, paresthesias, renal failure

frequently occurs, and thrombopenia may be severe owing to storage of up to 90% of the circulating platelet mass. The term "hypersplenism" should be avoided, because it obscures the complex function of the spleen, which destroys some elements, stores some, and has no effect on others.

MALIGNANCIES

Malignancies of the MMS are rare {#73}. Because of the resistance of monocytes and macrophages to chemotherapy, these malignancies carry poorer prognoses than the lymphomas or myeloproliferative disorders. Patients with acute mono-cytic leukemia {#100} often have soft tissue invasion (e.g., gingiva, central nervous system, liver, skin) and shorter remissions than those with other kinds of acute leukemia.

LIPOIDOSES AND POLYSACCHARIDOSES

The lipidoses and polysaccharidoses are rare diseases, and many are due to a lack of the enzymes necessary to degrade normal breakdown products of cells. For example, the patient with Gaucher's disease lacks the enzyme glucocere-brosidase, which cleaves glucose from a glycolipid, glucocerebroside. This gly-colipid is a normal breakdown product of leukocytes and erythrocytes. The indigestible glycolipid fills the macrophage, producing the peculiar "ball of string" appearance {#76}. New macrophages, equally incompetent, are recruited to degrade the glycolipid. Work hypertrophy leads to accumulation of large masses of glucocerebroside-filled cells in the bone marrow, liver, and spleen. It is a waste management problem. These massive accumulations of macrophages lead to liver and marrow failure and ultimately to the patient's death. Other storage diseases are briefly summarized in Table 13-3.

SUMMARY POINTS

The monocytes/macrophages originate in the bone marrow and pass through the blood to spend their lives dispersed in the tissues. They are a hidden system of the body economy. The antigen-presenting role is a frontier of study. Monocytes are clinically noticed most frequently when they become malignant or when failure of one of their enzymes leads to illness.

CHAPTER 14

Lymphocytes and Lymphoma

Archie A. MacKinney, Jr.

OBJECTIVES

- Be familiar with morphologic and functional differences that distinguish different lymphocyte populations and disorders.
- Understand why infectious mononucleosis is called a self-limited lymphoma.
- Describe the triad of clinical disorders that accompany chronic lymphocytic leukemia.
- Understand the clinical differences between Hodgkin's and non-Hodgkin's lymphomas.
- Understand Burkitt's lymphoma as a model malignancy.
- List some risk factors for lymphomagenesis.

As recently as 40 years ago, the functions of lymphocytes were unknown. Twenty-five years ago, medical writers were discussing "the lymphocyte." Currently, lymphocytes are a complex group of blood cells, with five or six types easily recognized by light microscope, 17 to 20 by immunologic markers, and literally millions based on antigen recognition. At least 60 surface markers have been identified on lymphocytes. The lymphocytes are discussed together because they are a highly integrated system. In this chapter, we discuss some of the different kinds of lymphocytes, their interactions, and three illustrative diseases—infectious mononucleosis, chronic lymphocytic leukemia (CLL), and lymphoma—and give an overview of other lymphoid malignancies.

NORMAL LYMPHOCYTES

Numbers

About 35% of peripheral blood leukocytes are lymphocytes. The normal range in adults is 1300 to 4200 per μL of blood. Unlike the granulocytes, the number of lymphocytes in blood do not remain constant throughout life. Newborns have about 5000/μL; the count drops to 2000 by age 10, remains constant to age 40, and then slowly declines to 1500/μL by age 80 (Fig. 14-1). These changes are due

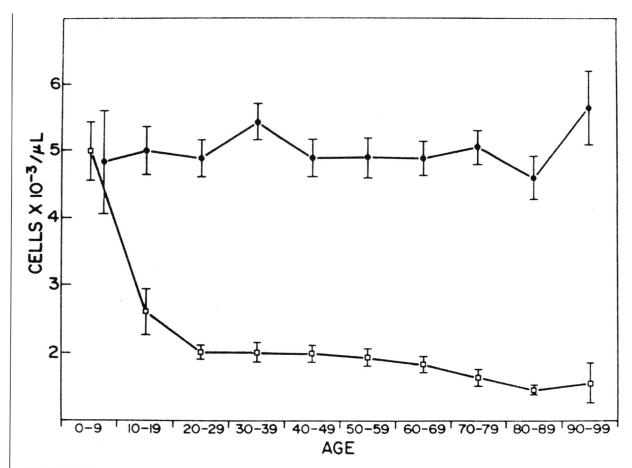

FIGURE 14-1.
Changes in the absolute lymphocyte count compared with the absolute neutrophil count over 10 decades in 2568 patients. Upper line: granulocytes; lower line: lymphocytes. Bars indicate 95% confidence limits.
(From MacKinney AA. Effect of aging on the peripheral blood lymphocyte counts. *J Gerontol* 33:213).

to the loss of T cells, especially CD4 helper cells, with minor increases in B cells and cytotoxic CD8 cells as the child matures into an adult.

An absolute lymphocyte count below 1000/μL is **lymphopenia**. Lymphopenia occurs in those with aplastic anemia, AIDS, and certain immunodeficiency diseases as well as those with lymphomas, especially the advanced stages of Hodgkin's disease. Counts above 5000/μL are called **lymphocytosis**. In children, lymphocytosis occurs in acute infectious diseases. In an adult, a persistent lymphocytosis greater than 6000/μL is highly suggestive of CLL.

Morphology

Traditional morphology classifies lymphocytes as small, medium, or large; mature, prolymphocytic, or lymphoblastic; and normal, atypical (reactive), or plasmacytoid. These designations are useful for defining diseases. For example:

- Small- or medium-sized mature-appearing lymphocytes {#63, 64} are characteristic of CLL and the lymphocytosis of pertussis and other acute infections of childhood.
- Lymphoblasts are poorly differentiated cells {#65} found in acute lymphocytic leukemia, the most common acute leukemia of children.
- Atypical lymphocytes are characteristic of the immune responses to infectious mononucleosis, infectious hepatitis, cytomegalovirus infections, and some drugs. Atypical lymphocytes have a large polygonal nucleus and abundant watery-blue cytoplasm with few granules {#61, 62}.
- Large granular lymphocytes (natural killer [NK] cells) are also seen in viral illness, drug reactions, and autoimmune disorders. These cells have a kidney-bean–shaped nucleus and a dozen large red granules {#103, 105} and are naturally cytotoxic to tumor cells.
- Plasmacytoid lymphocytes, with features of both lymphocytes and plasma cells {#62}, synthesize IgM and are characteristic of Waldenström's macroglobulinemia.
- Plasma cells, although rarely seen in peripheral blood, are easily recognized {#11} by their deep blue cytoplasm, perinuclear halo (Golgi), and eccentrically placed nucleus; they synthesize and secrete immunoglobulins IgG, IgA, IgD, or IgE. They are seen in blood during viral infections and advanced multiple myeloma.

Although these morphologic labels on the differential count orient the physician to a diagnosis, the information is soft compared with the immunologic details of lymphocytes that can be gathered using flow cytometry. Resting B and T cells, for example, are small round lymphocytes and can be separated only by immunologic markers (Table 14-1).

Cell Markers

A combined morphologic/immunologic classification of leukemias and lymphomas generates many new disease labels under morphologically similar cell types (Fig. 14-2). The key events in the development of T cells and B cells are rearrangements of DNA encoding the T-cell receptor and immunoglobulins. B cells originate in the bone marrow and undergo selection and maturation in lymphoid tissue. T cells also come from the bone marrow, but undergo selection and maturation in the thymus.

TABLE 14-1. Lymphocytes Found in Peripheral Blood

Types	% ± SD	CD Markers	Other Markers
B cells			
Mature	9 ± 5	CD19$^+$ CD20$^+$ CD24$^+$	Surface Ig, Epstein-Barr virus receptor
Plasma cell	Rare	CD23$^+$ CD25$^+$	Cytoplasmic Ig
T cells			
Suppressor	25 ± 4	CD3$^+$ CD8$^+$	
Helper	57 ± 10	CD3$^+$ CD4$^+$	HIV receptor
Natural killer	4 ± 2	*CD16$^+$ CD56$^+$*	

Physiology

The division of lymphocytes into B cells, T cells, and NK cells separates them into humoral and cellular immune functions, respectively. Humoral immunity is mediated by immunoglobulins G, A, M, D, and E. Cellular immunity is the product of effector T lymphocytes and NK cells, which are involved in graft-versus-host reactions, delayed hypersensitivity reactions, tumor cytotoxicity, and control of infection. We may think of T cells as inducible effector cells. The NK cells, on the other hand, have been described as the "natural immune system," since they require no previous exposure to the foreign antigen they attack.

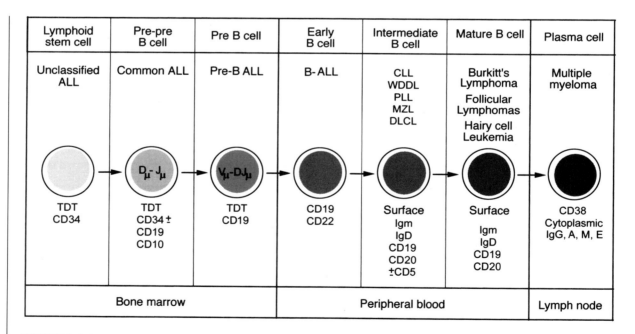

FIGURE 14-2.

Development of normal B cells and their compartments. Surface markers (CD classification), immunoglobulin evolution, and isotype switches are indicated. Malignant diseases are found at all levels of B-cell maturation. Aggressive diseases are not limited to the primitive cell types. Burkitt's lymphoma is one of the most highly malignant diseases known. (ALL, acute lymphocytic leukemia; CLL, chronic lymphocytic leukemia; DLCL, diffuse large cell lymphoma; MZL, marginal zone lymphoma; PLL, prolymphocytic leukemia; TDT, terminal deoxynucleotidyl transferase; WDDL, well-differentiated diffuse (small round cell) lymphomas.

The enormous diversity necessary for B and T cells to meet foreign antigens depends on recombination and mutation. In B cells, the heavy-chain locus rearranges, and more than 100 *V* region genes combine with 12 or more *D* region genes and 6 *J* genes (Fig. 14-31*A*). When combined with a similar diversity of *κ* (Fig. 14-3*B*) or *λ* light-chain gene, an estimated million (10^6) combinations of antibody molecules can be generated. In addition to these recombinations, mutations also are introduced into the hypervariable regions by several mechanisms. The lability of the B cell, due to both recombination of genes and mutation, may explain its peculiar vulnerability to the development of malignancy. Eighty percent of lymphomas come from the B-cell line. In many

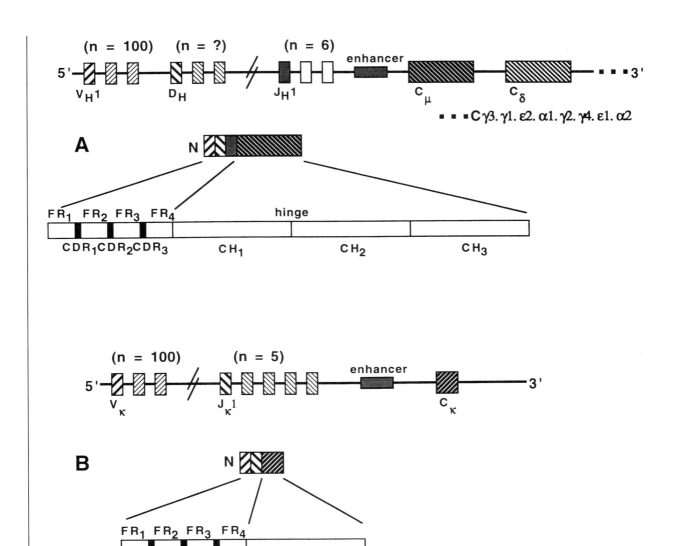

FIGURE 14-3.

(**A**) Organization of H-chain gene. The germline DNA is rearranged so that V-D-J joining results in a *V* region. In the mRNA, the *V* region is joined to one of the *C* genes, which encodes a complete H chain. (**B**) Organization of *κ*-chain gene. The germline DNA is rearranged in a *κ*-producing cell so that one *V* region is brought together with one *J* region. The mRNA that encodes the protein has the C region adjoined to the V-J region and yields a complete *κ* chain. An alternate scheme in which there are six prejoined J, C cassettes (not shown) is used in the organization of *λ* chains. T-cell receptor *β* subunits arise from a process like immunoglobulin heavy chains, whereas *α* subunits arise like *κ* light chains. (CDR, hypervariable regions; FR, framework regions.)

cases, the heavy-chain gene has been translocated, suggesting a vulnerable site for the development of malignancy. However, since the T cell has a similar genetic structure and diversity due to recombination, the reason for fewer T-cell lymphomas is not known.

There are two kinds of helper T (Th) cells (Fig. 14-4). Th1 cells are responsible for cell killing, protection against viral and parasitic infections, and delayed hypersensitivity. Th1 cells secrete interferon-γ, interleukin–2 (IL-2), and lymphotoxin. Th2 cells assist B cells and are involved with antibody production. Th2 cells secrete IL-4, IL-5, and IL-6. Through these lymphokines, Th1 and Th2 cells

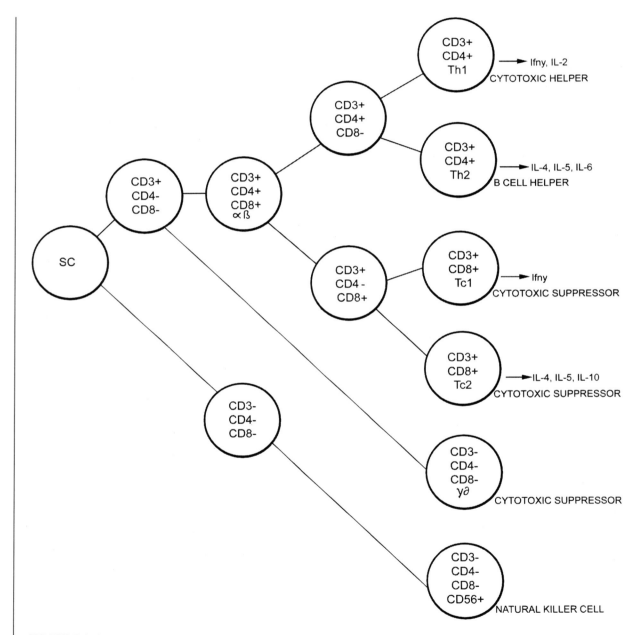

FIGURE 14-4.
Lineage of normal T cells and NK cells. Most T cells have $\alpha\beta$ T-cell receptors (TCRs). The function of cells with $\gamma\delta$ TCR is less well understood. NK cells are morphologically similar to T cells but have neither CD4 nor CD8 markers and are believed to derive from a separate pathway. (SC, stem cell; Th1, Th2, classes of helper cells; Tc1, Tc2, classes of cytotoxic cells; IFN-γ, interferon-γ; IL, interleukin.)

stimulate their own growth and inhibit the growth of their counterparts. A comparable division of cytotoxic T cells (Tc1, Tc2) is based on similar patterns of interleukin secretion. Th1, and Th2 cells are also susceptible to outside influences such as HIV infection or ultraviolet radiation, which can reduce their numbers and unbalance their functions. It is also possible that a B-cell lymphoma could skew the balance of these cells: if the Th1 cells (cytotoxic) were suppressed by the lymphoma; that is, if the tumor secreted IL-6 and the Th2 cells (B-cell stimulators) were enhanced by this cytokine secretion, the tumor would have secured an advantage in its own growth.

T-cell deficiency is associated with an increased incidence of fungal and viral infections. Selective loss of B cells, with loss of γ-globulin production, is associated with recurrent bacterial infections. Acquired agammaglobulinemia, however, may be caused by several mechanisms, such as loss of helper T cells, excessive activity of suppressor T cells, or loss of B cells.

Circulation

In contrast to other white cells, lymphocyte physiology is characterized by unusual kinetics of circulation and proliferation and a profusion of secretory functions. Unlike every other blood cell, lymphocytes recirculate in and out of the blood, moving from the marrow and thymus through the blood to lymph nodes. Lymphocytes leave the nodes via lymphatics and reenter the circulation through the thoracic duct and so return to the node again. Such recirculation allows the lymphocytes to localize to nodes draining areas of active inflammation, where the generation of effector clones can be carried out. Homing receptors and specialized endothelial cell molecules are in part responsible for the paths of lymphocyte migration. For instance, the $\alpha_4\beta_1$-integrin receptor localizes lymphocytes to the endothelium of Peyer's patches in the gut.

Lymphocyte Birth and Death

Lymphocytes divide and proliferate in response to a wide variety of antigens and other stimuli that cross-link receptors on the lymphocyte surface. The normal circulating small lymphocyte is a resting cell rather than a differentiated cell in a terminal state like the granulocyte. Consequently, a lymphocyte's age is related to its place in the mitotic cycle, not the time since it emerged from the stem cell pool. A "young" lymphocyte is close to mitosis; a "mature" lymphocyte is probably not in the mitotic cycle. All lymphocytes have nucleoli; those that are visible are in lymphocytes that probably have been activated and are in the mitotic cycle. This activation occurs in benign diseases such as infectious mononucleosis and infectious hepatitis, as well as in malignancies such as lymphomas and leukemia. The time lymphocytes spend between divisions varies from 1 day to more than 10 years. Rapidly dividing lymphocytes are found in the marrow, spleen, and thymus. Slowly dividing lymphocytes are found in lymph nodes.

Both cell life and death are elaborately programmed. The four phases of the cell cycle are well known:

- G0/G1—the resting phase that precedes DNA synthesis
- S—the period of active DNA synthesis
- G2—the premitotic rest phase
- M—mitosis, subdivided into prophase, metaphase (when the chromatids separate from each other), anaphase (when the chromatids come to the aster ends of the spindle and resume a nuclear appearance), and telophase (when the cytoplasmic membrane is reformed, dividing the daughter cells)

The cell cycle is important to understand because chemotherapy drugs act in different phases of the cycle. The best programs combine drugs that can strike the malignant cell in several phases at once. Vincristine and vinblastine, for example, are active in M phase and arrest cells in mitosis. Purine and pyrimidine analogues such as 6-mercaptopurine and cytosine arabinoside attack the cell in S phase. Alkylating agents such as cyclophosphamide attack nonspecifically and are active against cells in G0/G1.

The progression of B and T cells through the cell cycle is closely monitored at various check points in the cell cycle to control autoimmunity, regulate the size and variety of immunologic responses, and block the emergence of aberrant clones. **Cyclins** (A-E) are proteins that regulate the cell cycle. Cyclins are modified by cyclin-dependent kinases and inhibitors (e.g., p21, p27) as dia-

Mammmalian Cell Cycle

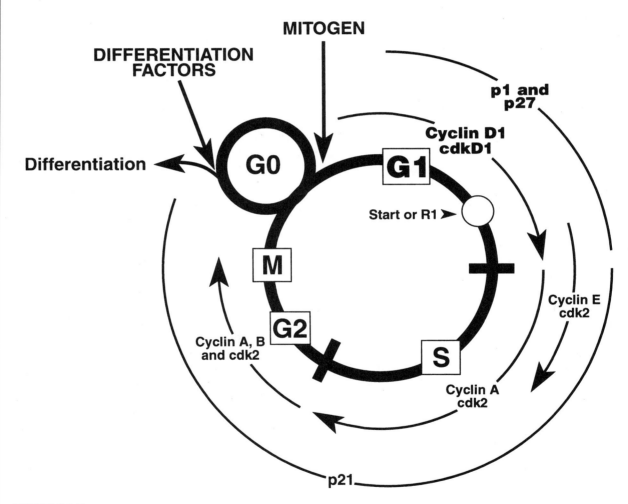

FIGURE 14-5.

Some biochemical details of the mammalian cell cycle. G1, S, G2, and M are the phases of the cell cycle. Cdk(s) form a complex with cyclins p21 and p27 regulatory proteins and other proteins expressed at specific times during the cell cycle to modulate progression of cells through the cycle by phosphorylation of critical substrates. Mitogenic substances such as cytokine growth factors stimulate progression through a series of commitment steps (e.g., R1) in G1. Differentiation factors induce a resting state (G0). (Courtesy of Paul Bertics, University of Wisconsin Medical School, Department of Biomolecular Chemistry.)

grammed in Figure 14-5. Cyclin D dysregulation (specifically cyclin D1, also known as *Bcl-2*) is currently the best example of a tumor-related abnormality in this system. *Cyclin D1* gene translocation and loss of mitotic regulation has been implicated in mantle cell lymphoma and multiple myeloma.

One clinically important director of the cell cycle is *p53* (Fig. 14-6). *p53* is a tumor suppressor gene that monitors DNA damage and governs the cellular decision to repair DNA and proceed into the mitotic cycle or undergo programmed death. If **p53** function is lost because of mutation, the risk of malignancy is increased because cells are allowed to progress rather than being destroyed. Altered **p53** is found in half of all human malignancies studied.

Programmed cell death is called **apoptosis** and is a critical part of the lymphocyte life cycle. In apoptosis, nuclear DNA is degraded by endonucleases, easily identified by a ladder pattern of uniform DNA fragments seen on gels. Apoptosis is responsible for the high rate of T-cell death found in the normal thymus; it regulates B-cell numbers as well. Apoptosis is also the means by which NKs destroy abnormal cells such as Epstein-Barr virus–infected B cells. Radiation, oxidants, corticosteroids, and many chemotherapeutic agents kill by inducing apoptosis (Fig. 14-7). Attachment of Fas, a transmembrane glycoprotein, to its natural ligand leads to lymphocyte death. In the case of HIV, an activated monocyte expressing Fas ligand may attach to the Fas on the CD4+ lymphocyte and initiate apoptosis of the CD4 helper cell. Engagement of the T-cell receptors, deprivation of interleukins or a pulse of glucocorticoid can also give the cell a death signal. A group of mitochondrial proteins (e.g., *bcl-2*) is critical for processing of this signal. *Bcl-2* is a protooncogene product that blocks apoptosis. *Bcl-2* is upregulated in CLL and follicular lymphomas and is implicated in these malignancies because the prevention of cell death allows the accumulation of the malignant cells.

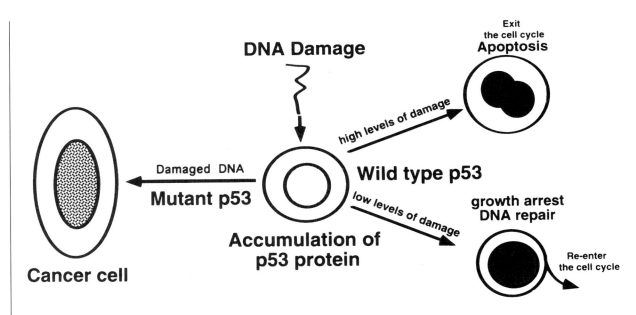

FIGURE 14-6.

The p53 pathway. DNA damage leads to apoptosis or repair by p53. If p53 is mutated, injured cells are allowed to continue and may become malignant. (From Prokocimer M, Rotter V. Structure and function of p53 in normal cells and their aberrations in cancer cells: projection on the hematologic cell lineages. *Blood* 84:2391–2411, with permission.)

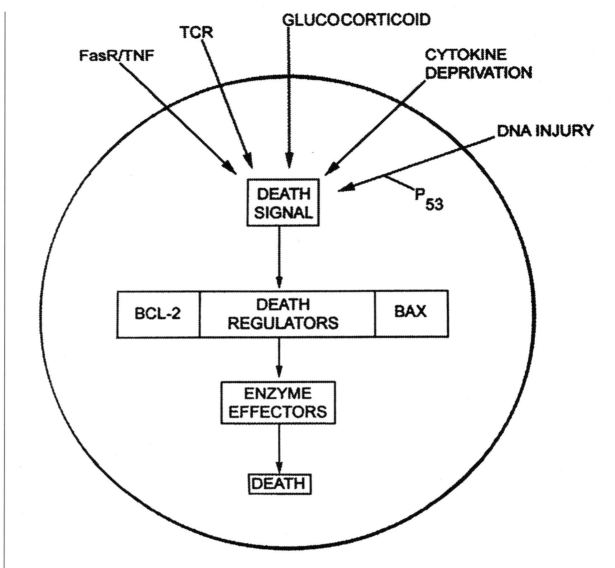

FIGURE 14-7.

The signaling pathway in apoptosis is activated by Fas ligation, attachment of the T-cell receptor, deprivation of cytokines, a pulse of corticosteroid, or DNA injury. The signal is modified by the BCL and Bax/Bak systems and effected by enzymes attacking specific substrates. (BAX, a positive regulator of apoptosis at the mitochondrial level; BCL-2, a negative regulator of apoptosis at the mitochondrial level; FasR, Fas receptor; TCR, T-cell receptor; TNF, tumor necrosis factor.)

Secretion

Lymphocytes secrete chemical mediators called **cytokines**. Cytokines are medium-sized molecules (15,000 to 90,000 molecular weight) that signal macrophages to come and go, activate lymphocytes or induce their growth or death, suppress virus replication, or stimulate the breakdown of bone (osteoclast activating factors). See Chapter 2 for a list of some of the important cytokines and their actions.

ABNORMAL LYMPHOCYTES

In this chapter, we illustrate lymphocyte physiology by the description of three diseases: infectious mononucleosis, CLL, and the lymphomas.

Infectious Mononucleosis

Clinical Features

Infectious mononucleosis is a viral illness of children and young adults. Symptoms and signs are impressive in young adults: fever, sore throat, enlarged lymph nodes in the neck and axillae, rash, splenomegaly, and, less often, hepatomegaly. Symptoms usually last 1 to 4 weeks. Some of these clinical features also may be found with cytomegalovirus and toxoplasma infections. More complicated manifestations such as splenic rupture, aseptic meningitis, respiratory distress as a result of enlarged tonsils, and severe hepatitis can be seen but are rare. There is no specific treatment for infectious mononucleosis. Aside from being an important cause of morbidity among college students, infectious mononucleosis is important to study as a model of self-limited lymphoid proliferation.

Etiology

Infectious mononucleosis is caused by infection with the Epstein-Barr virus (EBV); the virus is also pivotal in Burkitt's lymphoma and nasopharyngeal carcinoma. In young children, EBV infection is a trivial upper respiratory illness that is seldom recognized. In young adults who have been protected from casual exposure during childhood, infection comes from kissing, since EBV is shed abundantly in pharyngeal secretions long after the illness subsides.

Immunologic Response

B lymphocytes are preferentially infected by the virus because they express CD21, the cell surface receptor for C3d, which has been subverted by the virus for use as the EBV receptor. EBV gains entrance to the host by infecting the epithelial cells of the oropharnyx via a CD21 homologue. Infected B lymphocytes are given a stimulus to multiply by the virus. But infected B cells also express new antigens on the cell surface and evoke a series of responses in the host, beginning with an attack by NK cells and atypical lymphocytes.

The NK cells, a subset of normal cells that are erroneously termed "atyical," are the SWAT team of the immune system. They recognize new antigens on the infected B cell and kill them. Proliferation of infected B cells is held down while the rest of the force is being mobilized. The more specific CD8 suppressor/cytotoxic cells (also atypical lymphocytes) come in like a swarm of hornets, stinging and killing infected B cells, pulling away to sting and kill again. They work mainly during the first week of the illness. Meantime, the third line of defense, the antibody-secreting cells, are turned on and make an astonishing array of immunoglobulins.

Antibodies are made against viral capsid antigen, viral nuclear antigens (Epstein-Barr nuclear antigen [EBNA] 1, 2, 3A, 3B, 3C), and latent membrane proteins. The B cells also pour out a variety of biologically irrelevant but clinically useful IgM antibodies, called heterophile antibodies, because they agglutinate the red cells from many animals including ox, sheep, horse, and monkey. Autoantibodies are common as well.

Infectious mononucleosis has been described as a "self-limited lymphoma." When biopsies are done, atypical lymphocytes are found, especially in the lymphocytic and phagocytic organs of the body: lymph nodes, liver, and spleen. Lymph nodes show a marked proliferative response. The nodal architecture is preserved, but there is a great increase of cells in the paracortical T-lymphocyte–dependent area of the nodes, and the sinuses are engorged with atypical lymphocytes and macrophages. Even in mild cases, lymph node pathology may resemble a lymphoma. Reed-Sternberg cells similar to those found in Hodgkin's disease have been described.

The barrier between infectious mononucleosis and lymphoma can be lost in immunocompromised patients. In X-linked lymphoproliferative syndrome (Duncan's syndrome), males are immunologically incapable of controlling the primary EBV infection and develop B-cell lymphomas or polyclonal lymphoma-like tumors. Transplant recipients whose T suppressors are inhibited by drugs are also at risk for EBV-positive lymphomas. Thus, in immunologically incompetent persons, the B-lymphocyte proliferation in infectious mononucleosis may not be self-limited. It is our cytotoxic lymphocytes that stand between us and disaster from EBV.

The susceptibility of African children to malignancy by EBV may be related to immunosuppression of the T-cell system by malaria. Moreover, recent information suggests that the immunogeneic EBV antigens (EBNA 3A, 3B, 3C) are not expressed by the virus in patients with Burkitt's lymphoma. Perhaps virus as well as cell mutation will turn out to be important factors in malignancy.

Laboratory Findings

Many hematologic changes are associated with infectious mononucleosis. Initially, there may be leukopenia. Lymphocytosis with a preponderance of atypical lymphocytes (>25%) is most frequently seen several days into the clinical illness. Anemia is rare (in 3% of cases) and is probably related to anti-i hemagglutinin. The Coombs' test results may be positive. A mild reduction in platelet number is found in 25% of patients, owing to antibody-mediated thrombocytopenia. Elevation in liver enzymes is found in 80%, indicating mild hepatitis.

Testing Procedures

The heterophile antibodies are the basis for simple clinical tests. Agglutination of horse cells or hemolysis of ox cells is used as a rapid but not completely specific clinical test (Monospot). Heterophile antibodies may also be increased in viral hepatitis and serum sickness. Other antibodies that increase in infectious mononucleosis are cold hemolysins, anti-i antibodies, anti–smooth muscle antibodies, rheumatoid factors, and antinuclear antibodies.

Specific tests for infectious mononucleosis involve assaying for antibodies against components of EBV. Early in the infection, there is a rise in the IgM viral capsid antigen and the so-called early antibody. Later, the IgG V viral capsid antigen appears and remains for life. In addition, several other complement-fixing and neutralizing antibodies develop. Antibody against EBNA develops after several weeks.

Other Diseases of Cytotoxic Lymphocytes

The cytotoxic lymphocytes system that stands between us and death from EBV infection may be the rogue in other situations. The large granular lymphocyte syndrome was described in 1985 in patients with arthralgias, positive rheumatoid factor, severe neutropenia, and atypical lymphocytosis. In this syndrome, the suppressor cell population expands and neutrophil production fails; occasionally, decreased red cell production also occurs. Decreased immunoglobulins and autoimmune antibodies have been reported. The atypical lymphocytes appear to be responding to some unknown antigen, since they are polyclonal in many cases. However, the clinical situation is a troublesome, sometimes life-threatening neutropenia, which may persist for years. Eventually, the atypical lymphocytosis may become monoclonal and aggressive, a true malignancy.

Chronic Lymphocytic Leukemia

CLL is the most common and can be the most benign of the leukemias. Symptoms may be so minimal at the outset that CLL is often diagnosed by accident when the patient is being seen for some other problem. It is a disease of the older age group: 90% of patients are over 50 years, and the incidence reaches 25 per 100,000 at age 70. Radiation exposure is not an etiologic factor as it is for chronic myelocytic leukemia, but some families have a genetic predisposition.

In the peripheral blood, blood smears show large numbers of normal-appearing small lymphocytes—from 6000 to more than 500,000/μL {#63, 64}. Smudged cells are prominent. The lymph node architecture can be effaced with uniform, mature lymphocytes meeting the description of a diffuse lymphoma {#115, 116}. The only known difference between CLL and diffuse small round cell lymphoma is that in CLL the cells circulate in significant numbers. Probably, there is a cell membrane receptor that determines distribution of CLL cells in blood.

CLL is immunologically a homogeneous disease. Ninety percent of CLL patients have the same immunologic markers. CLL cells typically exhibit a monoclonal B-cell surface marker, IgM ± IgD. CD5 and CD19 are also expressed. The full designation of CLL is CD5$^+$CD19$^+$SIgM ± (weak)SIgD ±. There are other malignant disorders that must be differentiated from the common variety of CLL. Immunologic markers have identified more than 10 rare variants with a similar appearance, such as T-cell leukemia, helper T-cell leukemia (Sézary's syndrome), and hairy cell leukemia. CLL cells have their normal counterpart in a minor population of lymphocytes, the B1 cells, committed to autoimmunity. Autoimmunity is vital for disposing of aged red cells, dead cells, out-of-date immunoglobulins, and aberrant cell clones, but it is not well controlled in CLL.

CLL cells respond weakly to mitotic stimulants and synthesize immunoglobulin poorly in vitro. In general, the cells behave as if they were inert. Few of them (0.1%) are in the mitotic cycle in vivo, although the proportion of cells in cycle increases as the disease becomes aggressive. Apoptosis is inhibited by the overexpression of *Bcl*-2.

Immune Dysfunction

Monoclonal B lymphocytes accumulate in CLL, and immunoglobulin production is poor. At least 50% of patients have a decrease in one or more immunoglobulins early in the course. This acquired hypoglobulinemia may be related to an increase in normal suppressor cells, since there is an inverse correlation between the number of suppressors and the concentrations of immunoglobin. CLL patients suffer from infection with bacterial pathogens as well as with viruses. Effects on cellular immunity are variable. Normal T cells in CLL patients divide poorly in vitro. High levels of soluble interleukin-2 receptor found in the serum of these patients may alter normal T-cell functions. Examples of decreased as well as exaggerated delayed hypersensitivity have been reported. Some patients react to mosquito bites with 3 to 4 cm wheals and skin necrosis.

Patients with CLL have an increased risk of autoantibody-mediated immune phenomena such as acquired hemolytic anemia, thrombocytopenic purpura, Sjögren's syndrome, and rheumatoid arthritis. Second malignancies, such as carcinoma of bowel, lung, skin, prostate, or bladder, are also more common than in normal populations and reach 30% in some series. This propensity for second malignancies may be related to a decrease in NK cells, which are normally in the front line of defense against foreign cells.

In summary, CLL is a disease in which a monoclonal B cell overruns the immune system, accompanied by an increase in suppressor cells and a loss of some T- and NK-cell functions. The disease is accompanied by a clinical triad of **immune incompetence, autoimmunity**, and **cancer**.

Staging

Lymphomas, as described later in this chapter, are staged by the distribution of pathologic lymphoid tissue. A different staging system is used for CLL, since cells are in the blood at the time of diagnosis. Table 14-2 classifies CLL by simple criteria (a modified Rai classification) and also correlates changes in the white cell count and immunoglobulins. Patients found at stage 0 progress through the stages, acquiring the prognosis of the stage into which they move. A natural history of the disease is suggested: as the lymphocytes increase in the blood, there also is an increase in lymphoid tissue—first the nodes, then the spleen, and finally the marrow {#95}—to the point of suppressing normal marrow function, leading to anemia and thrombocytopenia. Thus, the stage is a rough index of lymphoid mass. Note that circulating immunoglobins are often reduced, which may predispose to infection.

Outcome

In spite of the many advances in chemotherapy in general over the last 30 years, there has been no improvement in life expectancy of CLL patients. The median survival of all patients is 39 months. CLL patients usually die from infection, the result of low granulocyte numbers, poor immunoglobulin production, and the effects of treatment on the immune system. Poor red cell and platelet production are signs of advanced disease. Pulmonary infections are common and may be complicated by the infiltration of lymphocytes into mediastinal nodes and peribronchial lymphatics. In 3% to 10%, the disease transforms into an aggressive, primitive lymphoma that does not respond well to treatment (Richter's syndrome). Transformation into acute leukemia, which is usual in chronic myelogenous leukemia, does not occur in CLL.

Lymphomas

Lymphomas are solid tumors of lymphocytes arising usually in lymphoid tissue. They are recognized clinically by enlargement of neck, axillary, inguinal, or abdominal lymph nodes. Extranodal lymphomas arise from lymphoid tissue in the wall of the stomach or intestine or skin. Rarely, lymphoma can be found elsewhere in the body.

TABLE 14-2. A Staging Classification of Chronic Lymphocytic Leukemia*

Stage	Criteria	Average WBC $\times 10^{-3}/\mu L$	Fraction of Patients with Decreased Ig	Prognosis
0	>15,000/μL lymphocytes in blood; >40% lymphocytes in marrow	19	13/16	Indefinite
1	Enlarged nodes	36	9/11	101 mo
2	Enlarged spleen and/or liver	76	10/10	71 mo
3	Hematocrit <33% or platelets <100,000/μL	225	10/11	19 mo

*This classification is a hybrid of the Binet and Rai classification.

Pathogenesis

The pathogenesis of lymphomas in humans is becoming fairly well understood. There are four important factors: **virus infection, chromosome translocation, oncogene expression**, and **immunosuppression**. These four factors may be independent, and not all may be required. For example, virus infection is found in only a minority of cases. In humans, three viruses have been implicated: EBV, the human T-cell lymphotrophic virus (HTLV-I/II), and Kaposi's sarcoma–associated herpes-type virus. Oncogene expression may be the result of virus infection or chromosome translocation. In Burkitt's lymphoma, all four of these factors have been implicated.

Usually, EBV infection results in infectious mononucleosis, as described. EBV, however, has been strongly associated with the cause of Burkitt's lymphomas in African children. In cases of Burkitt's lymphoma occurring outside of Africa, however, EBV association has not been frequently found. EBV also has been found to have a positive association with nasopharyngeal carcinoma, a rare tumor with a high incidence in Asia. EBV is found in 50% of those patients with Hodgkin's disease.

A second herpesvirus, Kaposi's sarcoma–associated herpes-type virus, has been found to infect marrow stromal cells in about 50% of patients with multiple myeloma, also a B-cell neoplasm. However, in this case, the virus infection does not contribute directly to the growth of malignant cells, because it does not infect them. Instead, it may cause stromal cells to secrete interleukins such as IL-6, which stimulate tumor growth.

HTLV-I, a retrovirus, is associated with adult T-cell lymphoma and leukemia in Japan and the Caribbean. This is a weak virus, causing disease infrequently. HTLV-I/II also causes tropical spastic paraparesis. It immortalizes helper T cells.

In 75% of Burkitt's lymphoma cases, a chromosomal defect is also found, with part of the long arm of chromosome 8 translocated onto the long arm of chromosome 14, t(8;14). This attaches the oncogene, c-*myc*, of chromosome 8 to the heavy-chain gene for immunoglobulin (Fig. 14-8). An alternate translocation attaches the c-*myc* oncogene to the κ light-chain gene on chromosome 2, t(8;2) or the λ light-chain gene on chromosome 22, t(8;22). The malignant cell usually expresses the immunoglobulin gene that has been disturbed. Lymphomas of the mouse and rat have also be identified with the same translocations, indicating the biologic importance of this event.

Translocation involving c-*myc* is only one step in lymphomagenesis, since cells carrying this translocation are not necessarily malignant, but are immortalized; that is, they proliferate indefinitely in vitro. Probably another oncogene (B-*lym* or N-*ras*) must also be activated for overt malignancy to be expressed.

The fourth event that sets the stage for lymphoma is immunosuppression. Three groups are especially susceptible: boys with X-linked immune deficiency syndrome, African children with malaria (which strongly suppresses T-cell immunity), and transplant recipients who are given immunosuppressive drugs to prevent transplant rejection. All three develop EBV-related lymphomas. Transplantation patients who develop EBV-related lymphomas do not have the typical histology of the Burkitt's lymphoma found in African children, and the translocation is typically t(2;19). AIDS and various kinds of hereditary immune deficiency disorders also predispose to lymphoma; most of these tumors have not been linked to EBV.

In conclusion, most lymphomas do not yet have a viral cause, but most have translocations that are undoubtedly important. The frequency of translocation of chromosome 14 at the heavy-chain site is striking for many of the B-cell malignancies (Table 14-3). More than 85% of follicular lymphomas manifest translocation of the heavy-chain gene site to the *Bcl-2* locus, leading to dysregulation of the apoptosis pathway. Presumably, the prolonged life span of the follicular cells contributes to the pathogenesis of the disease.

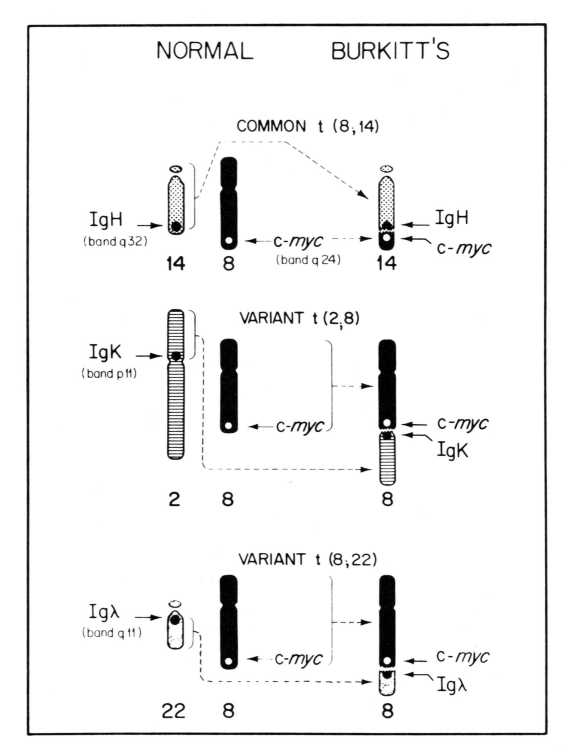

FIGURE 14-8.
The common t(8;14) and variant t(2;8) and t(8;22) chromosomes in Burkitt's lymphoma. c-*myc* is indicated in white dots and the immunoglobulin genes in black dots. The normal chromosomes are illustrated on the left and the abnormal c-*myc*-bearing chromosomes on the right. The second abnormal chromosome produced by each translocation (which may contain nonfunctional fragments of c-*myc* or immunoglobulin genes) is not represented, nor is the normal chromosome of each pair, which does not participate in the translocation. (From Aisenberg AC. New genetics of Burkitt's lymphoma and other non-Hodgkin lymphomas. *Am J Med* 77:1083).

TABLE 14-3. Critical Translocations in Lymphoproliferative Diseases

Tumor	Virus	Translocation	Comment
Follicular lymphoma		t(14;18): IgH + Bcl-2	Decreased apoptosis
Large cell lymphoma		t(3;14): IgH + Bcl-6	Decreased apoptosis
Multiple myeloma	[KSHV]*	t(14;–): IgH + many sites	
Plasmacytoid lymphoma		t(9;14): IgH + PAX-5	p53 repressed
Mantle cell lymphoma		t(11;14): IgH + cyclin D	Decreased apoptosis
Burkitt's lymphoma	[EBV]	t(8;14): IgH + c-*myc*	Immunosuppression an underlying factor
		t(2;8): Igκ + c-*myc*	
		t(8;22): Igλ + c-*myc*	
T-cell leukemia/lymphoma	HTLV-I		Environmental factors
Hodgkin's disease	[EBV]		

EBV, Epstein-Barr virus; HTLV-I, human T-cell lymphotrophic virus type I; KSHV, and Kaposi's sarcoma-associated herpes-type virus.
Bracket indicates that the virus role is variable or in doubt.

Clinical Presentation

Lymphomas have been divided into Hodgkin's and non-Hodgkin's lymphomas, because of distinctive differences in histopathology, clinical behavior, mode of spread, and response to treatment. Non-Hodgkin's lymphomas are about three times more common than Hodgkin's disease. In both diseases, there is a male preponderance, which is more pronounced in children although the diseases are rarer in children. For Hodgkin's disease, there is a characteristic bimodal age/incidence curve, with 50% of the cases of Hodgkin's disease occurring between the ages of 20 and 40 years and a second peak between the ages of 50 and 60. The peak incidence period for non-Hodgkin's lymphomas is later than that for Hodgkin's disease; about 25% of cases develop between the ages of 50 and 59 years.

Both Hodgkin's disease and non-Hodgkin's lymphomas may present as a painless unilateral swelling of the lymph nodes in the neck {#119}. Any group of nodes may be involved, but the anterior and posterior cervical nodes are most frequently observed. Enlarged lymph nodes are especially common in children as a response to infection, but persistent unilateral posterior cervical, supraclavicular, or axillary node measuring more than 2 × 2 cm despite treatment with antibiotics is a clue to malignancy.

After the history and physical examination, the third step in diagnosis of lymphoma is surgical biopsy. Not all biopsies are diagnostic, but the larger the node (i.e., >2 cm), the more likely it is to be abnormal {#120}. Lymph node pathology is a challenging discipline because of the potential curability of several types and the uncertainties of classification. The diagnosis of malignant lymphoma has been incorrectly assigned on occasions when pathologic changes in the node have been due to infections such as histoplasmosis or cat-scratch disease or due to phenytoin therapy. In these conditions, the lymph node pathology may mimic lymphoma.

Non-Hodgkin's Lymphoma

Classification

Non-Hodgkin's lymphoma is the subject of intensive study. According to the simplest classification, lymphomas are divided into follicular (the lymph node is replaced by giant germinal centers {#117} and diffuse (when the node architecture is effaced by sheets of lymphoma cells), {#115, 116} and then into small cell, large cell, and mixed cell types. These subdivisions are further classified according to the morphology of the lymph node. Eighty percent of lymphomas are of B-cell origin, and 50% originate from the germinal center cell. T-cell lymphomas arise within the paracortical areas and medullary cords of the lymph node {#118} (Fig. 14-9). Pure T-cell lymphomas, including mycosis fungoides, Sézary syndrome, adult T-cell leukemia/lymphoma and the T-cell immunoblastic lymphomas, are not common. The aggressiveness of lymphomas is related in part to the proportion of cells that is dividing.

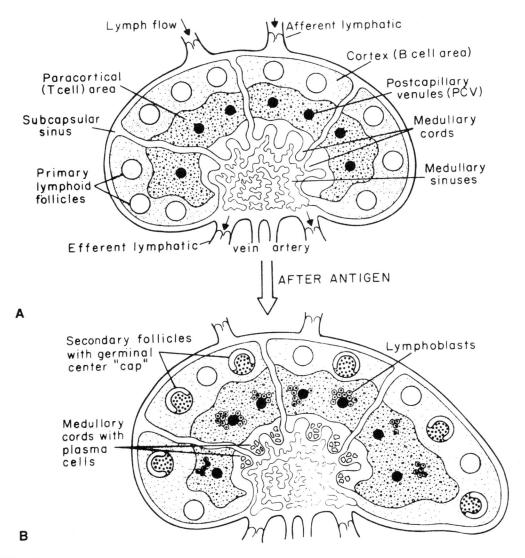

FIGURE 14-9.
Diagrammatic representation of the human lymph node. (**A**) Quiescent, (non–antigen-stimulated) lymph node. Lymphocytes migrate through the node through the postcapillary venules or through the afferent lymphatics. They exit the node by way of the efferent lymphatics, where they may travel to the next node in the chain. (**B**) Morphologic changes that occur in an antigen-stimulated lymph node. The B-cell–dependent follicular regions in the cortex transform into secondary follicles containing germinal centers—areas of lymphocyte proliferation. In the T-cell–dependent paracortical regions, many lymphoblasts are observed. Plasma cells can be found accumulating in the medullary cord region. These events serve to expand the pool of effective T and B lymphocytes and to increase the size of the node. (From. Hoffman R, Benz EJ Jr, et al. *Hematology*, 2nd ed. Edinburgh: Churchill Livingstone, 1995:170.)

The length of life for those with untreated lymphoma divides the tumors into low, intermediate, and high grades (Table 14-4). The irony is that tumors labeled low grade may carry a poorer survival rate than those labeled high grade, because high-grade tumors can be cured by intensive chemotherapy. However, when treatment is unsuccessful, the patients die in short order. Low-grade lymphomas are treatable, and patients live longer in general, but remissions are unusual and most patients die of their disease. Also, T-cell lymphomas have a poorer prognosis than B-cell lymphomas, partly because B-cell lymphomas are more sensitive to chemotherapy.

In practice, two lymphomas make up about 80% of clinical cases: follicular, small cleaved cell lymphoma and diffuse large cell lymphoma.

Clinical Features

More than two thirds of patients with non-Hodgkin's lymphoma have disseminated disease at diagnosis. Such patients are prone to extranodal disease, especially in the bone marrow and gastrointestinal tract. The incidence of circulating lymphoma cells and central nervous system involvement, particularly in children, also is high.

Immunologic abnormalities may be found in patients with non-Hodgkin's lymphomas, especially in those with CLL (diffuse small round cells). These abnormalities include Coombs'-positive hemolytic anemia, IgG deficiencies, and monoclonal gammopathies. Patients with non-Hodgkin's lymphomas are more prone to bacterial than fungal or viral infections, in contrast to patients with Hodgkin's disease.

TABLE 14-4. A Classification of Non-Hodgkin's Lymphomas

Working Formulation	Comments	Cell of Origin	Median Life Expectancy in Years
I. Low Grade			
A. Diffuse, small round cells	Cells commonly circulate as CLL	90% B	5.8
B. Follicular, small cleaved cells	Cells may circulate as "lymphosarcoma cell leukemia"	All B	7.2
C. Follicular, mixed small and large cells		All B	5.1
II. Intermediate Grade			
A. Diffuse, small cleaved cells		Usually B	3.4
B. Follicular, large cells		All B	3.0
C. Diffuse, mixed small and large cleaved cells		Usually B	2.7
D. Diffuse, large cell		Usually B	1.5
E. Large noncleaved			
III. High Grade			
A. Diffuse, large cell			1.5
1. Immunoblastic		50% B, 50% T	1.3
2. Lymphoblastic (ALL-like)		Usually T	2.0
B. Diffuse, small noncleaved cells		Usually B	0.7
T cell			
Mycosis fungoides	Cutaneous T-cell lymphoma	T cells	8.0
Sézary's syndrome	Cutaneous T-cell lymphoma with circulating cells (leukemic phase)		1.5

Staging

Stages of non-Hodgkin's lymphoma are defined as follows:

- Stage I disease involves one group of nodes on either side of the diaphragm.
- Stage II disease involves two groups of nodes—noncontiguous—on the same side of the diaphragm.
- Stage III disease involves nodal groups on both sides of the diaphragm.
- Stage IV disease extends outside the lymph nodes and spleen into any organ, such as the liver or bone marrow.

Subscripts A or B are added to indicate whether the patient has constitutional symptoms (B) or not (A). The subscript E is added to stages I, II, and III if a single extralymphatic site is involved, potentially curable by radiation therapy; for example, lung involvement contiguous with bilaterally enlarged mediastinal lymph nodes is stage II_E

Clinical assessment of a patient with aggressive non-Hodgkin's lymphoma includes a careful search for disease in the bone marrow and central nervous system. Computed tomography (CT) scans of chest and abdomen are used to determine the extent of disease. Since most non-Hodgkin's lymphomas are disseminated from the beginning, rigorous staging is not usually necessary. Staging laparotomy is almost never done.

Treatment

Therapy for non-Hodgkin's lymphoma is individualized according to the patient's age and the clinical course and natural history of the disease. In some forms of low-grade lymphoma—localized nodular lymphoma, for example—patients may have an indolent clinical course without therapy. Therapy for these patients can often be postponed. For solitary lymphomas, radiation therapy to a diseased node is the treatment of choice. For intermediate- and high-grade tumors, combinations of drugs such as cyclophosphamide, vincristine, doxorubicin, and prednisone can induce remissions in the majority of patients, and some patients can be cured.

In children with non-Hodgkin's lymphomas, diffuse lymphoma is much more common than follicular variants. At diagnosis, children have disseminated disease more commonly than do adults, and in the past children have had a rapidly fatal course. In recent years, a more aggressive approach to the therapy of disseminated lymphomas in children, using central nervous system treatment along with combination chemotherapy, has resulted in a remarkable improvement in survival.

Prognosis depends on age (patients >60 respond less well), pathology, immunology, stage and mass of disease, growth rate, site (brain lymphoma is associated with a very bad prognosis), lactic dehydrogenase, symptoms, and performance status (the patient's health and ability to do regular activities).

Hodgkin's Disease

Differences from Non-Hodgkin's Lymphoma

Hodgkin's disease differs from the non-Hodgkin's lymphomas for the following reasons:

- Hodgkin's disease is curable in about 70% of patients, even though it is considered a slow-growing tumor. It is believed to begin in one focus and to spread contiguously to adjacent nodes.

- In Hodgkin's disease, there is a polycellular response of neutrophils, eosinophils, plasma cells, and fibroblasts in the lymph node.
- The malignant cell—the unique Reed-Sternberg cell—is a minor but crucial component of the pathology of Hodgkin's disease.
- T-cell immune function is poor in Hodgkin's disease, whereas humoral immunity is more likely to be deficient in the non-Hodgkin's lymphomas.

Pathogenesis

Current opinion holds that Hodgkin's disease involves the autonomous proliferation of a malignant B lymphocyte, the Reed-Sternberg cell, with suppression of T-cell function (poor generation of IL-2) and an inflammatory reaction of neutrophils, eosinophils, and plasma cells in response to this malignant cell. The cause is unknown, although EBV is found in 50% of cases. It is not known whether EBV is a passenger virus or whether it is important in the pathophysiology.

Immune Dysfunction

Abnormalities in cellular immunity, such as skin test anergy and decreased levels of circulating T-cells, are found in patients with Hodgkin's disease. These defects are common in more advanced stages and may persist after treatment. Consequently, patients with Hodgkin's diseases are more susceptible to fungal and viral infections, such as cryptococcosis and herpes zoster. Immunoglobulin production is preserved.

Pathology

The distinctive Reed-Sternberg cell in the presence of an unusual cellular background is the hallmark of Hodgkin's disease. In tissue sections, the Reed-Sternberg cell is a large binucleate (owl-eyed) or multinucleate cell with a large eosinophilic nucleolus in each nucleus {#122}. Reed-Sternberg cells also may be seen in lymph node sections from other diseases, such as infectious mononucleosis, adenocarcinoma, and multiple myeloma, and therefore are not sufficient to make the diagnosis of Hodgkin's disease. The diagnosis requires a correlation of pathology with other clinical data.

Hodgkin's disease is divided into four pathologic types. Each type is characterized by loss of the normal lymph node architecture and the presence of the Reed-Sternberg cell in a distinctive cellular background.

- **Lymphocytic predominance**. A few Reed-Sternberg cells are found in a lymph node diffusely replaced by small lymphocytes and occasional histiocytes. It has the best prognosis.
- **Nodular sclerosis**. More Reed-Sternberg cells are found as well as large birefringent bands of collagen traversing the node {#121}. Large histiocytes and Reed-Sternberg cells are surrounded by clear-space fixation artifact (the so-called lacunar cells). Nodular sclerosis accounts for 50% of cases and is more common in children.
- **Mixed cellularity**. Reed-Sternberg cells are found in a more heterogeneous cell population composed of plasma cells, eosinophils, lymphocytes, and histiocytes.
- **Lymphocytic depletion**. Bizarre Reed-Sternberg cells are found in a heterogeneous cell population characterized by lack of lymphocytes. Lymphocytic depletion is the rarest type and has the worst prognosis.

Stages of Hodgkin's disease (I-IV) are further divided into "A" or "B," depending on the presence of systemic symptoms. A indicates absence of systemic symptoms; B indicates fever, night sweats, or unexplained loss of 10% body weight within a 6-month period. B symptoms have an adverse affect on prognosis of Hodgkin's disease, regardless of the stage of the disease.

Since Hodgkin's disease appears to spread in a nonrandom fashion and treatment is designed according to extent of disease, it is most important to know the disease stage before initiating treatment. Staging for Hodgkin's disease usually includes the chest x-ray, chest and abdominal CT, and, in a few cases, staging laparotomy. Laparotomy is done for early-stage disease, in which radiation therapy is a possible treatment, to prove the extent of disease before treatment. Staging laparotomy is a major surgical procedure in which the surgeon carefully examines the lymph nodes in the entire abdomen, taking biopsy samples of any suspicious nodes. Even small nodes may be involved. Splenectomy is routinely performed because splenic involvement may be detected only microscopically. A liver biopsy is performed, as well as bone marrow biopsies. Recent advances in diagnosis and treatment are making the laparotomy uncommon.

In many series of patients with Hodgkin's disease, the clinical stage was increased or decreased in up to one third of patients as a result of the information gained at the staging laparotomy. If a patient presents with extensive disease above {#120} and below the diaphragm (stage III) or outside of lymph node areas (stage IV), staging laparotomy would not affect therapy decisions and therefore would not be done.

Treatment

Treatment for Hodgkin's disease depends on the stage of the disease. Radiation therapy is the main mode of therapy for patients in stage I and IIA. Radiation therapy is delivered to known areas of disease and beyond to a limited extent, taking into account the known contiguous spread of the disease. For more advanced disease, combination chemotherapy is used.

The prognosis for patients with Hodgkin's disease has greatly improved with modern therapy. The prognosis for 5-year survival is:

- Stage I and II—up to 80% to 90%
- Stage III—60% to 70%
- Stage IV—possibly up to 30% to 40%

Children do as well as adults, although Hodgkin's disease is rare in children under 10 years of age. With the improvement in prognosis, less aggressive treatment regimens are now being tried in an attempt to decrease the amount of therapy given to patients with favorable prognosis. This is because of the long-term side effects from therapy (e.g., sterility, growth abnormalities in children, and other organ dysfunction from radiation therapy). Acute myelogenous leukemias and second lymphomas are being reported with increasing frequency in patients treated for Hodgkin's disease, particularly if they have been treated with both radiation therapy and chemotherapy.

SUMMARY POINTS

Lymphocytic diseases as illustrated in this chapter cover a wide spectrum of pathophysiology. Infectious mononucleosis is a viral disease and not a malignancy so long as host defenses are adequate. CLL is a minimum-deviation tumor of a minor population of lymphocytes often committed to autoimmune functions. The failure of apoptosis leads to accumulation of one clone of cells and embarrassment of the host. Immune failure and bone marrow failure are causes of death. The lymphomas are mostly of B-cell origin and kill by their invasive properties. Treatment of lymphoid malignancies is tailored to the pathologic classification and biologic behavior.

SUGGESTED READINGS

Hirama T, Koeffler HP. Role of the cyclin-dependent kinase inhibitors in the development of cancer. *Blood* 1995;88:841–854.

Prokocimer M, Rotter V. Structure and function of p53 in normal cells and their aberrations in cancer cells: projection on the hematologic cell lineages. *Blood* 1994;84:2391–2411.

Yang E, Korsmeyer SJ. Molecular thanatopsis: a discourse on the BCL2 family and cell death. *Blood* 1996;88:386–401.

CASE DEVELOPMENT PROBLEM: CHAPTER 14

History and physical examination: A 19-year-old white garage mechanic presented to the clinic with a 4×5 cm left posterior cervical node enlargement. He had no other symptoms. He did not appear ill, and the physical examination was otherwise negative.

1. What diagnoses would you consider from this abbreviated list of diseases that are associated with lymph node enlargement?

   a. Cat-scratch disease
   b. Tuberculous lymphadenitis (scrofula)
   c. Acne with regional lymphadenitis
   d. Infectious mononucleosis
   e. Lymphoma
   f. Pseudolymphoma associated with phenytoin (Dilantin) therapy
   g. Metastatic carcinoma
   h. Syphilis
   i. Hyperthyroidism
   j. Lymphogranuloma venereum
   k. Bubonic plague
   l. Sarcoidosis
   m. AIDS

2. What other questions would you like to ask?
3. The questions confirmed the lack of symptoms and the absence of smoking history. What is your next diagnostic maneuver?
4. There was destruction of architecture with replacement by an infiltrate of lymphocytes, plasma cells, eosinophils, fibroblasts, and monocytes around primitive giant cells with bilobed nuclei and prominent pink nucleoli. There were dense bands of fibrosis. What is your impression?
5. Does this disease spread by contiguity or by hematogenous dissemination?
6. What does the position of the lymph node indicate about other possible sites of involvement?
7. Nodes in the abdomen are usually not palpable. What methods can be used to demonstrate enlarged lymph nodes in the chest and abdomen?
   The patient was seen after studies demonstrated that periaortic nodes were positive and that there was no disease in the liver. Bone marrow was negative.
8. What stage of disease does the patient have?
9. Before the workup was completed and treatment was started, the patient began to complain of night sweats, fever, and itching. What is the likely cause of these symptoms?
10. What do symptoms such as fever indicate regarding prognosis? What is the stage now?
    The white blood cell count was 17,000/μL, 89% neutrophils, 6% monocytes, 3% lymphocytes, and 2% eosinophils.
11. (a) What information does the differential count give regarding the patient's immune status? (b) What does this abnormality indicate about the prognosis?

12. (a) What kind of lymphocyte is defective in this disease? (b) What kinds of functions are served by these cells?
13. (a) What bedside test of function of these cells can you perform? (b) What would the results be?
14. (a) What kinds of disease is the patient unusually susceptible to? (b) What is the therapeutic strategy for this patient?
15. Which agents from the following list are effective in the treatment of this disease?

BCNU (carmustine)	Prednisone
Bleomycin	Procarbazine
Cyclophosphamide	Triethylene melamine
Doxorubicin	Vinblastine
Imidazole carboxamide (DTIC)	Vincristine
Nitrogen mustard	

16. Is one agent better than three or four agents combined in the treatment?
    The patient was treated with chemotherapy. He remained well for 3 years and then suffered relapse with chills, fever, and widespread lymph node disease as well as a sclerotic lesion at the second lumbar vertebra.
17. (a) What is the disease stage now? (b) What treatment should be given now?
    The patient tolerated chemotherapy well and went back into remission. He remained in remission for 4 months.
18. What would you advise him to do?
    a. Come back to your clinic every 3 to 4 months regardless of symptoms.
    b. Come back when he felt sick.
    c. Come back if he felt an enlarged node.
    d. Consider himself cured.
    e. Consider intensive chemotherapy with an autologous bone marrow transplantation to attempt to cure the disease.

CASE DEVELOPMENT ANSWERS

1. The list of causes of small lymph-node enlargement (0.5 to 2 cm) is very long. The list of causes of large nodes like this one is very short. A neck mass of this size eliminates virtually all of the possibilities except lymphoma and metastatic carcinoma.
2. Have you lost weight recently? Do you sweat at night? Do you smoke or use smokeless tobacco?
3. Lymph node biopsy.
4. Nodular sclerosing Hodgkin's disease.
5. Usually by contiguity.
6. The left posterior cervical chain receives flow from the tongue and mandible, as well as from the abdomen and the left side of the thorax.
7. Chest x-ray; computed tomography of the chest and abdomen; laparotomy (surgical exploration of the abdomen).
8. Stage IIIA, because he has involved nodes above and below the diaphragm, without symptoms.
9. These symptoms commonly accompany Hodgkin's disease, although infection must be considered. The cause of fever in Hodgkin's disease is unknown. It is not due to any known infection. Antibiotics are not effective.
10. The prognosis is poorer with symptoms, and the patient must now be staged IIIB.
11. (a) He has lymphopenia. The absolute lymphocyte count is $510/\mu L$. (b) The prognosis is worse when the patient has lymphopenia.
12. (a) T lymphocyte. (b) Delayed hypersensitivity, graft rejection, graft-versus-host reactions, helper and suppressor cell functions.

13. (a) Delayed hypersensitivity skin tests to tuberculin, mumps, *Candida*, and *Histoplasma* infections. (b) All negative.

14. (a) Mycobacteria infection; deep fungi, for example cryptococcus; viruses such as herpes zoster; and protozoans such as *Pneumocystis carinii* infection. (b) Eradicate disease-containing lymph nodes. Destroy all malignant cells.

15. Hodgkin's disease has probably the broadest spectrum of drug sensitivity of any tumor. All of these agents have been used successfully in the treatment of Hodgkin's disease.

16. The body tolerates nearly full doses of agents acting at different biochemical sites. Tumor cell kill and remission duration appear improved by the use of multiple agents. The best protocols include four to seven drugs.

17. (a) Stage IVB, because of disease above and below the diaphragm as well as in nonlymphoid tissue—the bone—and symptoms. (b) More chemotherapy.

18. The correct answer is e. This is a difficult decision. To decrease chance of further relapses, that is, maximize chance of a cure, hematopoietic stem cells can be harvested, intensive chemotherapy given, and an autologous bone marrow transplantation done. This is a relatively low-risk procedure.

Plasma Cell Disorders

Deane F. Mosher

CHAPTER 15

OUTLINE

OBJECTIVES

- Understand how plasma cells and "plasmacytoid" lymphocytes are generated from B lymphocytes.
- Understand how the three immunoglobulin gene loci are rearranged from their germline configurations to encode functional genes.
- Understand the roles of hypermutation and heavy-chain switching in maturation of the immune response.
- Understand the tests that would allow you to distinguish whether an elevated IgG of 2000 mg/dL is due to a monoclonal or polyclonal proliferation of plasma cells.
- Distinguish monoclonal gammopathy of unknown significance, Waldenström's macroglobulinemia, and multiple myeloma.
- Understand how multiple myeloma can destroy bones and kidneys.
- Know which measurements of serum and urine are necessary to evaluate a patient with multiple myeloma.

Although prehistoric skeletons with the characteristic bone lesions of multiple myeloma have been unearthed, little was known about this disease until the middle of the 19th century, when a urine sample from a patient with a destructive bone disease and "animal matter" in his urine was referred to Dr. Henry Bence Jones. The abnormal urine was found to contain protein with the unusual property of precipitating at 56° C and dissolving at the boiling point. This protein later was shown to be isolated light chain of the immunoglobulin molecule. In the last 40 years, understanding the structure of immunoglobulins, the generation of the immune response, and the kinetics of growth of the myeloma cell have made myeloma an excellent pathophysiologic model. Multiple myeloma is one of the most frustrating tumors we know, relatively resistant to treatment and often resulting in devastation to the patient's bones. Like a termite-ridden old house, sometimes the first sign of trouble is the collapse of a supporting timber.

PLASMA CELLS

Plasma cells make up less than 3% of the nucleated cells in normal bone marrow. As the differentiated effector B cells of the humoral immune apparatus, plasma cells manufacture and secrete antibodies in response to antigenic stimulation. This secretory activity is reflected by deep-blue RNA-rich cytoplasm, prominent Golgi apparatus manifested as a clear perinuclear halo, and frequent occurrence of cytoplasmic vacuoles. The nuclear chromatin is frequently clumped toward the margin, producing the "cartwheel" or "clock face" nucleus.

Plasma cells are terminally differentiated B lymphocytes (Fig. 15-1). There are two populations of plasma cells: those in the lymph node that are short-lived (2 to 3 days) and those in the bone marrow that are longer-lived (about 1 month). The difference between the two populations is that the precursor surface IgM-/IgD-bearing lymphoblast enters the germinal center and is subject to hypermutation of the rearranged *VDJ* segment and isotype switch so as to secrete IgG or IgA (or, rarely, IgD or IgE) before assumption of residency in the bone marrow. IgM-secreting cells tend to remain in the lymph node and morphologically are a hybrid with the nucleus of a lymphocyte and a Golgi apparatus reminiscent of a plasma cell.

IMMUNOGLOBULINS

Structure

A plasma cell produces a quantity of one specific (idiotypic) antibody. Each idiotype is unique. The basic immunoglobulin unit, called an **immunoglobulin monomer**, consists of four peptide chains—two heavy chains and two light chains—linked by disulfide bridges and noncovalent bonds (Fig. 15-2). The heavy chains (H chains) and light chains (L chains) are arranged symmetrically with respect to the long axis of the molecule. There are five possible heavy-chain classes (α, γ, μ, δ, and ϵ) and two light-chain classes (κ and λ). However, in each individual immunoglobulin molecule, the two heavy chains and two light chains are identical. The N-terminal ends of a light and a heavy chain together form the antigen-binding sites, which is divalent because there are two such regions per immunoglobulin molecule. The antigen-binding fraction of an immunoglobulin is called the Fab (fragment, antigen-binding) region. Papain, an enzyme that cleaves the immunoglobulin molecule in the midsection, produces two such fragments. The third fragment produced by papain proteolysis is termed the Fc fragment (for "crystallizable fragments"); it contains the carboxy-terminal remnants of the two heavy chains connected by disulfide bridges.

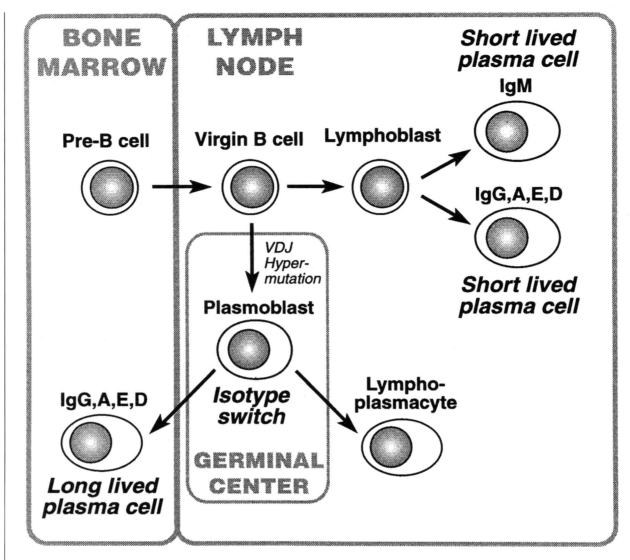

FIGURE 15-1.

Generation of plasma cells and immunoglobulins. Long-lived plasma cells responsible for the most specific humoral immunity are derived from plasmablasts that have undergone VDJ hypermutation and isotype switch in response to antigenic stimulus and T-cell help in the germinal center.

Five classses of immunoglobulins have been identified, based on the five chains: IgG has γ heavy chains, IgM has μ heavy chains, and so on; κ and λ light chains are found in all five classes (Table 15-1). Thus, an IgA molecule will be composed of either $\alpha_2\kappa_2$ or $\alpha_2\lambda_2$, whereas an IgG molecule would be $\gamma_2\kappa_2$ or $\gamma_2\lambda_2$. Other structural differences exist among the immunoglobulin classes, and many are listed in Table 15-1. For review of B-cell antibody generation, see Chapter 14.

Laboratory Tests of Immunoglobulins

Total Serum Protein

The total serum protein is a refractometer or colorimetric measurement of all proteins, including the immunoglobulins in the serum. Although not specific, it is a rapid screen for increased serum protein.

Serum Protein Electrophoresis

Serum protein electrophoresis is a more informative laboratory test than the total serum protein. For this study, the serum is applied to cellulose acetate or agarose, and an electrical current is applied. At pH 8.2 to 8.6, all serum proteins except IgG are negatively charged and migrate toward the anode. The IgG remains at the origin or migrates toward the cathode. After the separation, a protein-binding dye is applied, and five major groups of proteins can be identified: albumin and the α_1, -α_2-, β-, and γ-globulin groups (Fig. 15-3[3-1]). A semiquantitative assessment of the groups can be made by measuring the amount of dye bound to each band and expressing it as a percentage of the total serum protein. If a monoclonal immunoglobulin is produced, an intensely stained narrow band or spike is found, usually in the γ-globulin region (Fig. 15-3[3-3 and 3-4]). Much of the IgA and IgM and some of the IgG migrate in the β or α_2 regions, so that occasionally spikes are found there. Hence, the serum protein electrophoresis quantifies the amount of monoclonal protein, but does not identify it exactly. When polyclonal hyper-globulinemia occurs (i.e., an increase in immunoglobulin production by many different clones of plasma cells), a broad, diffuse γ-globulin band is seen on the protein electrophoresis (Fig. 15-3[3-2]).

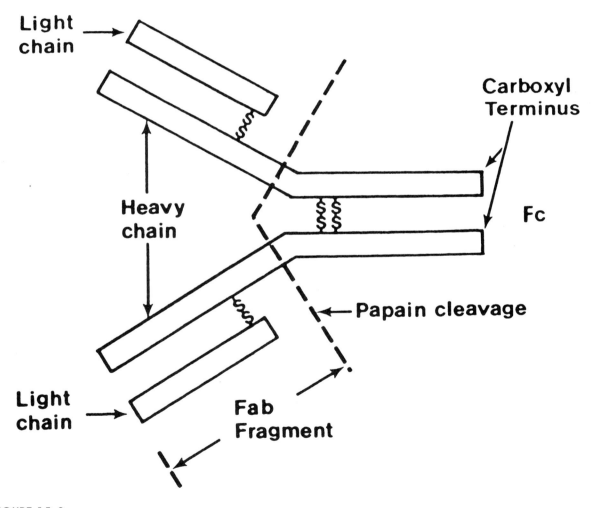

FIGURE 15-2.

Diagram of the immunoglobulin molecule. The terminal portion of the Fab fragment is the antigen-combining site. Monocytes and other cells have receptors for the Fc portion of the molecule.

TABLE 15-1. Comparative Properties of Human Immunoglobulins

	IgG	IgA	IgM	IgD	IgE
Serum concentration mg/dL	800–1,400	100–300	60–200	2–4	.02–.04
molecular weight	150,000	160,000	900,000	180,000	190,000
sedimentation constant	6.7S	7S, 9S, 11S, 15S	19S	7S	8S
carbohydrate (%)	3	5–10	12	10–12	1
biologic half-life (days)	23	5.8	10	2.8	2.3
fixes complement	+	0	+++	0	0
crosses placenta	yes	no	no	no	no
heavy chain	γ	α	μ	δ	ϵ
light-chain frequency (κ:λ ratio)	2:1	1:1	3:1	1:4	UK

+,++,+++: Intensities of fixation.
UK: Unknown

Immunoelectrophoresis

To analyze serum proteins further, immunologic precipitation can be used. Immunoelectrophoresis uses a polyvalent antiserum from a laboratory animal immunized with normal human serum. This antiserum is capable of reacting with 20 or more serum proteins. The patient's serum is electrophoresed in agar or on cellulose acetate to separate the proteins. Next, the polyvalent antiserum is allowed to diffuse at right angles toward the path of electrophoretic migration. A series of precipitin lines appears, identifying the major serum proteins. If a monoclonal protein is present, a characteristic bowing of the precipitin arc of that immunoglobulin class will be present (Fig. 15-4). Follow-up immunoelectrophoresis studies using antisera specific for κ and λ light chains and the various classes and subclasses of heavy chains allow an exact characterization of the myeloma protein.

Quantitative Measurements of Immunoglobulins

Immunoprecipitation also makes it possible to quantify each immunoglobulin class. Serum is reacted with constant amounts of specific anti-immunoglobulin antibodies and yields a precipitate proportional to the amount of antigen in the sample. The reaction can be done in an agar plate (radial immunodiffusion) or cuvette (immunonephelometry). Although this technique is reproducible and accurate at the low and normal ranges (when anti-immunoglobulin antibody is in moderate excess), there is some variability at very low and high levels, when the test is most needed. Furthermore, the value reported does not indicate whether the protein is monoclonal or polyclonal. For example, a report of 2000 mg/dL of IgG could reflect an increased polyclonal IgG, such as that seen in chronic infection, or a monoclonal IgG produced by a plasma cell tumor.

In practice, serum protein electrophoresis is used to establish the presence of a monoclonal protein and to follow its course, and the immunoprecipitation test is used to identify the class of the monoclonal protein.

Other Tests

In some cases of multiple myeloma only a light chain is produced by the malignant plasma call clone. This appears in the urine as a Bence Jones protein, where it can be detected by electrophoresis (Fig. 15-3 [3-5]). The serum of such cases contains little detectable γ-globulin (Fig. 15-3 [3-6]).

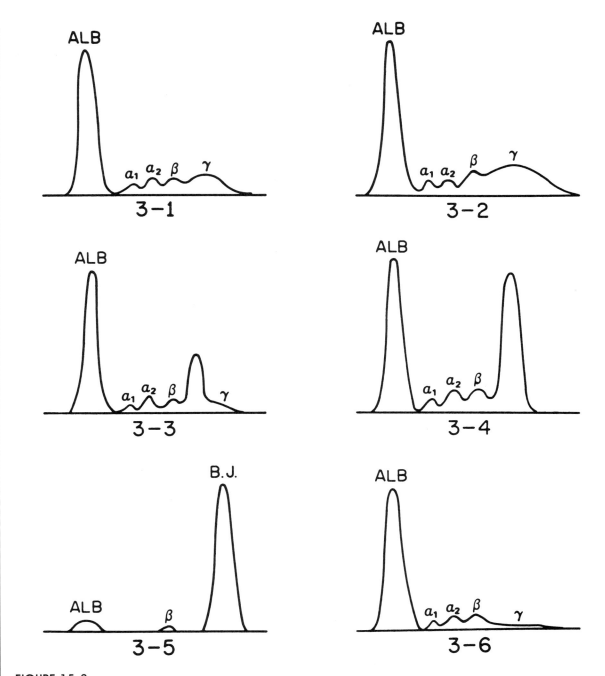

FIGURE 15-3.
Serum protein electrophoresis. (3–1) Normal serum protein electrophoresis. (3–2) Polyclonal increase in γ-globulin. (3–3) Macroglobulinemia (the test is not specific for IgM). (3–4) Multiple myeloma. Note the monoclonal spike in the γ region. (3–5) Urine electrophoresis in light-chain myeloma (Bence Jones protein). No spike is found in serum. (3–6) Serum protein electrophoresis in light-chain myeloma with the characteristic decrease in normal immunoglobulins. Alb, albumin.

Other laboratory tests, although less specific, may be useful in hyper-immunoglobulinemic states. The erythrocyte sedimentation rate may be elevated owing to the tendency of the increased immunoglobulins to cause rouleaux of red cells, or it may be depressed when IgM is elevated. Serum viscosity may be increased; it is measured by the rate of flow of serum through a calibrated capillary tube.

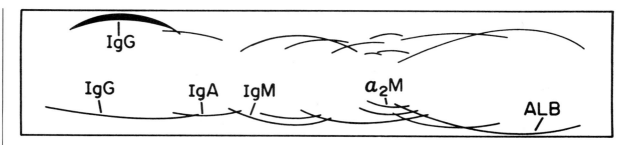

FIGURE 15-4.

Immunoelectrophoresis. Normal pattern is below; IgG myeloma with a heavy arc of IgG is shown above. Alb, albumin.

PLASMA CELL PROLIFERATIONS AND MALIGNANCIES

Monoclonal Gammopathy of Unknown Significance

Not all patients with monoclonal serum immunoglobulins have a malignant disease. Three percent of those over age 60 have a monoclonal immunoglobulin that is either stable or transient. In the latter situation, it is frequently associated with an infectious disease. Such cases are therefore considered benign disorders with low risk (2% to 3% of cases per year) of evolving into myeloma. Such patients should be evaluated thoroughly and then followed up for progression of disease, but not treated. The monoclonal protein usually does not exceed 2.5 g/dL. Bone destruction does not occur.

Analysis of such patients over time has demonstrated the appearance and disappearance of clones of cells and differences in the sequences of the hypervariable region of the heavy chain. Thus, the monoclonal protein is not strictly monoclonal but a population of closely related proteins with the same VDJ heavy chain and VJ light-chain rearrangements. The related clones of plasma cells presumably arise from a single clone of lymphoblasts that has a growth advantage and pumps offspring through the germinal center and into the bone marrow (Fig. 15-5).

Multiple Myeloma

Autonomous proliferation of plasma cells is associated with the elaboration of a monoclonal protein—either an intact immunoglobulin or a light chain (Bence Jones protein). The immunoglobulin has been shown to have antigenic specificity in rare cases, as one would predict from the way normal plasma cells behave. The clinical features of plasma cell malignancies are dominated by the following:

- Pathophysiologic effects of the abnormal protein
- Production of cytokines by plasma cells resulting in bone destruction

Epidemiology

Multiple myeloma is a relatively rare disease, but its incidence has been gradually increasing for reasons that are unclear. In the United State, there are 2 or 3 new cases per 100,000 population per year, which is similar to the incidence of Hodgkin's disease and chronic lymphocytic leukemia. Myeloma accounts for 1% of all malignancies. Although the age range of those affected is wide (30 to 80 years or older), myeloma tends to be a disease of older people, with the peak

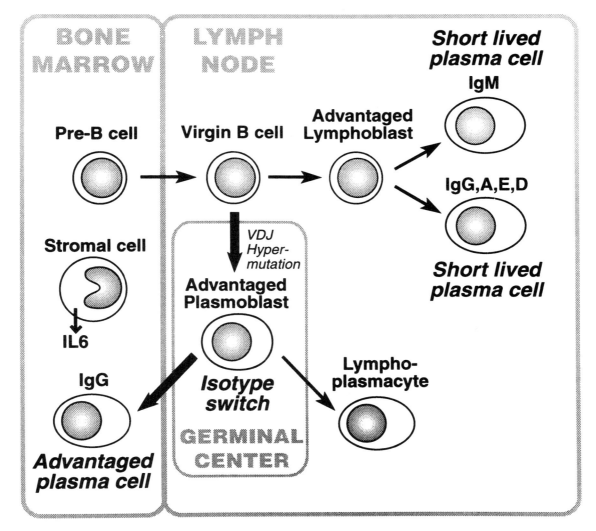

FIGURE 15-5.

Monoclonal gammopathy of unknown significance. A lymphoblast is hypothesized to have a growth advantage, perhaps because of translocation between a heavy-chain locus and an oncogene (e.g., *myc, cyclin D1*) and thus to give rise to offspring that dominate the plasma cell population. These offspring secrete large amounts of a protein that appears monoclonal unless detailed studies are performed to demonstrate that different *VDJ* sequences were introduced during exposure to the "mutator" in the germinal center.

incidence in the seventh decade. Men are affected slightly more frequently than women, and the disease is more common among blacks than those of other races.

Etiology

Radiation exposure and antigenic stimulation are involved in the cause of multiple myeloma. Atomic bomb exposure in Japan resulted in a fivefold increase in risk. The spontaneous development of plasma cell tumors in mice is known to be reduced when animals are maintained in a germ-free environment. In addition, intraperitoneal deposition of mineral oil in these animals produces a granulomatous inflammatory response, frequently followed by intra-abdominal plasma cell tumors that produce monoclonal immunoglobulin. Chronic antigenic stimulation is therefore is considered a probable causative feature in the mouse. In humans, a history of chronic antigenic stimulation is not usually found. Information about karyotypes of malignant cells has been limited because of the

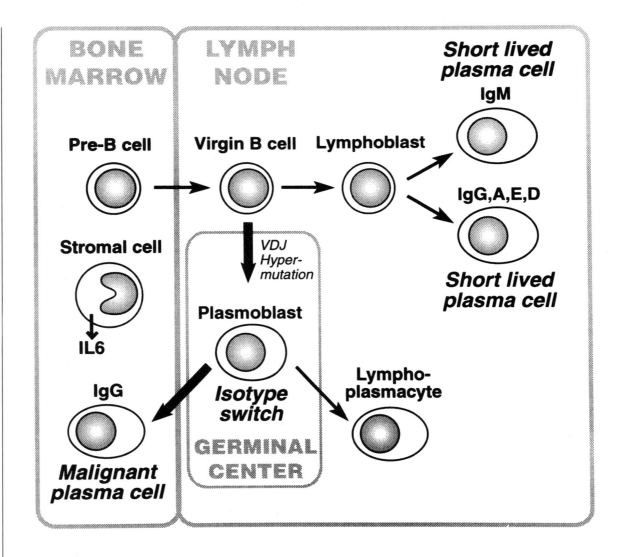

FIGURE 15-6.

Multiple myeloma. The malignant plasma cell clone proliferates semiautonomously in the bone marrow under with the stimulation of interleukin-6 (IL-6). Normal generation of plasma cells is lost.

low growth fraction. It is likely, however, that translocation of the heavy-chain locus to another site is a regular event. Partners in the translocation include *cyclin D1, myc,* and the receptor for fibroblast growth factor 4. In cases in which whole immunoglobulins are secreted, the second heavy-chain allele is used. Additional genetic changes are likely to occur, which allow the plasma cell clone to grow in the marrow, which is a rich source of interleukin-6 (IL-6) (Fig. 15-6).

Recent evidence that marrow stromal cells of myeloma patients are infected with human herpesvirus 8 has been reported. This virus was identified originally in Kaposi's sarcoma. The virus encodes a viral version of IL-6, which causes proliferation of plasma cells. This finding, if confirmed and extended, may be a key to understanding how multiple myeloma is initiated and progresses.

Protein Abnormalities

About 75% of patients with myeloma have a circulating monoclonal immunoglobulin in the serum. Of this group, approximately two thirds are IgG,

TABLE 15-2.   Plasma Cell Disorders

Disease	Immunoglobulin	Incidence (%)	Prognosis (months)*
Multiple myeloma	IgG	52	29–35
	IgA	21	19–22
	IgD	2	9
	IgE	<0.01	Unknown
	Light chains	11	10–28
Waldenström's macroglobulinemia	IgM	12	50

Median survival.

with one-third IgA and approximately 2% IgD (Table 15-2). In 20% of myelomas, the neoplastic plasma cells produce only the light-chain portion (Bence Jones protein) of the immunoglobulin. The light chains (molecular weight 20,000) are filtered rapidly by the kidney and are not present in the serum unless renal failure develops (Fig. 15-3[3-5 and 3-6]). Excess light chains also may be produced by plasma cells that are producing unbalanced amounts of light and heavy chains. "Non-secretors," who make up less than 1% of all patients with myeloma, have no recognizable serum or urine monoclonal protein.

Pathophysiology

PROBLEMS DUE TO INCREASED QUANTITIES OF ABNORMAL PROTEINS IN SERUM AND URINE

When the first malignant plasma cells emerge, the immune system may hold them in check. Normal immunoglobulin synthesis is countered by the synthesis of anti-idiotypic antibody and the expansion of suppressor T cells to downregulate the plasma cells. This mechanism probably explains why some patients develop monoclonal gammopathy of unknown significance, which does not increase beyond 2.5 g/dL and may remain constant for years. Eventually, 25% of these patients go on to typical myeloma.

If the myeloma plasma protein concentration increases to 4 g/dL, the levels of normal, functional immunoglobulins will be low. Malignant plasma cells make humoral mediators that bind to macrophages; the macrophages in turn suppress normal B cells but do not disturb T cells. The result of poor B-cell function is increased susceptibility to bacterial infection, especially of lung and urinary tract, whereas resistance to viral and fungal diseases is preserved.

Many features of myeloma are due to the high concentration of serum protein. Hyperglobulinemia produces similar effects, whether it is polyclonal or monoclonal. Plasma becomes viscous when the IgM exceeds 2 g/dL (as seen in Waldenström's macroglobulinemia), but also in IgA myeloma if IgA polymerization occurs, and occasionally with high levels of IgG. Hyperviscosity decreases cerebral blood flow, producing headache, nausea, visual impairment, and mental clouding. Decreased renal blood flow may contribute to the renal failure so common in multiple myeloma. The blood volume expands and congestive failure may develop. The high concentrations of serum protein interact with erythrocyte membranes and cause coin-like stacking of red cells known as **rouleaux** {#43}. Rouleaux can be seen in scleral vessels as "box carring." Coating of platelets by immunoglobulin results in diminished aggregation and purpura. The high protein level also may interfere with coagulation by forming complexes with specific coagulation factors or by inhibiting fibrin polymerization. Bleeding may result.

Light chains are filtered by the kidney and, to a variable extent, are reabsorbed by the proximal tubule and secreted by the distal tubule. Crystals of light-chain protein have been demonstrated in the tubular cells, and protein casts often are seen in tubular lumens. These findings are associated with renal tubular dysfunction and overt renal failure in many patients with myeloma. Monoclonal λ light chains are more likely to produce tubular injury than κ light chains. Renal injury may explain the poorer prognosis of λ (11 months) compared with κ (28 to 30 months) light-chain disease. Kidney function in patients with myeloma also may be impaired by six other factors: dehydration, hyperviscosity, hypercalcemia, hyperuricemia, infection, and amyloidosis. Therefore, even in the absence of Bence Jones proteinuria, renal failure can occur. Occasionally, renal failure occurs after injection of an iodine-containing dye used for x-ray studies; these dyes are to be avoided in the patient with myeloma or one with symptoms and signs that may indicate myeloma.

OSTEOCLAST ACTIVATING FACTORS PRODUCED BY THE MALIGNANT PLASMA CELLS

Approximately 70% of patients with myeloma initially complain of bone pain. X-rays reveal either localized punched-out lytic lesions or diffuse osteoporosis, usually in bones with active hematopoietic tissue. The discrete lytic lesions characteristically have no evidence of new bone formation {#69–71}. The lytic areas are characterized by large and numerous osteoclasts on the bone-resorbing surface. Myeloma cells grown in culture secrete interleukins (IL-1, tumor necrosis factor [TNF]-α, TNF-β, IL-6) that stimulate osteoclastic bone resorption. This set of interleukins make up the so-called osteoclast activating factor. Thus, bone destruction in myeloma appears to be a normal process, exaggerated by the secretion of mediators from excess plasma cells. The demineralization may be so extreme that the bone not only looks like Swiss cheese, but can be cut as easily. In some cases, a vertebra all but disappears, with devastating consequences. The use of bisphosphonates such as pamidronate, inhibits osteoclastic activity, reduces bone resorption, and has a highly favorable effect on bone pain, performance status, quality of life, and survival. (See Bataille and Harousseau.)

With bone demineralization due to osteoclast activation and with decreased activity because of pain, hypercalcemia may be expected. The symptoms of hypercalcemia (drowsiness, confusion, nausea, and thirst) are nonspecific, but their occurrence should alert the physician to investigate this possibility. Cardiac arrhythmias, renal insufficiency, and profound central nervous system depression can develop if the hypercalcemia progresses.

TUMOR EXPANSION

In the early stages of multiple myeloma, up to 10^{11} malignant plasma cells may occur in clusters in the marrow. A single bone marrow sample may not reveal the abnormal cells, despite positive serum or urine tests. As the disease evolves, however, a random-marrow aspirate characteristically reveals large numbers of plasma cells {#66–68} as the total mass approaches 10^{12} cells. The normal hematopoietic tissue decreases, and in most cases a normochromic, normocytic anemia develops with moderate neutropenia and thrombocytopenia. Plasma cells also may form a tumor mass that erodes and destroys vertebrae, causing collapse. Extrusion of the mass into the epidural space leads to spinal cord compression. Infiltration in the liver, spleen, lung, and other vital organs can occur but usually does not compromise their functions. Occasionally, plasma cells are found in the peripheral blood.

IgE myeloma presents a distinct clinical entity—plasma cell leukemia—which, in contrast to multiple myeloma, is characterized by greater tissue and organ involvement, less bone destruction, and a more rapid course. It resembles acute

PATHOPHYSIOLOGY OF MULTIPLE MYELOMA

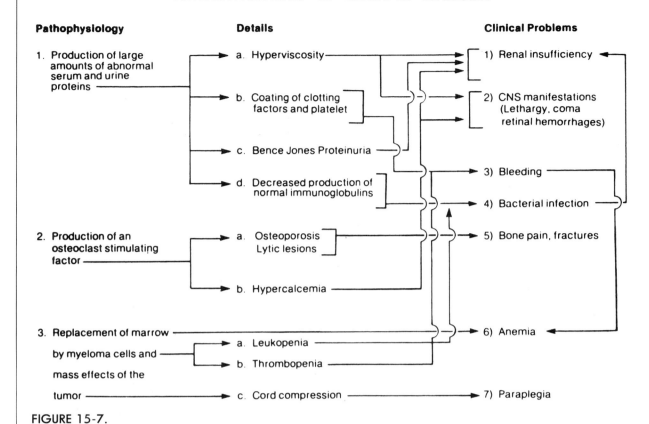

FIGURE 15-7.
Flow diagram of the pathophysiology of multiple myeloma.

leukemia more than multiple myeloma. The pathophysiology of multiple myeloma is summarized in Figure 15-7.

Diagnosis

The diagnosis of multiple myeloma is based on the triad of plasma cell infiltration of marrow, lytic lesions of bone, and a monoclonal protein in serum or urine.

Multiple myeloma occurs primarily in older patients. In a large series, only 2% of patients were less than 40 years of age, and the greatest incidence was in those in their seventh decade. Bone pain is the most common symptom, reported by 70% at presentation; however, fatigue, weakness, and recurrent infections also may cause the patient to seek medical attention. Occasionally, incidental myeloma is found in a patient examined for other medical problems. Such a patient generally develops overt myeloma, although this presymptomatic period is variable and may last 20 years or longer. Death from infection, renal failure, or hypercalcemia occurs when the tumor burden reaches 3×10^{12} cells.

The bone marrow aspirate or biopsy characteristically reveals more than 20% plasma cells, many of which are large, immature, and multinucleated {#66–68}.

Management and Therapy

Effective treatment for multiple myeloma patients includes chemotherapy, radiation therapy, and aggressive use of supportive measures. The current standard chemotherapy is intermittent oral melphalan (phenylalanine mustard) and prednisone. Cyclophosphamide, nitrosoureas (BCNU), doxorubicin, and vincristine all have been used, either alone or in combination, with variable success. More than 90% reduction in myeloma cells is unusual, and cures do not occur. Focal radiation therapy is used to relieve pain and to decrease risk of fracture.

The log-kill theory has been applied to the evaluation and treatment of patient's with multiple myeloma. Multiple myeloma is a model malignancy in which an estimate of tumor mass is aided by the presence of secreted protein, the monoclonal immunoglobulin. Myeloma cells secrete immunoglobulin in vitro so that the rate of synthesis of protein per unit number of cells can be calculated. The rate of disappearance of protein from the vascular space also can be measured by isotopic labeling a typical calculation is:

$$\text{Total myeloma cell number} = \frac{\text{total body protein synthetic rate}}{\text{protein synthesis rate per cell}}$$

$$= \frac{\text{Plasma volume} \times \text{immunoglobulin concentration} \times \text{fractional catabolic rate}}{[12] \times 10^{-12} \text{ g/cell/day}}$$

$$= \frac{3 \text{ L} \times 40 \text{ g/L} \times 0.1/\text{day}}{[12] \times 10^{-12} \text{ g/cell/day}}$$

$$= \frac{12}{[12] \times 10^{-12}} = 10^{12} \text{ cells}$$

Such data have made possible the following clinical observations.

- Multiple myeloma can be recognized by a detectable serum protein spike when 2×10^{11} myeloma cells are present in the body. Patients with less than 10^{12} cells usually do not have symptoms. The presence of more than 2×10^{12} cells is associated with osteolytic lesions, fractures, hypercalcemia, and poor diagnosis. Death usually occurs before the tumor reaches 10^{13} cells (10 kg).
- Estimates of tumor doubling indicate that 10^{12} cells require 1 to 2 years of growth.
- Alkylating agents lead to a stable number of cells after 1.0 to 1.5 logs have been killed, so that continuing the same treatment program does not yield further benefit. If the growth fraction (the number of cells in cycle) increases as the total number of cells decreases, therapeutic strategy indicates that cycle-specific agents, such as those used in acute leukemia, may now be used to advantage. Alkylating agents are effective at the beginning of therapy, when very few of the cells are in the mitotic cycle, because they attack the cell at several sites.

Bisphosphanate should be given to minimize bone resorption. Measures designed to maintain activity and hydration are also important. Analgesics, orthopedic surgery, and orthopedic supports facilitate mobilization. With adequate mobilization and fluid intake, the symptom complex of hypercalcemia, dehydration, and renal failure often can be prevented. Objective response to chemotherapy currently approaches 70%, and median survival for new patients is approximately 36 months, a prognosis similar to that for patients with chronic myelogenous leukemia.

Recently, allogeneic and autologous stem cell transplantations have been attempted in younger patients with multiple myeloma. The hope is that additional log-kills of cells will occur during intensive chemotherapy for the transplantation. The presence of allogeneic transplants also may lead to graft-versus-myeloma effect.

Other Gammopathies

Waldenström's Macroglobulinemia

Waldenström's macroglobulinemia is due to proliferation of a neoplastic clone of IgM-producing cells called "lymphocytoid plasma cells" (Fig. 15-1). Bone destruction is not a feature. In many respects, macroglobulinemia resembles a well-differentiated lymphocytic lymphoma, with infiltration of the marrow by lymphocytes or lymphocytoid plasma cells. Lymphadenopathy and splenomegaly are common.

The presence of a circulating monoclonal macroglobulin (IgM) appears to explain much of the pathophysiology (Fig. 15-7). The macroglobulin coats platelets and interferes with clotting. Marked expansion of the plasma volume leads to spurious anemia and may result in congestive heart failure. The hyperviscosity syndrome is common.

Therapy is directed at both the proliferating malignant clone of cells and the abnormal circulating protein. Alkylating agents such as chlorambucil (Leukeran) have proved effective in prolonging survival. If hyperviscosity causes symptoms, plasmapheresis can produce dramatic, although temporary, relief. Plasmapheresis is effective in macroglobulinemia because 90% of the protein is in the vascular space. In contrast, 40% to 50% of smaller IgGs and IgAs are in the extravascular space.

Heavy-Chain Disease

Heavy-chain disease is a rare malignancy characterized by the proliferation of plasma cells, which produce an abnormal monoclonal heavy chain without associated light-chain synthesis. Like macroglobulinemia, heavy-chain disorders resemble lymphoma more than myeloma. Bone disease does not occur, but lymphadenopathy and hepatosplenomegaly are common. γ, α, and μ heavy-chain diseases have been described. α Heavy-chain disease is usually associated with lymphoma involving the gastrointestinal tract with malabsorption, whereas μ heavy-chain disease is associated with longstanding chronic lymphocytic leukemia. γ Heavy-chain disease is a lymphoma that histologically resembles Hodgkin's disease.

Amyloidosis

Amyloidosis is a heterogeneous group of disorders characterized by the deposition of insoluble protein as β-pleated sheets in tissues with eventual compromise in function of the involved organs. Several different proteins have been identified in deposits, but two are common. In type I amyloid, the principal protein component is immunoglobulin light chains, whereas in type II, a nonimmunoglobulin protein serum amyloid A is found. In both types, the proteins form noncovalent polymers in a fibrillar pattern, which can be recognized by electron microscopy. Different patterns of tissue distribution are associated with the types of protein deposited.

When amyloidosis is associated with plasma cell dyscrasia (type I), amyloid deposits are found primarily in the muscles (including heart and tongue), gastrointestinal tract, and skin. In conditions associated with serum amyloid A deposition (e.g., chronic infections, rheumatoid arthritis, and familial Mediterranean fever), amyloid deposition involves kidney, spleen, liver, and adrenals. Mixed patterns, however, are common, and the representing site of involvement is not sufficient to classify the type of amyloid involved.

SUMMARY POINTS

The pathophysiology of multiple myeloma is dominated by the action of inter-leukins—osteoclastic activating factors that destroy bone—and IL-6, which appears to drive tumor growth. The pathophysiology of its sister disease, macroglobulinemia, is based principally on the secretion of viscous protein and its effects on the circulation. The treatment of both of these diseases remains unsatisfactory because of their resistance to chemotherapy.

SUGGESTED READINGS

Attall M, Harousseau JL, Stoppa AM, et al. A prospective, randomized trial of autologous bone marrow transplantation and chemotherapy in multiple myeloma. *N Engl J Med* 1996;335:91–97.

Bataille R, Harousseau JL. Multiple myeloma. *N Engl J Med* 1997;336:1657–1664.

Berenson JR, Lichtenstein A, Porter L, et al. Efficacy of pamidronate in reducing skeletal events in patients with advanced multiple myeloma. Myeloma Aredia study group. *N Engl J Med* 1996;334:488–493.

Clamp JR. Some aspects of the first recorded case of multiple myeloma. *Lancet* 1967;2:1354.

Hallek M, Bergsagel L, Anderson KC. Multiple myeloma: increasing evidence for a multistep transformation process. *Blood* 1998;91:3–21.

CASE DEVELOPMENT PROBLEM: CHAPTER 15

History: A 51-year-old construction worker and father of seven children suffered from low back pain after a pipe fell on him. In the following months, pain progressed to the point where he required crutches for walking. His weight dropped from 220 to 180 lb. His medical history revealed exposure to radiation during atomic bomb testing 25 years before admission. For years he had been having intermittent fever that had not been satisfactorily explained. He had a family history of cancer in two of seven siblings.

1. Is it possible to make a diagnosis from these data?

Physical examination: The patient was a drowsy, confused man without focal neurologic deficits. He had "box carring" of the scleral vessels, a retinal hemorrhage, and dried blood in the nares. There was tenderness to percussion over the lower spine. His ribs were tender to compression (barrel-hoop sign), and he had pain in the left arm on local pressure.

2. Can you narrow the choices from these data?
3. Select from the following list of laboratory data the tests you think are appropriate for diagnosis. Order by group. Then, look at the answers for the group and use the information to choose tests from the next group.

Routine analyses
A1 Hematocrit
A2 White blood cell count and differential
A3 Platelet count
A4 Urinalysis
A5 Reticulocyte count

Tests of blood and body fluids
B1 Urine culture
B2 Total serum protein
B3 Serum protein electrophoresis

B4   Spinal fluid examination
B5   Pleural fluid examination
B6   Prothrombin time
B7   Blood urea nitrogen
B8   Creatinine
B9   Serum calcium
B10 Uric acid
B11 Stool guaiac

Special immunology and hematology tests
C1   Hemoglobin electrophoresis
C2   Red cell protoporphyrin
C3   Urine urobilinogen
C4   Quantification of B and T cells in the peripheral blood
C5   Blood typing and cross-match
C6   Immunoelectrophoresis
C7   Bence Jones protein in the urine
C8   Leukocyte alkaline phosphatase
C9   Serum viscosity
C10 Quantitative immunoglobulins

Radiography
D1   Bone scan
D2   Bone survey (x-rays of skull, vertebrae, femurs, humeri)
D3   Chest x-ray
D4   Liver-spleen scan

Biopsies
E   Bone marrow aspiration
E2   Lymph node biopsy
E3   Liver biopsy

4. State the diagnosis.
5. List in words the clinical problems that are derived from these data, such as anemia, metabolic acidosis.
6. Describe the mechanism of each problem.

The patient was treated with intravenous fluids and a diuretic (furosemide) to aid in calcium excretion; allopurinol to decrease uric acid; and prednisone, vincristine, and cyclophosphamide to kill myeloma cells. He was given transfusions of packed red blood cells. His left humerus was pinned with an orthopedic prosthesis to prevent it from fracturing. On the next outpatient visit, he was walking with crutches and complained of pain in the left fourth rib and low lumbosacral spine. He had gained 10 lb. There was no evidence of bleeding.
Repeat laboratory values: HCT 34%; Creatinine 1.2 mg/dL; blood urea nitrogen 30 mg/dL; calcium 10.5 mg/dL; prothrombin time, 14 seconds; γ-globulin spike reduced from 7.5 to 5.1 g/dL; urine culture, clean.

7. Interpret the latter data.
8. (a) Estimate the cell kill. (b) Is this a satisfactory result?
9. Collate the clinical problems into three pathophysiologic processes; list the different detailed effects and the clinical problems that result.

CASE DEVELOPMENT ANSWERS

1. No.
2. The presumptive diagnosis of multiple myeloma would now be the first choice. However, many other diseases are possible.

3. A1 Hematocrit 21%

   A2 White blood cell count 4200/μL; differential, 50% segmented neutrophils, 2% bands, 30% lymphocytes, 14% monocytes, 2% eosinophils, 2% atypical lymphocytes; rouleaux formation seen

   A3 Platelet count 218,000/μL

   A4 Urinalysis: protein less than 100 mg/dL; no glucose or acetone; many white cells, some bacteria

   A5 Reticulocyte count 1.0%

   B1 Uriine culture: *Escerichia coli* >100,000 colonies/mL

   B2 Total serum protein 12.1 g/dL

   B3 Serum protein electrophoresis: 60% γ-monoclonal spike

   B4 Spinal fluid examination: not applicable

   B5 Pleural fluid examination: not applicable

   B6 Prothrombin time 16 seconds (international normalized ratio = 1.6)

   B7 Blood urea nitrogen 49 mg/dL

   B8 Creatinine 3.3 mg/dL

   B9 Serum calcium 12.6 mg/dL

   B10 Uric acid 11.3 mg/dL

   B11 Stool guaiac-positive

   C1 Hemoglobin electrophoresis: not applicable

   C2 Red cell protoporphyrin: not applicable

   C3 Urine urobilinogen: not applicable

   C4 Quantification of B and T cells in the peripheral blood: not applicable

   C5 Blood typing and cross-match: done

   C6 Immunoelectrophoresis: monoclonal IgG (κ-type)

   C7 Bence Jones protein in the urine: trace, κ chains

   C8 Leukocyte alkaline phosphatase: not applicable

   C9 Serum viscosity: 3.8

   C10 Quantitative immunoglobulins: IgG 7500 mg/dL; IgA 50 mg/dL; IgM 33 mg/dL

   D1 Bone scan: not applicable

   D2 Bone survey: multiple lytic lesion in skull, ribs, spine, and pelvis; left humerus shows a large lytic lesion and fracture appears imminent

   D3 Chest x-ray: an extrapleural mass

   D4 Liver-spleen scan: not applicable

   E1 Bone marrow aspiration: many (57%) abnormal plasma cells

   E2 Lymph node biopsy: not applicable

   E3 Liver biopsy: not applicable

4. Patient has IgG multiple myeloma, κ-type with an estimated 3×10^{12} plasma cells.

5. (a) Anemia; (b) uremia (renal insufficiency); (c) hypercalcemia; (d) bone destruction; (e) urinary tract infection; (f) bleeding disorder; (g) delirium.

6. (a) Anemia is due to marrow replacement by 57% plasma cells and bleeding in the gastrointestinal tract. Hemodilution (expanded plasma volume) may also contribute.

   (b) Uremia may be due to hypercalcemia (calcium may precipitate in the kidney), hyperuricemia (uric acid may precipitate in the kidney), and/or increased viscosity that may interfere with renal blood flow. Urinary tract infection may also contribute to uremia. Since the patient did not have significant Bence Jones protein or albumin in the urine, light-chain nephrophty and amyloi-dosis are unlikely.

   (c) Hypercalcemia: The osteoclast-activating factors secreted by plasma cells stimulate osteoclasts to resorb bone. Immobilization due to pain and weakness further accelerates bone resorption and raises the serum calcium. Nausea, somnolence, elevation of the blood urea nitrogen and creatinine, and muscle weakness develop.

(d) Gross bone destruction is associated with a large tumor burden. Bone destruction is found close to plasma cell concentrations, indicating a local effect of the osteoclast activating factors.

(e) The urinary tract infection is due in part to poor production of normal immunoglobulin. Cell-mediated immunity is better preserved.

(f) The bleeding disorder is due to protein coating of platelets and inhibiting their aggregation, as well as interference with factors I, II, V, VII, and VIII. Interference with factors is probably the cause of the prolonged prothrombin time.

(g) Cerebral symptoms are in part the result of hypercalcemia and hyper-viscosity.

7. The patient remains anemic. The uremia has been corrected, suggesting that only the reversible hypercalcemia, hyperuricemia, hyperproteinemia, and dehydration were important. He now has a normal serum calcium and uric acid. The prothrombin time is almost normal. He has had a small decrease in the total serum protein.

8. (a) The cell kill is proportional to the reduction in the γ-globulin concentration. In this case, 2.4 g/dL decrease over a 7.5 g/dL initial concentration represents approximately 30% cell kill (70% remaining). (b) The reduction of $3 \times 10^{12} \times 7 \times 10^{-1} = 2 \times 10^{12}$ is not satisfactory. The treatment was continued with five drugs, then with other schedules, totaling six drugs to which the tumor was exposed. The total serum protein never fell below 9 g/dL and the patient died uremic, hypercalcemic, and hyperproteinemic 9 months later.

9. Consult Figure 15-7.

SUMMARY OF HEMATOLOGIC MALIGNANCIES

Investigations of hematologic malignancies have contributed much to our knowledge about malignancies in general. A cancer is a population of mono-clonal cells that dominates and displaces its normal counterparts and leads to extinction of normal tissues. This section summarizes information from Chapters 12 through 15.

There are three broad classes of hematologic malignancies: leukemias, lymphomas, and myelomas.

- Leukemias (literally, white blood) are a group of diseases in which the malignant cells are found primarily in the blood. Leukemias may be myeloid or lymphoid and chronic or acute.
- Lymphomas (literally, tumor of the lymph node) are tumors of the lymphoid system. Lymphomas are divided into Hodgkin's and non-Hodgkin's lymphomas. The non-Hodgkin's lymphomas are further divided into follicular and diffuse, into small and large cell types, and prognostically into low grade, intermediate grade, and high grade. In general, the larger the cell, the more malignant the disease and the higher the grade.
- Myelomas (literally, tumor of the bone marrow) are tumors of terminally differentiated plasma cells that actively secrete the products of immunoglobulin genes. These are considered separately from other B-cell malignancies because the monoclonal proteins can dominate the clinical picture and the pathophysiology is distinctive. Waldenström's macroglobulinemia behaves like a low-grade lymphoma but also secretes an immunoglobulin.

The broad classification depends on both the clinical appearance of the malignancy and its pathology at the time of clinical recognition. In chronic lymphocytic leukemia, the malignancy may present purely as a leukemia or purely as a lymphoma. As a disease advances, the pattern may shift, so that lymphoma cells may appear in the blood late in the course (lymphoma cell leukemia), and rarely even the myelomas may become leukemic (plasma cell leukemia). Conversely, leukemic cells can invade lymph nodes and give the clinical appearance of a lymphoma.

Hematologic malignancies have given us valuable insight into the biology of cancer, mainly because of the identification of translocations that fuse two genes together and give rise to oncogenic proteins. We have learned to think of leukemogenesis and lymphomagenesis as a multiple-step process with the primary lesion being the translocation that confers a survival advantage. Progression is due to accumulation of additional genetic lesions. Molecular lesions can be classed under three headings: those that lead to defective DNA, those that drive cell growth, and those that inhibit programmed cell death.

Factors That Lead to Defective DNA

- The risk of genetic accidents is proportional to the number of mitoses. Although mutation is a rare event, populations such as stem cells, when forced to divide more rapidly than normal, are more vulnerable to error. Normally, 90% of the stem cell population is dormant and only 10% of the cells are replicating. In situations such as myelodysplasia, cell division is increased and cell death is also increased. The stem cell population is driven to higher division rates. Myelodysplasia patients have a high risk of leukemia. Patients with immunodeficiency similarly drive their dysfunctional immune systems and have an increased risk of lymphoid malignancy. HIV is associated with massive death of lymphocytes as well as intense immune stimulation. In this high turnover situation, the risk of lymphoma is greatly increased.

- Inborn errors of DNA synthesis and repair such as ataxia telangiectasia lead to increased risk of lymphoma. Fanconi's syndrome carries a high risk of leukemia.

- Chemical and radiologic modifiers of DNA lead to deletions and mutations. Patients treated with both radiation and chemotherapy for Hodgkin's disease, for example, have an increased risk for acute leukemia or a second lymphoma, although they may be cured from their original disease. Atomic bombs or reactor accidents and radiation therapy of nonmalignant conditions (ankylosing spondylitis) all confirm the risk of increased malignancy from x-ray and nuclear radiation.

Factors That Drive Cell Growth

- **Viruses**. Epstein-Barr virus (EBV) immortalizes B cells and allows them to grow autonomously. The mechanism is not known. In some patients in whom virus cannot be eliminated or adequately suppressed, ongoing immune stimulation may drive (overdrive) the immune system. Hepatitis C is an example. Autoimmune phenomena are common in hepatitis C and are associated with polyclonal B-cell proliferation and the development of lymphomas.

- **Translocations**. Lymphomas in general are characterized by translocations in which promoters for the immunoglobulin heavy or light chains or the T-cell receptors cause aberrant expression of genes. The vulnerability of the heavy-chain locus 14q32.33 to translocation in B-cell malignancies is particularly important. For instance, in the t(11;14) translocation, the heavy-chain locus causes overexpression of cyclin D1, a mitotic cycle control protein. This translocation is found regularly in mantle cell lymphoma and in some cases of myeloma. The t(8;14) found in Burkitt's lymphoma links the c-*myc* oncogene to the heavy-chain locus, leading to sustained proliferation. Similarly evidence that the translocation t(9:22) is the cause of chronic myelogenous leukemia is strong.

- **Cytokine stimulation**. Although we think of the immune system as inhibiting cancer, it is likely that the immune system drives some malignancies. Interleukin-6 (IL-6), for example, is believed to sustain the growth of myeloma. One of the current controversies is whether IL-6 driving myeloma cells is from marrow dendritic cells infected by Kaposi's sarcoma herpes-like virus, also called human herpesvirus 8.
- **Suppression and enhancement**. A suppression of the Th1 (cytotoxic helper) system and enhancement of the Th2 (B cell-stimulatory) system favor the malignant lymphoma. This imbalance may precede the appearance of malignancy as in the case of AIDS, in which the HIV preferentially destroys the Th1 cells. A second possibility is that the tumor itself secretes lymphokines that suppress the Th1 cells and release the Th2 cells that would favor its growth.

Factors That Inhibit Cell Death

- **Inhibition of apoptosis**. *Bcl-2* is one of a family of genes that regulate apoptosis. *Bcl-2* itself blocks apoptosis. The t(14;18) translocation activates *Bcl-2*, which inhibits germinal center cell death and contributes to the growth of follicular lymphomas. When *Bcl-2* blocks apoptosis, mutant forms may continue to replicate and increase the likelihood of a crucial error. Inhibition of apoptosis also confers chemotherapy resistance, since most anticancer drugs depend on apoptosis to kill cells.
- **Loss of immune surveillance**. Organ transplant recipients must be given immunosuppressive drugs to inhibit the cytotoxic T cells and avoid rejection of the transplant, but this leads to increased risk of lymphoma. The cytotoxic cell population is an external monitor of cell quality. It attacks foreign antigens on the transplant or on malignant cells. The immunosuppressive drugs cut both ways: permitting the transplant to survive, but allowing a tumor to escape. Many of these lymphomas contain EBV.
- **Loss or mutation of internal cell monitors**. The *p53* gene is a tumor suppressor gene (one of at least six tumor suppressor genes). It monitors the quality of DNA and presides over the apoptosis pathway to destroy defective cells. For example, the large cell lymphoma that may emerge in advanced chronic lymphocytic leukemia (Richter's syndrome) is associated with the mutation of *p53*. *p53* mutations are also associated with disease progression in a number of other cancers as well as in hematologic neoplasms.

PART IV
CLOTTING

Hemostasis and the Vascular Phase of Hemostasis

Bradford S. Schwartz, Deane F. Mosher

OUTLINE

OBJECTIVES

- Understand how endothelium normally prevents clotting.
- Visualize the sequence by which bleeding is stopped in a wound.
- Know the cell that generates platelets and the name of humoral mediators of platelet production.
- Explain how a large spleen can cause thrombocytopenia.
- Know how aspirin affects platelets.
- Explain why patients with von Willebrand's disease have prolonged bleeding times and hemophiliacs do not.
- Define purpura, petechiae, ecchymosis, and hematoma.
- Know the most common cause of bleeding in humans.
- List five drugs most commonly associated with thrombocytopenia.
- List disorders of supporting tissue, endothelium, and intravascular space that lead to purpura.

INTRODUCTION TO HEMOSTASIS

The mechanisms that turn blood from a fluid to a gel and prevent blood from escaping from injured blood vessels are referred to as hemostasis. Normal hemostasis requires vascular, cellular, and humoral components. At the moment of injury, the blood vessel contracts, narrowing the lumen. Injured tissue exposes blood to substances that cause adhesion and aggregation of platelets. Platelet plug formation occurs almost instantly (Fig. 16-1). A network of soluble coagulation factors is activated, causing prothrombin to convert to the master clotting enzyme thrombin and within 5 minutes to produce a fibrin gel. The definitive hemostatic plug consists of irreversibly aggregated platelets stabilized by a fibrin network. The hemostatic plug serves as a nidus for the migration and growth of repair cells into the site of injury. When healing is established, the plug is lysed by cell-based fibrinolytic activators.

Abnormal bleeding may result from:

- Thrombocytopenia (lack of platelets)
- Defective platelet adhesion
- Defective platelet aggregation
- Defective fibrin formation
- Excessive fibrinolysis

Abnormal thrombosis may result from:

- Inappropriate activation of hemostasis
- Failure to localize hemostasis
- Failure of fibrinolysis

Inasmuch as a working knowledge of platelets, coagulation, and fibrinolysis is required for almost every area of medicine, it is worth learning about blood coagulation mechanisms in some detail.

The study of balanced hemostasis can be organized around a series of questions:

1. What normally keeps blood in a liquid state?
2. What starts the blood clotting process?
3. What amplifies and intensifies clotting?
4. What prevents the hemostatic plug from propagating into other vessels?
5. What becomes of the redundant clot?
6. What limits clot lysis?

This chapter is concerned with questions 1 and 2. Subsequent chapters deal with questions 3 through 6.

VASCULAR AND CELLULAR PHASES OF HEMOSTASIS

Endothelial Cells

The intact endothelial cell lining of blood vessels inhibits clotting by at least two mechanisms:

First, endothelial cells present a nonthrombogenic array of glycoproteins, proteoglycans, and glycolipids to the luminal surface, different from the basal surface of endothelium that abuts the collagen-containing internal elastic membrane (Fig. 16-2). In cell culture, endothelial cells show the same polarity, and it is

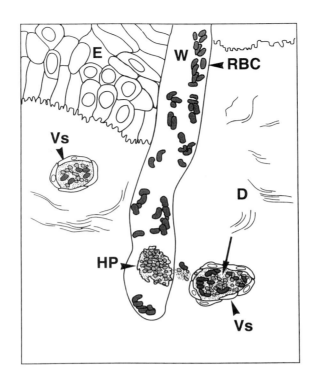

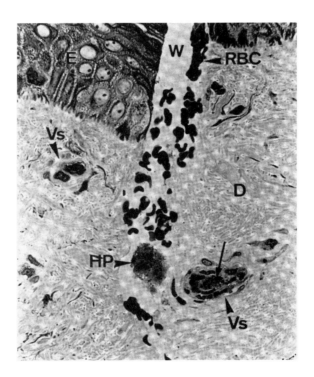

FIGURE 16-1.

Schematic and photograph of a skin wound made for the determination of the bleeding time. A biopsy specimen was excised at 30 seconds. The bleeding time stylet created the wound (W) through epidermis (E) into dermis (D). Red cells pour into it from transected vessels (Vs). A hemostatic plug (HP) consisting of aggregated platelets adheres to collagen on the dermis (D). Part of the hemostatic plug remains in the vessel (*arrow*). Fibrin formation will develop over the next several minutes. (From Wester J, Sixma JJ, Geuze JJ, Van der Veen J. Morphology of the human hemostatic plug. *Lab Invest* 1978;39:298.)

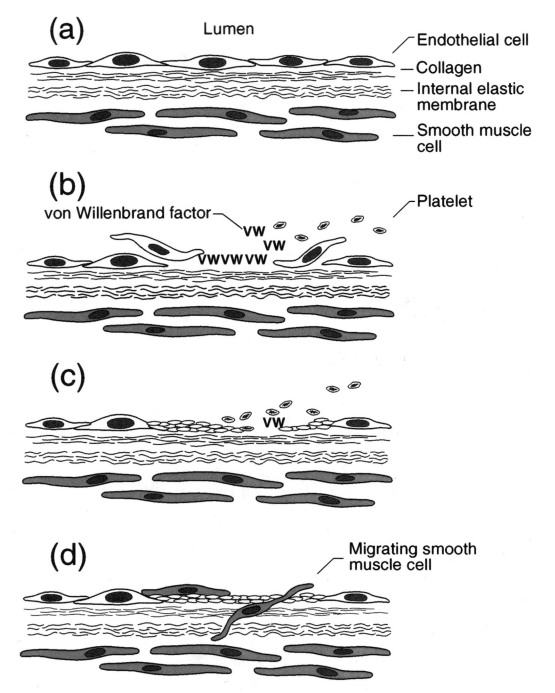

FIGURE 16-2.
Sequence of events after damage to endothelial cells. In a classic experiment, rabbit aortas were injured by inserting a balloon catheter through the femoral artery, blowing up the balloon, and stripping off endothelial cells. At various times after injury, animals were sacrificed and their aortas examined histologically. When the intact endothelial cell layer was removed (a), platelets adhered to the subendothelium (b) and formed a monolayer (c). Later, smooth muscle cells migrated through the internal elastic membrane to form nests of cells on the luminal side of the internal elastic membrane (d).

only when the monolayer is disrupted and the extracellular matrix proteins are exposed that the platelets adhere to endothelium.

Two proteins on the endothelial surface modify the activity of any thrombin that diffuses from other sites. Thrombomodulin has a high-affinity binding site for thrombin and changes its enzymatic specificity so that it has anticoagulant rather than procoagulant properties. Heparan sulfate proteoglycan, a heparin-like material on the endothelial surface, binds the natural circulating inhibitor of thrombin (antithrombin) as well as thrombin itself and thus enhances antithrombin inactivation of thrombin.

Second, stimulated endothelial cells convert arachidonic acid to **prostacyclin** I_2, a powerful inhibitor of platelet aggregation, which causes blood vessels to dilate and platelets to disaggregate. In contrast, **thromboxane A_2**, generated by platelets, causes platelets to aggregate and blood vessels to contract.

An additional protection against thrombosis is the rapid flow of blood, which disperses activated clotting factors. Areas of stasis, such as varicose veins of the leg, are prone to thrombosis, even where the endothelium is not disturbed. Once thrombosis has occurred and blood flow is impaired, the risk of further thrombosis is increased. Patients with thrombophlebitis of the leg are prone to repeated episodes.

Platelets

Platelets are the smallest of the formed elements of human blood and appear in blood smears as anucleate, granular bodies, 2 to 4 μm in diameter. Because platelets were easily confused with microscopic debris, microscopists did not agree on the existence of platelets until the latter half of the 19th century, long after the advent of microscopy. It soon became clear that platelets are important for hemostasis and platelet function. Most of the physiologic and biochemical details of platelet function have come to light since 1960.

Platelet Kinetics

Each microliter of normal blood contains 1.5 to 4×10^5 platelets compared with 4 to 5×10^6 red cells and 4 to 10×10^3 white cells. Ten percent of platelets are replaced daily, generated by cytoplasmic fragmentation of polyploid megakaryocytes. The megakaryocytes are the largest cells in the marrow (~50 μm) {#47}. They are derived from diploid (2n) megakaryocyte precursors by repeated endomitosis. Under normal conditions, megakaryocytes reach the 8 n, 16 n, or 32 n ploidy class before endomitosis ceases and the cytoplasm is mature. At this point, fragmentation channels develop, dividing the cytoplasm into 1000 to1500 platelets.

A specific cytokine, **thrombopoietin** (TPO), is the major mediator of platelet production. TPO is believed to act on the stem cell and throughout proliferation and differentiation. Inflammatory mediators such as interleukin (IL)-6 and IL-11 also act on differentiated megakaryocyte precursors to increase platelet counts. TPO is a 31-kd protein that binds to circulating platelets. Such binding may regulate platelet production by simple feedback: If the platelet mass is low, the amount of free TPO is increased and megakaryocyte differentiation is stimulated. If the platelet mass is high, free TPO is low and megakaryocyte differentiation decreases.

With a limited ability to synthesize proteins, platelets age rapidly in the circulation and are removed by the spleen in about 10 days, if not consumed in clotting reactions. About 30% of circulating platelets are normally sequestered in the spleen and can be released in response to epinephrine. Sequestered platelets are a special part of peripheral blood pool. Larger than normal spleens store platelets in proportion to their mass. No hyperplasia of megakaryocytes results. On the other hand, platelets that are coated with antibody are rapidly destroyed by the spleen. Megakaryocyte hyperplasia is expected under this condition.

Molecular Anatomy

Platelets are motile, nonnucleated cells that are capable of phagocytosis and granule secretion. They are analogous in this respect to granulocytes. The molecular anatomy of the platelet is complex (Fig. 16-3). Electron microscopy shows that most platelets are disc-shaped. A circumferential band of microtubules just inside the external membrane seems to serve as a skeletal frame to hold the discoid shape. Platelets also contain large amounts of actin and myosin, which, upon activation of the platelet, organize to form contractile cytoskeletal elements called **microfilaments**. Channels within platelets are connected with one another and with the surface, much like the channels of a sponge. Platelets also contain a membranous system that sequesters Ca^{2+}, similar to the T system of muscle.

Platelets contain mitochondria, glycogen-containing granules, lysosomes, and two types of granules that are specific for platelets—dense granules and α granules. Dense granules contain serotonin, calcium, adenosine diphosphate (ADP), and adenosine triphosphate (ATP). α Granules contain proteins that are also found in plasma, including fibrinogen, von Willebrand factor, fibronectin, coagulation factor V, and proteins that are specific for α granules, including platelet factor 4, β-thromboglobulin, thrombospondin, and platelet-derived growth factor (PDGF, a fibroblast and smooth muscle growth stimulant). The cytoplasm of platelets is also rich in coagulation factor XIII, the precursor of an enzyme that cross-links fibrin.

On the surface of platelets are a number of glycoproteins. Many of the glycoproteins have been given Roman numeral names based on their mobility in gel electrophoresis. Glyprotein Ib (GpIb) is the receptor for von Willebrand factor.

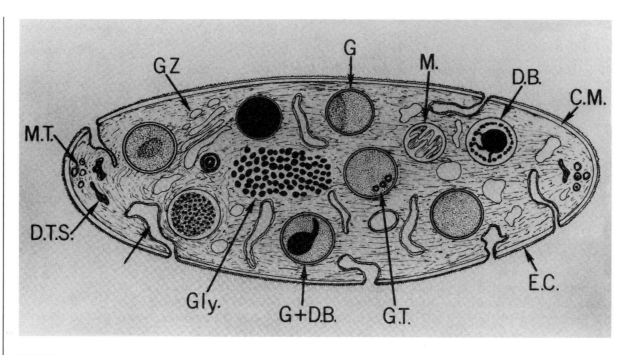

FIGURE 16-3.

Discoid platelets cut in cross-section. Components of the peripheral zone include the external coat (E.C.) and trilaminar unit membrane (C.M.). The matrix of the platelet contains the circumferential microtubular band (M.T.) and glycogen granules (Gly). The membrane systems include the canalicular system (CS), which connects to the surface (*unlabeled arrow*), and the dense tubular system (D.T.S.). Formed elements include mitochondria (M), granules (G), Golgi zone (GZ), and dense bodies (D.B.). (From Colman RW, et al. *Hemostasis and Thrombosis*. Philadelphia: JB Lippincott, 2nd ed. p. 344).

GpIIb-IIIa is the receptor for the sticky proteins, fibrinogen, fibronectin, and vitronectin. The glycoproteins also have names in the CD nomenclature, such as CD42 for GpIb and CD41/61 for GpIIb-IIIa. The membrane of α granules contain membrane glycoproteins that are expressed on the surface of activated platelets after externalization of the platelet. The most important granule membrane protein is p-selectin (CD62p).

Reactions

Platelets plug holes in two ways. First, they fill defects between normal endothelial cells. Purpura occurs as soon as platelets disappear, at sites where no trauma has occurred. Red cells can be seen leaving normal-appearing capillaries by diapedesis when platelets are absent.

The second function of platelets is to plug holes in injured vessels. When blood is exposed to injured tissue or a foreign surface, a striking transformation of platelets takes place. The shape changes from discoid to spherical, and long processes protrude from the body of the platelet. Sequestered Ca^{2+} is released. Receptors for factor V and fibrinogen/fibrin appear on the surface. The microtubular ring contracts, and the contents of dense and α granules are secreted (Fig. 16-4).

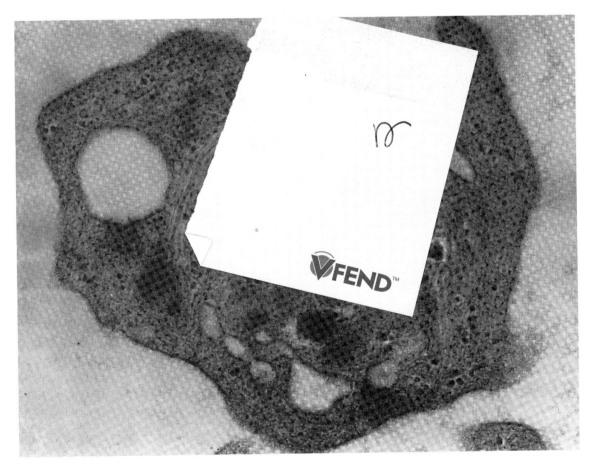

FIGURE 16-4.
Platelet shortly after exposure to thrombin. The cell has lost its discoid shape and has bulky pseudopods. The organelles are crowded to the center, encircled by the band of microtubules. Discharge of the granules will follow shortly. (From Colman RW, et al. *Hemostasis and Thrombosis*. Philadelphia: JB Lippincott, 2nd ed. p. 353).

Arachidonic acid, a fatty acid in platelet membrane phospholipids, is liberated and converted into endoperoxides by cyclooxygenase. The endoperoxides, in turn, are converted to thromboxane A_2, a potent aggregating agent. Platelets aggregate and fuse to form an amorphous mass that plugs the hole in the vessel. Plug formation is enhanced by reflex contraction of the vessel, which narrows the lumen. Platelets are quickly enmeshed, along with red cells, in a network of fibrin.

The contractile elements of the platelets pull together the fibrin strands to which the platelets have adhered, trapping the red cells and forcing out serum (plasma minus fibrinogen, platelets, factors V, and VIII); this phenomenon is called "clot retraction." Retraction of a clot formed from shed blood in vitro is a simple bedside measure of platelet function. Physiologic activators of human platelets include:

- Collagen and microfibrillar glycoproteins, present in the subendothelium of damaged vessels
- ADP, released from damaged red cells and secreted by activated platelets
- Thromboxane A_2, synthesized by activated platelets
- Platelet activating factor, a phospholipid produced by activated basophils
- Epinephrine, which circulates at times of stress
- Thrombin, activated during blood coagulation

Other substances are fortuitous activators, but have proved valuable in the clinical laboratory. Ristocetin is an antibiotic that induces aggregation of human platelets in the presence of human von Willebrand factor and can be used to assay for the presence of this protein in plasma.

The inhibitors of platelet activation used clinically are aspirin, ticlopidine, and clopidigrel. Aspirin inhibits platelet cyclooxygenase irreversibly. Ticlopidine and clopidogrel inhibit ADP-mediated platelet aggregation. Both drugs are useful in stroke prevention, and aspirin is also widely used in prevention of myocardial infarction. Newer agents that inhibit the platelet IIb/IIIa receptor such as the antibody Abciximab are useful in the treatment of acute coronary syndromes.

Platelet Adhesion and Aggregation

It is useful to distinguish between platelet adhesion and platelet aggregation: adhesion is attachment of platelets to another surface; aggregation is the attachment of platelets to each other. As shown in Figure 16-1, platelets are thought to adhere in vivo to exposed collagen and microfibrillar glycoproteins, to become activated, to release dense and α-granule contents, and thus to induce other platelets to aggregate. Adhesion is mediated by von Willebrand factor diffusing from plasma and released by platelet α granules. The presence of p-selectin on the platelet surface also enhances adhesion.

Platelet aggregation in platelet-rich citrated plasma can be studied semiquantitatively in a platelet aggregometer, an instrument that has a 37° C heating block, a magnetic stirrer, a light source, and photo cell. As platelets aggregate, the turbidity of the suspension clears. Thus, characteristic curves are generated with stimulators of aggregation such as ADP, epinephrine, and collagen (Fig. 16-5). A distinction is made between "first-wave" aggregation, in which some of the platelets are induced to aggregate, and "second-wave" aggregation, in which some of the platelets release substances (Ca^{2+}, ADP, serotonin, thromboxane A_2 and α-granule proteins) that cause the rest of the platelets to aggregate. Fibrinogen is an essential cofactor for aggregation and bridges together activated platelets.

Congenital abnormalities have been identified in which platelets demonstrate abnormal aggregation; either because of abnormal first-wave aggregation

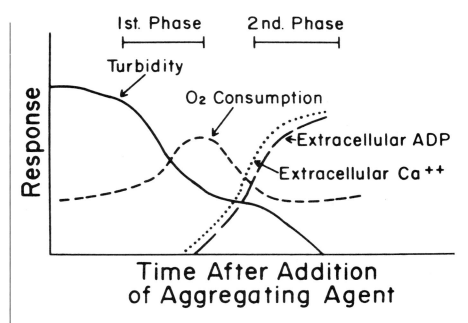

FIGURE 16-5.
Platelet aggregation in vitro. Platelet aggregation is studied semiquantitatively in a platelet aggregometer, a device with a 37° C heating block, magnetic stirrer, a light source, and a photo cell to measure turbidity. Aggregation is biphasic, and the second phase coincides with release of adenosine diphosphate (ADP) and Ca^{++} from dense granules. The rise in oxygen utilization is due to oxidation of arachidonic acid by cyclooxygenase.

(intrinsic inability of the platelets to aggregate) or abnormal second-wave aggregation (inability of platelets to release granules and propagate aggregation) (Table 16-1). Most noteworthy of the syndromes is Glanzmann's thrombasthenia ("weak platelets"!) in which GpIIb-IIIa, a dimer of the integrin class of adhesion receptors, is missing. GpIIb-IIIa binds fibrinogen when platelets are activated and thus is essential for platelet aggregation. Abciximab, a humanized monoclonal antibody that blocks GpIIb-IIIa, has proved to be a useful drug to stop thrombosis in coronary arteries after angioplasty, as have several other inhibitors of GpIIb-IIIa.

Platelets and von Willebrand Factor/Factor VIII Complex

Von Willebrand factor binds on the one hand to subendothelial connective tissue and on the other hand to platelets (by GpIb) and thus mediates the adhesion of platelets to subendothelium. Von Willebrand factor is synthesized by endothelial cells and megakaryocytes and is present in plasma and α granules of platelets. Von Willebrand factor is also the carrier for the protein that has factor VIII coagulant activity (Fig. 16-6). Von Willebrand factor is a multimer of identical subunits and, presumably, if half of the subunits are abnormal, then the whole multimer is abnormal. Thus, quantitative or qualitative abnormalities of von Willebrand factor are inherited as a dominant trait and cause von Willebrand's disease. Patients with quantitative or qualitative abnormalities of von Willebrand factor have prolonged bleeding times and increased bleeding, usually from mucous membranes, throughout life. Patients may be chronically iron-deficient and require many transfusions.

Citrated platelet-rich plasma of patients with von Willebrand's disease may aggregate poorly in response to ristocetin (Table 16-1). Patients with severe von Willebrand's disease also have deficiencies of factor VIII coagulant activity because they lack the carrier protein for factor VIII, that is, von Willebrand factor.

TABLE 16-1. Congenital Disorders of Platelets and Von Willebrand Factor

Disease	Inheritance	Primary Defect	Secondary or Additional Defect
Von Willebrand's disease	Autosomal dominant	Lack or abnormality of circulating von Willebrand factor	Lack of VIII activity, poor ristocetin-induced aggregation
Bernard Soulier disease	Autosomal dominant	Lack of surface glycoprotein Ib (von Willebrand factor receptor)	Mild thrombocytopenia; poor ristocetin-induced aggregation
Glanzmann's thrombasthenia	Autosomal recessive	Lack of surface glycoprotein IIb-IIIa complex	Abnormal first- and second-wave aggregation; poor clot retraction; defective binding of fibrinogen
Gray platelet syndrome	?	Lack of α-granule contents	Surprisingly few bleeding problems; poor aggregation
Dense granule syndromes	Heterogeneous	Lack of dense granules	Abnormal second-wave aggregation
a. Storage defect			Albinism and Wiskott-Aldrich syndrome
b. Release defect	Heterogeneous, autosomal recessive	Poor secretion of contents of dense granules	Abnormal second-wave aggregation

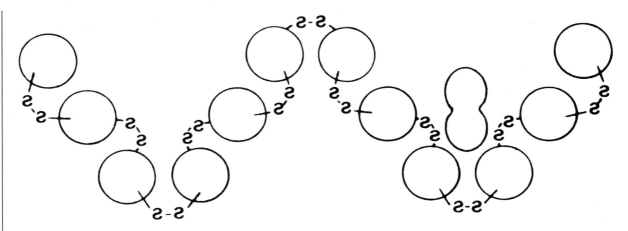

FIGURE 16-6.
Schematic of the von Willebrand factor-coagulation factor VIII complex. Von Willebrand factor is a multimer of 200,000-dalton subunits (*balls*) linked together by disulfide bridges (*S-S*). Bound noncovalently to the multimer is a second protein (*peanut shape*) exhibiting factor VIII coagulant activiity. Von Willebrand factor is quantitatively or qualitatively abnormal in von Willebrand's disease, whereas factor VIII coagulant protein is quantitatively or qualitatively abnormal in sex-linked hemophilia.

In contrast, patients with classic sex-linked hemophilia have normal ristocetin-induced platelet aggregation and normal or near-normal bleeding times because they have normal von Willebrand factor, even though they have severely depressed levels of factor VIII coagulant activity.

Because von Willebrand factor is the predominant protein in the von Willebrand factor/factor VIII complex, heterologous antiserum to the complex contains mainly antibodies to von Willebrand factor. Therefore, von Willebrand factor is sometimes referred to as "factor VIII-related antigen" or, incorrectly, as "factor VIII antigen."

Platelets and Atherosclerosis

Platelets have been implicated in the pathogenesis of subendothelial plaques, which are the basic lesion in atherosclerosis. When platelets adhere to de-endothelialized vessels and release growth factor (PDGF and transforming growth factor-β), smooth muscle cells in the media of arteries are induced to migrate through the internal elastic membrane and proliferate in the subendothelium. Normally, this "scar" regresses. When vascular injury occurs repeatedly, hemodynamically significant plaques can form. Recognized risk factors such as diabetes, hyperlipidemia, hypertension, nicotine abuse, and aggressive personality may act by making platelets hyperactive, causing excessive thrombus formation and interference with the orderly resolution of vascular injury. Clinical trials of drugs that inhibit platelet adhesion and aggregation have demonstrated benefit in patients with transient cerebral ischemic attacks and in prevention of myocardial infarction.

Platelet Count

The platelet count can be estimated in three different ways:

- From the blood smear. The normal platelet count is $3 \times 10^5/\mu L$, and platelets should number roughly 1 for every 10 red blood cells, since there are 4×10^6 red cells/μL. The normal blood smear has 10 to 15 platelets per oil immersion field. In severe thrombocytopenia, platelets are less than one per oil immersion field. This is a useful screening procedure.
- By lysing the red cells and counting the platelets in a chamber of known volume (hemocytometer) under a microscope.
- By using a sophisticated cell counter that can distinguish 2-μm platelets from 8-μm red blood cells and therefore can count the platelets in whole blood. This procedure is routine in most institutions.

Bleeding Time

The bleeding time is a simple test that has been used widely to screen for disorders of platelets and blood vessels. In the Ivy method, a standardized cut is made on the forearm while venous pressure is maintained at 40 mm Hg with a blood pressure cuff. The time to cessation of bleeding is determined by blotting the clot. If the cut is made parallel with the length of the forearm and if an adhesive bandage is used to snug up the edges afterward, the test should leave no detectable scar. However, one should ask the patient about a history of keloid formation before doing the test. The normal range of bleeding time is 2 to 8 minutes. Two aspirin tablets taken during the previous 24 hours significantly prolongs the test. As a test, bleeding time, despite its wide use, has performed poorly in prospective studies of sensitivity and specificity and in no way substitutes for a good personal and family history as a screening for bleeding during surgery, for example.

PURPURA

Purpura is the generic term for purple spots caused by hemorrhages in the skin. The smallest of these spots are **petechiae**, pinpoint hemorrhages most often found in areas of high hydrostatic pressure, such as the ankles and feet, but also around the eyes of infants (crying→Valsalva→high venous pressure in the head) and around constricting clothing. **Ecchymoses** are larger spots of hemorrhage. **Hematomas** contain enough extravasation of blood to form a mass and are usually painful.

Thrombocytopenic Purpura

Low platelet counts are due to one or more of the following:

- Decreased production (hypoproliferative or ineffective megakaryopoiesis)
- Increased destruction (by autoimmune or drug-related antibody)
- Increased utilization (consumption in clotting or vascular injury)
- Sequestration (in a large spleen)

These categories may overlap, so that a patient with chronic lymphocytic leukemia, for example, might have a large spleen, marrow replacement with lymphocytes, and an autoantibody against platelets.

Low platelets are the most common cause of bleeding and can be recognized easily by physical examination showing petechiae when the count is below 30,000/μL. The blood smear can be used as a quick screening, since there is 1 platelet per oil immersion field for every 10,000 to 20,000 platelets/μL (i.e., 10 to 15 platelets per field in the normal smear) {#45}. Further, if the platelets are larger than 3 μm {#46}, increased turnover (and therefore increased destruction) should be suspected. Thrombocytopenic bleeding occurs in the skin and mucous membranes, rarely in joints or brain.

Younger platelets seem to work better than older platelets; therefore, patients with rapid platelet turnover suffer fewer bleeding symptoms at a given low platelet count than patients with hypoproliferative thrombocytopenia. In patients with hypoproliferative thrombocytopenia, major procedures should not be performed if the platelet count is less than 50,000/μL, and prophylactic platelet transfusions are often given if the platelet count is less than 10,000/μL.

Idiopathic thrombocytopenic purpura (ITP) is the most common hematologic autoimmune disease in adults. It is due to autoantibody-coating platelets, with destruction in the spleen. The mechanism of antibody formation is unknown, but acute ITP occurs in children and is often self-limited, suggesting a sequel to viral infection. In adults, ITP is common in those with systemic lupus erythematosus, chronic lymphocytic leukemia, and AIDS, in which autoimmune phenonema are common.

The diagnosis of ITP requires four criteria:

- A low platelet count
- Increased megakaryocytes {#48}
- Negative drug history
- No other causes of thrombocytopenia, such as massive splenomegaly or microangiopathic hemolytic anemia

We do not have a convenient "Coombs' test" for platelet antibodies, although most patients have antibodies that react with platelet GpIIb-IIIa. Unfortunately, the reaction is with the cytoplasmic "tails" rather than the portion exposed on the cell surface. Thus, although ITP is also called "immune" thrombocytopenia, the best evidence for pathogenesis is some old and, in retrospect, frightening experiments in which infusion of plasma from patients into normal volunteers caused profound thrombocytopenia. Corticosteroids induce remissions in 25% of adults with ITP. Splenectomy is more effective: 50% of patients with splenectomy go into remission.

Drug-mediated thrombocytopenic purpura is important to distinguish from autoimmune purpura because the treatment is simple and obvious. Five drugs—quinine, quinidine, rifampin, heparin, and sulfonamides (TMP-S)—cause more than 50% of drug thrombocytopenias. Quinine used in tonic water can cause "cocktail purpura" and may be easily overlooked because it is not viewed as a drug. In most cases of drug thrombocytopenia, an antigen-antibody complex attaches to the platelet (innocent bystander mechanism) and leads to splenic trapping. The onset of thrombocytopenia is often sudden and drastic. Removing the offending drug is the obvious treatment.

Thrombocytopenias due to poor platelet production (hypoproliferative) are treated with platelet transfusions. Blood banks routinely harvest platelets from fresh blood. Platelet concentrates from 10 units of blood have a volume of approximately 300 mL and should raise the platelet count by approximately 50,000/μL when given to a 70-kg person. Repeated platelet transfusions, however, sensitize the recipient to human leukocyte antigens (HLAs). When this happens, only concentrates collected by platelet pheresis of HLA-matched donors are effective. Therefore, medical facilities that give treatments resulting in bone marrow aplasia, as in the treatment of acute leukemia or bone marrow transplantation, require the support of blood banks with rosters of willing, HLA-matched, potential platelet donors.

Nonthrombocytopenic Purpura

Nonthrombocytopenic purpura is much more complex than thrombocytopenic purpura, and we must take into account all the structures between the platelet and the skin. Beginning from the outside of the vessel inward, the connective tissue is a vital support structure for the capillaries. When collagen is poorly hydroxylated and stabilized, as in vitamin C deficiency (scurvy), bleeding around hair follicles and in the gums results. When collagen is poorly synthesized, as in old age or corticosteroid treatment, a benign, painless purpura (senile purpura) is seen, especially on the arms and trunk. Amyloid deposits in the skin may disrupt collagen and lead to striking purpura, especially around the eyes ("raccoon eyes"). Congenital defects of elastic tissue, such as Ehlers-Danlos syndrome, may cause cutaneous bleeding. Affected patients generally have long bleeding times.

Vascular anomalies include the rare congenital hemorrhagic telangiectasia (Osler-Weber-Rendu disease) and a common acquired form of gastrointestinal angiodysplasia in the elderly. Both are causes of recurrent, low-grade gastrointestinal bleeding.

Inflammation of the blood vessel (vasculitis) may be mediated by drugs, autoantibodies, or bacterial products, usually in the form of antigen-antibody complexes. A large number of acute and chronic illnesses are included under the term **vasculitis**, such as Henoch-Schönlein purpura, Goodpasture's syndrome, serum sickness, polyarteritis nodosa, meningiococcemia, and Rocky Mountain spotted fever. Different parts of the vascular tree may be attacked in these various diseases. For example, Goodpasture's syndrome is associated with bleeding from the pulmonary vessels, whereas polyarteritis nodosa attacks medium-sized arteries. Deposition of amyloid in the walls of blood vessels is associated with bleeding. Inside the vessel, high concentrations of γ-globulins, or uremia, may impair platelet function and lead to purpura.

SUMMARY POINTS

The initial phase of hemostasis must generate a platelet plug. It involves reflex vasoconstriction, the binding of platelets to the vessel wall with the aid of adhesive proteins, and the recruitment of other platelets to form a tissue mass. The failure of the system is demonstrated by petechiae and mucosal bleeding. It is most commonly caused by thrombocytopenia.

SUGGESTED READINGS

Aster RH. Pooling of platelets in the spleen. *J Clin Invest* 45:645.

George JN, et al. Drug-induced thrombocytopenia. *Ann Intern Med* 129:886.

Gernsheimer T, Stratton J, Bollem PJ, Slichter SJ. Mechanisms of response to treatment of autoimmune thrombocytopenic purpura. *N Engl J Med* 320:974–980.

Guerriero A, et al. Thrombopoietin is synthesized by bone marrow stromal cell. *Blood* 90:3444.

CASE DEVELOPMENT PROBLEM: CHAPTER 16

History:A 53-year-old machinist was seen in the outpatient department with chest pain, mild hypertension, and easy bruising. On further questioning, he said that he had noted easy bruising for the past 2 years. He was receiving hydrochlorothiazide to treat hypertension.

Physical examination: Negative except for purpura on the ankles. The spleen was not enlarged.

Laboratory values: Hematocrit (HCT) 42.7%; WBCs 4500/μL with normal differential count; platelets 22,000/μL.

1. No action was taken. Would you have done the same?
   Two years later, the patient returned for a second opinion of a diagnosis of prostate cancer, which had been found the previous year from a transurethral resection of the prostate. The platelet count was again low, 24,000/μL. Hydrochlorothiazide was stopped.
2. Why was this drug stopped?
   Treatment was recommended, but the patient refused.
3. What treatment would you have offered?
   Two weeks later, a bone marrow aspirate revealed normal cellularity with somewhat increased megakaryocytes (4 to 8 per low-power field). Bleeding time was 11 minutes. Prothrombin time and partial thromboplastin time are normal. Physical examination is normal, spleen was not palpable.
4. (a) How do you interpret the bone marrow data? (b) At what level of platelet count does the bleeding time become abnormal?
   Two months later, the patient had a second transurethral resection of the prostate. No cancer was found in the prostate chips. Bleeding in the urine continued for 6 days (normally 3 to 4 days). On the ninth postoperative day, ecchymosis was noted over the lower abdomen, penis, and scrotum. The patient was readmitted 10 days later with urethral bleeding. The hematocrit dropped from 34% to 25%. Transfusions of 3 units of packed red cells were given.
5. Can you comment on the management of the latter surgical procedure?
   The patient began treatment with prednisone 60 mg/day. A week later, his platelet count was 82,000/μL; the next week, 70,000; and the following week, 31,000. The prednisone dose was tapered and discontinued.
6. What is your interpretation of this treatment program?
   The patient returned with more bruising, and another procedure was performed. The platelet counts ($\times 10^{-3}$) are tabulated, beginning on the day of the procedure (day 0).
7. Can you guess what procedure was performed?
8. (a) What is your interpretation of the course? (b) Why did the counts go above normal?
9. What is the name of the patient's disease?
10. What could have been done if the surgery had been unsuccessful?
11. Can you make pathophysiologic sense of the various treatment options?

	PLATELETS $\times 10^{-3}/\mu l$		PLATELETS $\times 10^{-3}/\mu l$
Day 0	90	Day 6	893
Day 1	141	Day 7	950
Day 2	297	Day 8	1160
Day 3	439	Day 9	975
Day 4	639	Day 23	384
Day 5	784	Day 129	225

CASE DEVELOPMENT ANSWERS

1. The answer is "no", but a qualified "no". Many patients with platelet counts in the range of 20,000/μL do quite well. Others have symptomatic bleeding. The patient was believed to be minimally affected by his disease, and it was decided not to intervene. The problem is that the patient has unexplained thrombocytopenia, which has many causes, some requiring treatment. Thus, most physicians would establish why the patient has thrombocytopenia.
2. Hydrochlorothiazide is one of the compounds implicated in drug-mediated thrombocytopenic purpura. (It may also cause nonthrombocytopenic purpura.)
3. Prednisone is the drug of choice for treating idiopathic thrombocytopenic purpura (ITP), which seems the leading diagnostic possibility.
4. (a) The presence of increased megakaryocytes suggests an increase in platelet destruction rather than decreased production. Sequestration is excluded because the spleen is not large. There are no signs of accelerated coagulation, so that increased consumption is also excluded.
   The bleeding time increases linearly for platelet counts below 100,000/μL. The risk of bleeding increases similarly. However, ITP patients have shorter bleeding times for their degree of thrombopenia, apparently because their platelets are younger and more efficient. (b) Counts below 20,000/μL usually cause increased bleeding risk, regardless of mechanism.
5. The best test of the patient's platelets is a stress such as surgery. In retrospect, the patient's thrombocytopenia should have been corrected before surgery.
6. Prednisone was ineffective in inducing remission.
7. Splenectomy.
8. (a) The destructive process is interrupted. (b) Because production was increased over normal, we may expect the counts to overshoot.
9. Idiopathic (immune) thrombocytopenic purpura.
10. Immunosuppressive drugs would have been the next choice of treatment.
11. Stopping any suspicious drug is the first step in treating ITP. The traditional view is that corticosteroids act by interfering with macrophage immune adherence and phagocytosis. The likely pathway is downregulation of Fc receptors.
    Successful splenectomy removes the bulk of phagocytic cells and increases the life span of platelets. If splenectomy fails, labeled platelets are found in the liver. In this setting, splenectomy probably fails because the antibody density on the platelets was high enough to permit the liver, which is

much less efficient than the spleen at antibody detection and cell killing, to phagocytize platelets, so that destruction of platelets continues in the absence of the spleen. Note the parallels between ITP and autoimmune hemolytic anemia.

When splenectomy fails, immunosuppressive drugs designed to interfere with antibody synthesis are used.

Fibrin Clot Formation

Eliot C. Williams

CHAPTER 17

OUTLINE

OBJECTIVES

- Understand how various kinds of proteins interact in the coagulation cascade.
- Distinguish between the intrinsic and extrinsic systems and the tests used to assay them.
- Explain how the intrinsic and extrinsic systems are believed to interact in vivo.
- Know the roles of factors VIII and IX and the diseases caused by their deficiencies.
- Know the importance of tissue factor.
- Describe the role of platelets in the five-part reactions.
- Know the heparin cofactor.
- Know four mechanisms that prevent propagation of clotting.
- Know the importance of vitamin K for clotting.
- Know how coumarins cause anticoagulation.
- Know the importance of the protein C pathway.
- Know the physiologic importance of fibrinolysis.
- Know how plasminogen is activated in vivo.
- Know the clinical significance of fibrin degradation products.

To stop bleeding, a blood clot must form rapidly in the area of injury. At the same time, the clotting process must be limited to the site of injury. **Fibrinolysis** (degradation of the clot) is essential to wound healing, but it must not weaken the clot during the early stages of hemostasis or lyse the clot so rapidly that more bleeding occurs. Thus, clot formation and lysis are in a biochemical tug of war among several opposing forces, which must be exactly balanced to avoid bleeding or thrombosis. In the previous chapter, we considered why blood does not clot under normal conditions and how platelets initiate clotting. In this chapter, we will discuss the formation of the fibrin mesh, how fibrin formation is accelerated, what confines the clot to the site of injury, and how the clot is resorbed.

OVERVIEW

The fibrin clot is a protein mesh that forms in and around the platelet plug in about 5 minutes. Fibrin formation is the result of a series of linked enzymatic reactions (the coagulation cascade) that lead to the formation of **thrombin**. Thrombin is a serine protease that generates fibrin by cleavage of its precursor, **fibrinogen**. Fibrinolysis, on the other hand, requires formation of **plasmin**, another serine protease, which degrades fibrin. Fibrin formation and fibrinolysis involve a number of plasma proteins (Table 17-1). Most of these proteins are made by the liver. The most important exceptions are factor VIII, which may be made at other sites in addition to the liver; von Willebrand factor (discussed in Chapter 16), which is made by endothelial cells; and fibronectin, which is made by many cell types. Plasma proteins can be categorized as:

- Enzymes or proenzymes (zymogens), most of which activate or inactivate other proteins by proteolytic cleavage
- Helper or binding proteins, which bring reactants together
- Structural proteins, which form the substance of the clot or mediate adhesion of platelets or other cells to the clot
- Protease inhibitors, which neutralize active enzymes

THE COAGULATION CASCADE

Y Diagram

The coagulation cascade is usually depicted as two intersecting pathways—the intrinsic, starting with factor XII, and the extrinsic, starting with factor VII (Fig. 17-1A). This "Y-diagram" is an accurate description of how coagulation proceeds under laboratory conditions and thus is a valuable device for analyzing factors tested in vitro in the prothrombin time (PT) and partial thromboplastin time (PTT). PT is sensitive to deficiencies of factors VII, X, V, II, and I (fibrinogen). PTT is sensitive to deficiencies of prekallikrein, high-molecular-weight kininogen, and factors XII, XI, IX, VIII, X, V, II, and I (fibrinogen).

Physiologic Pathways

The Y diagram does not explain some important clinical observations. For example, the diagram suggests that deficiency of factor XII or other contact factors should lead to bleeding, as deficiencies of factor IX or VIII (lacking in patients with sex-linked hemophilia) do. But patients deficient in factor XII do not bleed abnormally. Recent advances in our understanding of coagulation provide an explanation for this puzzle. This explanation requires that we concentrate on the pathways that are initiated by tissue factor.

TABLE 17-1. Clotting and Fibrinolytic Proteins

Proteins	Size (kd)	Concentration* mg/dL (μM)	Kind of Protein†	Functions
Fibrinogen (factor I)	340	300 (9)	S	Forms the clot after proteolysis by thrombin (IIa)
Factor II	72.5	10 (1)	KZ	Activates I, V, VIII, XIII, platelets, and protein C
Factor V	350	2 (0.5)	H	Supports Xa activation of II
Factor VII	50	0.1 (0.02)	KZ, E	Activates IX and X
Factor VIII	350	0.1 (0.01)	H	Supports IXa activation of X
Factor IX	57	1 (0.2)	KZ	Activates X
Factor X	59	1 (0.2)	KZ	Activates II
Factor XI	160	0.5 (0.03)	Z	Activates XII and IX
Factor XII	75	2 (0.2)	Z	Activates XI and prekallikrein
Factor XIII, α subunit	80	2 (0.2)	Z	Covalently cross-links fibrin and other proteins
Factor XIII, β subunit	80	2 (0.2)	B	Binds α subunit of XIII
Von Willebrand factor	800	2 (0.05)	S, B	Binds factor VIII and collagen, mediates platelet adhesion
Prekallikrein and high-molecular-weight kininogen (HMWK)	88	2 (0.3)	Z	Activates XII plasminogen, cleaves HMWK
Plasminogen	85	10 (1.2)	Z	Lyses fibrin and other proteins
Fibronectin	400	40 (1)	S	Mediates cell adhesion, cross-links to fibrin
Protein C	62	0.4 (0.06)	KZ	Inactivates factors V and VIII
Protein S	80	3 (0.4)	KZ	Cofactor for activated protein C
α_2-Antithrombin	60	20 (3)	I	Heparin cofactor, inhibits IIa, IX, and other proteases
α_2-Antiplasmin	67	3 (0.5)	I	Inhibits Xa plasmin, cross-links to fibrin
TFPI	33	0.1 (0.003)	I	Inhibits VIIa and Xa

B, binding protein; E, active enzyme; H, helper protein; I, protease inhibitor; KZ, vitamin K-dependent zymogen; S, structural protein; TFPI, tissue factor protein inhibitor; Z, zymogen.
*For comparison, the concentration of albumin in plasma is 3500 mg/dL or 510 mM.
†For the proteins that are zymogens, the function after activation is given.

INITIATION AND PROPAGATION OF COAGULATION

Tissue Factor

In vivo coagulation is triggered when blood escapes from a vessel and encounters a lipoprotein called tissue factor. Tissue factor is a component of most cell membranes; the highest concentrations are found in brain, gut, and skin. It forms a hemostatic envelope or coat, having the greatest potential for activating coagulation in those tissues in which bleeding is most likely or could do the greatest harm. As expected, endothelial cells do not normally express tissue factor on their luminal surfaces, although they can be induced to do so in special conditions such as severe infection. Monocytes also express tissue factor when exposed to certain inflammatory cytokines.

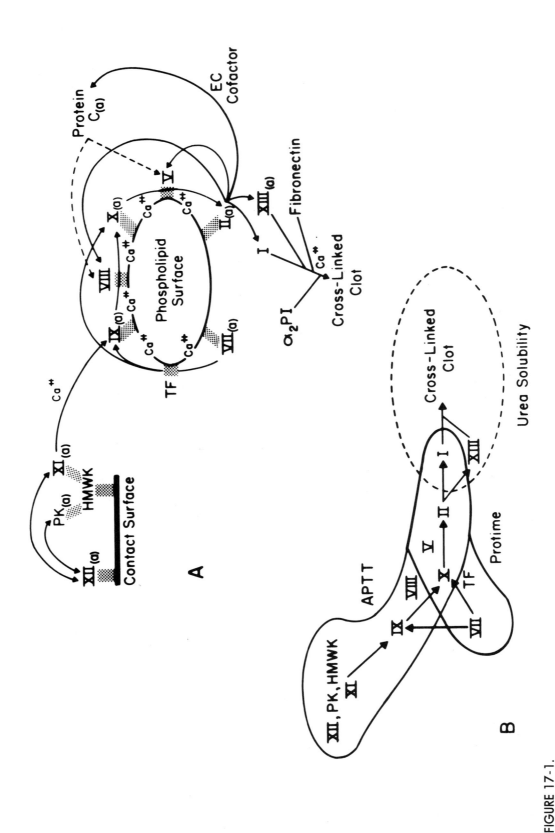

FIGURE 17-1.

Diagrams of interactions among coagulation factors. The top diagram is organized around the contact surface and the phospholipid surface. The bottom diagram (Y diagram) is organized around the three screening tests—activated partial thromboplastin time, prothrombin time and clot solubility tests. Solid arrows indicate activation. Broken arrows indicate inactivation. The stippled patches indicate binding of proteins to surfaces or to each other. The subscript (a) indicates proteins that are zymogens and can be converted to activate enzymes. Protime, prothrombin time; PK, prekallikrein; HMWK, high-molecular-weight kininogen; TF, tissue factor; α_2PI, α_2-plasmin inhibitor; EC cofactor, endothelial cell cofactor (thrombomodulin); APTT, activated partial thromboplastin time.

Propagation of Clotting Reaction

Exposure of blood to tissue factor starts a chain reaction of four enzymatic reactions. Each is characterized by the following features:

- A proteolytic enzyme generates a second enzyme by proteolytic cleavage of the proenzyme. The proenzymes are designated by Roman numerals: II (prothrombin), VII, IX, and X. The respective active forms (enzymes) are IIa (thrombin), VIIa, IXa, and Xa. (The numbers do not reflect the sequence of the reactions, but the order in which these proteins were discovered.)
- The reactions take place on a phospholipid surface, such as the platelet membrane. Binding of the enzyme and its proenzyme substrate to the membrane requires the presence of γ-carboxyglutamyl residues on both proteins. These residues bind calcium ions, resulting in a change in conformation of the protein that promotes membrane binding (Fig. 17-2).
- Each reaction requires the presence on the membrane of a third, helper, protein, which brings the enzyme and substrate proenzyme together. The three helper proteins are tissue factor, factor V, and factor VIII. Factors V and VIII are activated by trace amounts of thrombin or Xa, but tissue factor does not require activation.

The first reaction in the sequence is the cleavage of factor X (proenzyme) by factor VIIa (protease) and tissue factor (helper) to form factor Xa. Factor VII is unique among the clotting factors in that it possesses some intrinsic enzymatic

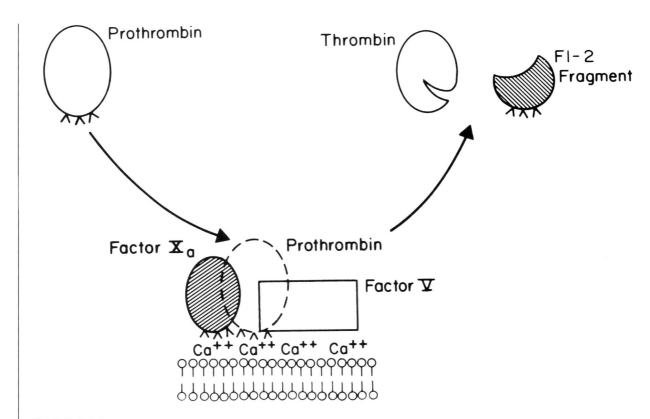

FIGURE 17-2.
Activation of prothrombin in a five-part complex. Prothrombin binds to the phospholipid surface to which factor Xa and V are bound. Prothrombin is cleaved, generating thrombin and fragment F1-2.

activity. This activity is greatly enhanced during the clotting sequence by cleavage to factor VIIa, which occurs as the result of a feedback loop involving factor Xa.

(1) VII (TF) + X → Xa [weak reaction]
Xa + VII → VIIa [feedback loop]
VIIa (TF) + X → Xa [strong reaction]

where TF = tissue factor.

The second reaction, which occurs in parallel with the first, is the cleavage of factor IX to IXa. This is also mediated by factor VIIa with tissue factor as helper. Note that this reaction is not included in the traditional Y diagram.

(2) VIIa (TF) + IX → IXa

The third reaction is the cleavage of factor X to Xa by factor IXa and its helper, factor VIIIa. Reactions (2) and (3) are critical to sustaining the clotting sequence, since the tissue factor-factor VIIa complex is inhibited quickly (see Propagation of Clotting Reaction), before it can generate much Xa. Reaction (3) is also the most efficient of all the reactions in the clotting cascade. These factors explain the importance of factors VIII and IX in the clotting process. Reaction (3) is augmented by a positive feedback loop whereby Xa activates VIII.

(3) IXa (VIIIa) + X → Xa
Xa + VIII → VIIIa (feedback loop)

The fourth reaction is the conversion of factor II (prothrombin) to IIa (thrombin) by factor Xa and its helper Va. Minute amounts of thrombin activate V and VIII to Va and VIIIa.

(4) Xa (Va) + II → IIa

This sequence can be likened to a controlled explosion: In this analogy, tissue factor is the "match" that ignites the process, and the IXa-VIIIa complex is the "fuse" that keeps it going, leading to the explosive, but contained, generation of thrombin.

FORMATION AND STABILIZATION OF THE FIBRIN CLOT

Fibrin Polymerization

Once formed, thrombin leaves the membrane surface. It converts fibrinogen (Fig. 17-3) to fibrin by cleavage of two pairs of peptide bonds near the N termini of the Aa and Bb chains of fibrinogen (marked α_N, β_N on the diagram), generating fibrin and two copies each of the small peptides, fibrinopeptides A and B. The reaction is very rapid.

Fibrinogen is by far the most abundant coagulation protein in the blood. It is a large elongated protein that consists of three globular domains, a central E nodule and two peripheral D nodules, linked by α-helical regions. Cleavage by thrombin of the fibrinopeptides, which have a strong negative charge, generates positively charged sites on the E nodule. These then associate with negatively charged sites on D nodules of other fibrin molecules, resulting in polymer formation (Fig. 17-4). The initial polymer contains a double chain of fibrin monomers (the **protofibril**). This protofibril then can participate in several other types of

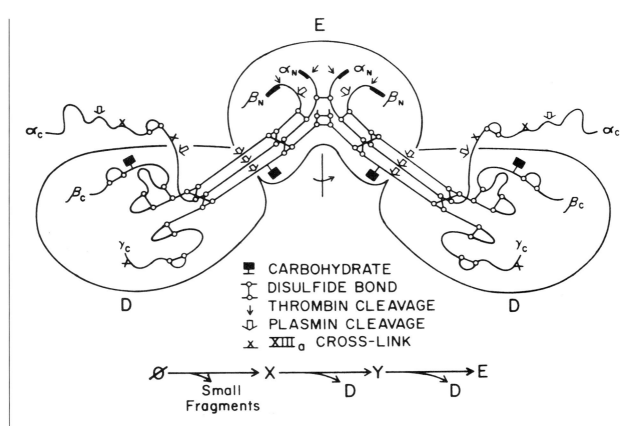

FIGURE 17-3.

The six chains of fibrinogen. Fibrinogen is seen in the electron microscope as a central nodule (E domain) and two peripheral nodules (D domains). One set of nonidentical chains, α, β, and γ, runs through half of the molecule and is bound to the other set by disulfide bonds in the E domain, where the amino termini of all six chains come together. The strands connecting the peripheral nodules to the central nodule contain all three chains, probably in an α-helical configuration. The carboxy-terminal regions of the three chains constitute the globular D domains. The end of the α chain extends out of the D domain as a coil. Thrombin releases fibrinopeptides A and B from the E domain (*small arrows*) to yield fibrin; plasmin cleaves the molecule between E and D (*wide arrows*).

fibrin-fibrin associations, which result in extensive branching so that the mature fibrin clot consists of thick fibrils arranged in a complex mesh.

Cross-linking of Fibrin

Fibrin polymerization is the product of ionic, noncovalent interactions among fibrin monomers. As fibrin polymerizes, however, covalent bonds that link the monomers also form very rapidly. This process is catalyzed by an enzyme called factor XIIIa. Factor XIII, like most other coagulation enzymes, circulates as an inactive precursor that is converted to the active form by thrombin. Factor XIIIa is a transglutaminase that causes formation of amide bonds between specific glutaminyl residues in fibrin and the ϵ-amino group of specific lysyl groups in a second fibrin molecule (Fig. 17-4), linking the two protofibrils together. This cross-linking process strengthens and stabilizes the clot.

Attachment of Fibronectin and α_2-Antiplasmin

In addition to cross-linking fibrin monomers together, factor XIIIa also cross-links at least two other molecules to the clot: fibronectin and α_2-antiplasmin.

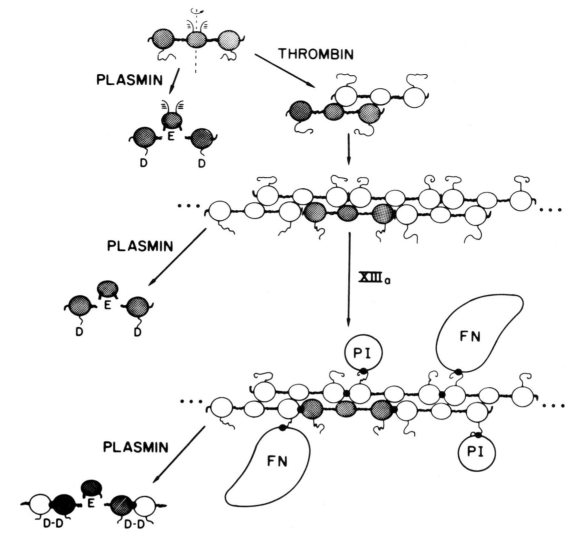

FIGURE 17-4.
Activation, assembly, cross-linking, and lysis of fibrinogen and fibrin. Both fibrinogen and fibrin are trinodular proteins. Clotting is initiated by release of the negatively charged fibrinopeptides from the E domain. Assembly is driven by noncovalent E–D interactions. XIII cross-links between γ chains and also attaches α_2-plasmin inhibitor and fibronectin to the α chain. Plasmin cleaves this portion of the α chain and separates the D and E nodules. PI, α_2-plasmin inhibitor.

Fibronectin is an adhesive protein that promotes the ingrowth of fibroblasts necessary for wound healing, whereas α_2-antiplasmin protects the clot from proteolysis by plasmin.

ROLE OF THE CONTACT SYSTEM (INTRINSIC PATHWAY)

Factors XII, XI, High-Molecular-Weight Kininogen, and Prekallikrein

Contact with foreign surfaces can start blood clotting in the absence of tissue factor. For example, blood clots spontaneously when placed in a glass tube. Clotting is initiated by four proteins known as contact factors: high-molecular-weight kininogen (HMWK), factor XII, prekallikrein (PK), and factor XI (Fig. 17-1A). When blood is exposed to a negatively charged surface (e.g., glass), HMWK and factor XII bind to the surface. HMWK then binds two other proteins, PK and factor XI. PK, HMWK, and factor XII undergo a series of reciprocal proteolytic cleavages that result in the formation of bradykinin, kallikrein and factor XIa. Factor XIa activates factor IX, which then leads to thrombin generation and fibrin formation as already described (Fig. 17-1). Thrombin also can activate factor XI, so it is possible that the physiologic function of factor XI is to participate in a positive feedback loop in which thrombin generates XIa, which in turn leads to further thrombin formation by activating factor IX.

Physiologic Significance

The role of the intrinsic pathway is uncertain, but it may initiate several wound-related processes. The pathway is known to be activated by contact of blood with negatively charged glycosaminoglycans found in connective tissue. Since complete congenital deficiency of PK, HMWK, or factor XII causes no apparent bleeding tendency (or other illness), this pathway appears to play at most a minor role in normal hemostasis. In contrast, deficiency of XI causes mild to moderate tendency to hemorrhage, confirming that its role in coagulation is independent of the other contact factors.

Kallikrein is a plasminogen activator and therefore can initiate fibrinolysis. Activated plasminogen can activate complement factors. Bradykinin plays a role in inflammation (pain and vascular dilation). Thus, the contact factors sit in a pivotal position where they may activate any of four processes: fibrinolysis, the complement pathway, kinins, or clotting.

REGULATION OF FIBRIN FORMATION

The coagulation cascade is an exquisitely regulated system. Two types of regulation have been defined: those that speed fibrin formation in an area of vascular injury and those that restrict coagulation to the injured area and turn off the clotting process once its mission has been accomplished. A working knowledge of these regulatory mechanisms is essential to understanding the clinical problems (bleeding or thrombosis) that may result when they fail to function normally.

Mechanisms that Enhance Fibrin Formation

The Cascade Effect

Each enzyme in the pathway creates many copies of the next enzyme in the sequence. For example, the molar concentration of prothrombin is 50 times greater than that of factor VII. Thus, beginning with a very small amount of tissue factor-VIIa complex, a large amount of thrombin is generated. It has been estimated that each step in the cascade may speed the rate of the overall reaction by as much as 100 times.

Catalysis by Platelet Membranes

Platelets accumulating at the injury site spread out to provide a large phospholipid surface on which the coagulation sequence can proceed. Platelet membranes have specific receptors that bind factors VIII and V.

Positive Feedback Loops

Factor Xa and thrombin can both promote their own formation. Factor Xa does this by converting factor VII to the more active VIIa; thrombin does so by activating factors VIII, V, and possibly XI.

Mechanisms that Localize and Restrict Fibrin Formation

Requirement for Platelet Membranes

Away from the area of injury where platelets are not adherent and activated, phospholipid support for the clotting cascade is limited.

Ability of Intact Endothelium to Inhibit Coagulation

Four endothelial cell products inhibit the coagulation process:

- **Prostaglandin I$_2$** inhibits platelet aggregation
- **Heparan sulfate** catalyzes inhibition of thrombin by antithrombin.
- **Thrombomodulin** favors activation of protein C by thrombin.
- **Nitric oxide** acts synergistically with prostaglandin I$_2$ as a vasodilator and an inhibitor of platelet aggregation.

Prostaglandin I$_2$ (also called prostacyclin) is synthesized by endothelial cell cyclooxygenase and secreted; heparan sulfate and thrombomodulin are expressed on the luminal surface of the endothelium. Nitric oxide is synthesized by endothelial cells (via oxidation of L-arginine) and secreted.

The Protein C Pathway

As shown in reaction 5, in the presence of endothelial cell thrombomodulin (TM), enzymatic activity of thrombin (IIa) is diverted to activate protein C (PC).

$$(5) \quad IIa\ (TM) + PC \rightarrow APC$$

As shown in reactions (6), activated protein C (APC) in the presence of protein S (S) inactivates factors Va and VIIIa.

$$(6) \quad APC(S) + Va \rightarrow Vi$$
$$APC(S) + VIIIa \rightarrow VIIIi$$

This is a powerful anticoagulant pathway because the two helper factors required for propagation of the coagulation cascade are destroyed. See also Figure 17-1B (4).

Inhibition of Tissue Factor-Factor VIIa

This reaction requires a plasma protein called **tissue factor pathway inhibitor**. This inhibitor binds factor Xa, forming a complex that binds to and irreversibly inhibits the tissue factor-factor VII complex (Fig. 17-1B). Thus, factor Xa initiates a negative feedback loop (as well as a positive one as previously described) extinguishing the "match" (tissue factor-factor VIIa) that ignites clot formation.

The fuse (factor IXa-VIIIa complex) keeps burning, however, generating more factor Xa until factor IXa is neutralized by antithrombin and VIIIa is destroyed by activated protein C.

THE ROLE OF VITAMIN K

To bind to the platelet membrane or other phospholipid surface, factors II, VII, IX, and X and proteins C and S must possess several γ-carboxyglutamyl residues. Conversion of glutamyl to γ-carboxyglutamyl residues is catalyzed by a liver enzyme, carboxylase. Vitamin K is an essential cofactor for this reaction. If vitamin K is limited or its action blocked by the anticoagulant drug warfarin (Coumadin), synthesis of these factors is decreased. The result of vitamin K deficiency or warfarin therapy is in most instances to make blood less coagulable because the activity of factors II, VII, IX, and X is decreased.

CONSEQUENCES OF CLOTTING FACTOR DEFICIENCY

Recessive Inheritance

Decreased blood level of a single procoagulant factor does not usually produce abnormal bleeding until the level drops below about 30% of normal. If we consider inherited factor deficiencies, a single normal gene will sustain blood levels of that factor at about 50% of normal. If values of other clotting factors are normal, no bleeding tendency exists. Most congenital factor deficiencies therefore cause symptoms only when both loci are affected, as a homozygous or mixed heterozygous deficiency. Such individuals are very rare. The exception to this rule is factor XI deficiency, for which there are three relatively common mutations (4.3% of factor XI genes are estimated to be mutant) in the Ashkenazi Jewish population.

Sex-Linked Inheritance

The most common deficiencies by far of clotting factors are those of factors VIII and IX (hemophilia A and B, respectively). Genes for these factors are on the X chromosome, so that the affected male patient has little or no factor VIII or IX. A large number of genetic defects, including large deletions, frameshift mutations, and point mutations have been described. Thus, these diseases, like the thalassemias and hemoglobinopathies, are genetically heterogeneous.

Deficiency of Several Factors

An exception to the rule that levels of coagulation factors must be lower than 30% to cause symptoms occurs when several clotting factor levels are low, as in liver disease or during warfarin treatment. When several factors are deficient, the effects are additive, so that a moderate or severe bleeding tendency results. Clinical details of clotting factor deficiency are given in Chapter 18.

Deficiency of Anticoagulant Proteins

Deficiency of any of the proteins that are anticoagulant, such as antithrombin, protein C or protein S, may result in a hypercoagulable state. In cases of inherited deficiency, this state may occur at blood levels lower than about 60% of normal, and so heterozygous deficiency may cause a thrombotic tendency (hypercoagulable state). The hypercoagulability is manifested by venous thrombosis at an early age (<40 years), repeated episodes of venous thrombosis, and thrombosis in unusual places (e.g., portal vein, sagittal sinus). A sizable percentage of the population (~5%) has a single-base polymorphism, which changes an arginine in factor V exactly where factor V is cleaved by APC. These people have "APC resistance"; their factor V is resistant to inactivation by APC. The risk of thrombosis in people who have both heterozygous deficiency of antithrombin, protein C, or protein S and the factor V mutation is greater than the risk in people having the deficiency state or the factor V mutation alone. This demonstration of how two genes can determine susceptibility to disease is an outstanding example of the general phenomenon of multigenic risk factors, which is likely to dominate future thinking about disorders such as hypertension, asthma, cancer, and atherosclerosis.

FIBRINOLYSIS

Plasminogen Activators

For a wound to heal properly, the fibrin clot must be broken down and replaced by connective tissue. Any fibrin that forms outside the wound must also be removed. Degradation of fibrin is caused by **plasmin**. Plasmin is a serine protease derived from the proenzyme plasminogen. Plasminogen may be converted to plasmin by one of several plasminogen activators (Table 17-2). The most important of these are tissue plasminogen activator (TPA) and urokinase (UK). Fibrinolysis in tissues is started by both TPA (made by endothelial cells) and UK produced by fibroblasts and many other cells. Most of the plasminogen activator activity that finds its way into the blood (and may be responsible for intravascular fibrinolysis) is TPA.

Fibrin Degradation Products

Plasmin cleaves fibrin in several places (Fig. 17-4), but the D and E nodules themselves are not degraded, so that complete digestion of a cross-linked clot yields E nodules and cross-linked D dimers. These fragments, as well as larger fragments resulting from incomplete clot lysis are known as fibrin degradation products. They can been measured in blood during episodes of thrombosis or in other conditions in which there is a significant activation of the fibrinolytic system.

Regulation of Fibrinolysis

Biologic Factors

Several mechanisms ensure that fibrinolysis proceeds at a controlled rate and that the fibrinolytic process remains confined to the area of the clot. TPA activates plasminogen much more efficiently when it is bound to fibrin, so that most plasmin is formed directly on the clot. The major inhibitor of plasmin is

TABLE 17-2. Activators of Plasminogen

Activator	Source	Characteristics
Tissue plasminogen	Vessel wall, most cells	Activates proteolytic plasminogen cleavage; binds to fibrin; activator activates plasminogen much better when both activator and plasminogen are bound to fibrin
Urokinase	Urine, kidney, most cells	Activates plasminogen in solution by proteolytic cleavage
Streptokinase	Streptococcus	Activates plasminogen in solution by forming 1:1 complex with plasminogen; the complex then can activate further plasminogen by proteolytic cleavage

α_2-antiplasmin; this protein is cross-linked to fibrin by factor XIII (see Role of the Contact System), helping to ensure that clot breakdown does not occur too rapidly. α_2-Antiplasmin also rapidly inactivates any plasmin that escapes into the blood. Any TPA or UK secreted in the blood is rapidly inhibited by circulating plasminogen activator inhibitors.

Pharmacologic Control of Fibrinolysis

Three plasminogen activators, TPA, UK, and the bacterial protein streptokinase are available to promote lysis of acute arterial or venous thromboses (Table 17-2). They are given intravenously to limit ischemic tissue damage due to vascular obstruction, as in myocardial infarction due to coronary thrombosis. Their use may cause bleeding, since they can overwhelm plasma fibrinolysis inhibitors and cause widespread activation of fibrinolysis and rapid clot lysis.

ε-Aminocaproic acid and transexamic acid are synthetic fibrinolysis inhibitors. These agents delay clot lysis by binding to a single site on plasminogen, preventing it from binding to fibrin. The agents are used to prevent minor bleeding in patients with defective hemostasis (hemophiliacs and thrombocytopenic patients) whose clots are small and weak.

Clinical Consequences of Abnormal Fibrinolysis

Accelerated fibrinolysis is seen in a variety of disorders, including disseminated intravascular coagulation (Chapter 18) and the administration of fibrinolytic drugs, and may cause severe hemorrhage. Diminished fibrinolysis, on the other hand, occurs in patients receiving fibrinolysis inhibitors, and may increase the risk of thrombosis.

SUMMARY POINTS

The task of the liquid phase of normal coagulation is to produce a fibrin clot around the platelet plug. This involves a cascade of amplifying enzyme reactions assisted by helper proteins and phospholipid surfaces, which takes about 5 minutes to complete. Elaborate controls accelerate and then extinguish the reaction, preventing it from being propagated throughout the vascular system. The fibrin clot is degraded by proteolysis as part of the tissue repair process. Failure of the system is demonstrated by tissue and joint bleeding.

SUGGESTED READING

Furie B, Furie BC. Molecular basis of hemophilia. *Semin Hematol* 27:270–285.
Mosesson MW. Fibrin polymerization and its regulatory role in hemostasis. *J Lab Clin Med* 116:8.

CASE DEVELOPMENT PROBLEMS: CHAPTER 17

Problem I*

History: A 72-year-old retired security guard with a long history of hypertension and congestive heart failure was admitted with a 1-week history of easy bruising and difficulty moving his elbow. He had bumped his elbow 1 week before admission and shortly thereafter noted bruising and swelling. He also noted a bruise on his thigh. When he saw a lump in his neck, he squeezed it, and it

---

* Some aspects of these problems are better understood after you read Chapter 18.

became much larger. He had no previous bleeding. The patient had stopped taking warfarin 4 weeks before admission. The drug had been given to prevent embolus from atrial fibrillation.

Physical examination: Found were 3 × 5 cm ecchymosis on the patient's neck, purpura on his arm, a tender mass on the radial aspect of his forearm, and limited movement of the arm. He had a large ecchymosis on the right thigh, no evidence of bleeding from mucous membranes, and no petechiae.

1. (a) From the patient's history, determine what possibilities are included and excluded? (b) From the pattern of bleeding, what are the diagnostic possibilities?

Laboratory data: HCT 35%, WBC 8600/μL, platelets 232,000/μL, PT 12 seconds, PTT 49.5 seconds. (normal, 20 to 32), fibrinogen 460 mg/dL. Bleeding time was 8 minutes. Fibrin degradation products were >40 (normal <10).

2. From the laboratory data, determine the diagnostic possibilities.
   The patient left the hospital against medical advice. He returned 10 days later with a 2 × 4 cm mass in his right thigh with extensive ecchymosis and weakness of the leg. He also had ecchymoses over the buttocks, and the neck ecchymosis was larger.
3. What additional laboratory studies would you recommend?
   The patient was treated with cyclophosphamide 100 mg/day and prednisone 60 mg/day. The following data were collected over the next 3 months in the outpatient clinic.
4. What treatment could be given?

	PTT	Comments
9/1	54	Cyclophosphamide 100, prednisone 60
9/7	50	
9/11	49	Taper prednisone
9/18	44	
10/2	38	
10/12	38	
10/19		Admitted for gastrointestinal bleeding; HCT dropped from 35% to 30%; no bleeding site found.
10/26	33	
11/16	31	Stop cyclophosphamide
12/21	26.6	Reduce prednisone to 15 mg every other day

5. What explanation can you offer for this therapy?

Problem II

History: An 8-year-old boy was referred in 1997 by a dentist. The dentist was about to administer nerve blocks before drilling and filling when he elicited a history of easy bruising. Birth and the immediate postpartum period were uneventful. Developmental milestones were normal. The boy's mother could remember at least eight episodes between ages 2 and 6 when the patient developed large bruises after trauma, including one instance in which he bled into his left knee. A brother died at age $1^1/_2$ years from intracranial hemorrhage after falling from a crib. (A detailed family history is diagrammed in Figure 17-5.)

Physical examination: Abnormal findings included dental caries and thickening of the left knee with loss of patellar motion.

Laboratory data: Blood counts, chemistry survey and urinalysis were normal. The platelet count was 280,000/μL, PTT, 58 seconds (normal <30), and PT 12.0 seconds (normal <13.0 seconds). Bleeding time was 7.5 minutes (upper limit of normal).

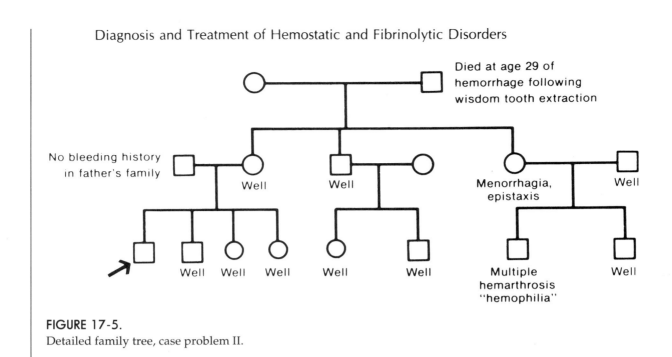

Diagnosis and Treatment of Hemostatic and Fibrinolytic Disorders

Died at age 29 of hemorrhage following wisdom tooth extraction

No bleeding history in father's family

Well

Well

Menorrhagia, epistaxis

Well

Well   Well   Well   Well   Well   Multiple   Well
                                        hemarthrosis
                                        "hemophilia"

FIGURE 17-5.
Detailed family tree, case problem II.

1. (a) What factors are likely to be deficient? (b) How would you choose between them?
   The patient's plasma mixed with normal plasma: PTT, 32 seconds. The patient's plasma mixed with Factor IX-deficient plasma: PTT 34 seconds. The patient's plasma mixed with Factor VIII-deficient plasma: PTT 55 seconds. The calculated level of the deficient clotting factor was less than 1%.
2. How should the patient be treated before dental work and in the future? Appropriate treatment was given.
3. (a) What treatment program would you offer the patient? (b) How and where should it be administered? (c) What complications of treatment might occur?
4. What activities would you advise this patient against?
   Despite medications and frequent medical attention, during the next 15 years the patient developed arthritis of elbows, wrists, hips, knees, and ankles. He required a long-leg left leg brace, crutches, and a wheelchair for mobility. He was unable to rest his left heel on the ground; both elbows had restricted movement. He developed a "claw hand" deformity.
5. (a) What is the pathogenesis of the patient's arthritis? (b) What is the cause of the claw hand?
   At the age of 15 he developed nausea, weakness, jaundice, and right upper quadrant pain. He was sick for 6 weeks.
6. (a) What disease do you suspect? (b) What other diseases is the patient likely to acquire?
   With an average of two exacerbations a month, he needed frequent pain medication. Acetaminophen with codeine was prescribed, but he frequently received meperidine and morphine in the emergency room. He also used street drugs and alcohol. With the help of Alcoholics Anonymous and rehabilitation programs, he broke out of the addictive pattern.
7. Could this problem have been prevented?
   At age 26, this patient noted that his treatment of exacerbations did not stop the bleeding. The laboratory found that a mixture of his plasma with normal plasma now gave a PTT of 58 seconds.
8. (a) What has caused this new development? (b) What can be done now?

CASE DEVELOPMENT ANSWERS

Problem I

1. (a) Since the onset is late in life, it is an acquired disease. Warfarin was recently used, so we must think of its duration of action and other drugs as well. (b) Looking at the distribution of the bleeding, factor deficiencies are more likely than thrombocytopenia. Von Willebrand disease seems less likely because there is no mucosal bleeding.

2. The long PTT and normal PT point to the intrinsic pathway and exclude warfarin as the explanation. The normal fibrinogen and platelets exclude disseminated vascular coagulation, and the elevated fibrin degradation products may be related to the large amount of subcutaneous bleeding.

3. Mixing studies. Mixing the patient's plasma with normal plasma 1-1 did not correct the PTT. Hence, an inhibitor was present. Subsequent studies demonstrated that the inhibitor was directed against factor VIII and he had 24 Bethesda Units of VIII antibody, that is, 1 mL of patient plasma neutralized factor VIII in 24 mL of normal plasma.

4. The clinical course precluded delay in treatment. Factor VIII replacement was unrealistic. Cytoxan and prednisone should be given.

5. An antibody against factor VIII was suppressed by chemotherapy over a 3-month period.
   The patient did not relapse and died of heart failure 1 year later.

Problem II

1. (a) Hemophilia A (factor VIII deficiency) or B (factor IX deficiency) are most likely based on the family history. (b) The mixing studies show that the PTT is long because the plasma lacks a factor rather than because it contains an inhibitor. They also identify which factor is lacking. Quantitative factor VIII assay (i.e., assaying the ability of the patient's plasma to correct the PTT of plasma of someone with known severe hemophilia A) revealed that the patient has 1% of the normal level of factor VIII. Factor VIII-related antigen (i.e., von Willebrand factor) also was measured and found to be 110% of normal.

2. The patient should receive intravenous factor VIII concentrate prophylactically if deep tissue injections of anesthetic are required for dentistry.

3. (a) The patient and his family should be taught about hemophilia A and encouraged to treat bleeding episodes early. (b) They should be provided with syringes and needles and factor VIII concentrate to use at home as soon as bleeding is suspected. Such treatment should minimize further damage to joints and prevent further bleeding episodes from becoming life-threatening. (c) AIDS, hepatitis B, and hepatitis C were three risks of factor VIII therapy.

4. He should not engage in sports or other physical activities in school other than walking.

5. (a) Arthritis is due to the effect of repeated bleeding into the joint. The pathogenesis is complex, but arthritis has been induced in normal dogs by repeated injection of blood into the joint space. The following mechanisms have been postulated: the generation of oxygen radicals by iron from degraded hemoglobin and the secretion of chondrolytic enzymes by macrophages activated by the products of hemoglobin breakdown. (b) The claw-hand is due to compression of the ulnar nerve by hematoma.

6. (a) The patient has acquired hepatitis B from blood products. (b) He is also susceptible to HIV, which 90% of severe hemophiliacs have acquired. Hepatitis C, human T-cell lymphotrophic virus type 1, cytomegalovirus, and Epstein-Barr virus are other possibilities.

7. Probably not. Chronic pain is difficult to manage. Physicians tend to be both too lenient and too stringent in their use of narcotics, more likely too lenient in the young person with a chronic problem and too stringent in the old person with terminal cancer.
8. (a) VIII antibody has developed. (b) This antibody can be overridden by intense VIII treatment, bypassed by IX infusion, mitigated by DDAVP (desmopressin) use and possibly negated by cyclophosphamide and prednisone.

Diagnosis and Treatment of Hemostatic Disorders

Deane F. Mosher

CHAPTER 18

OUTLINE

OBJECTIVES

- Know the three components of hemostasis and how defects in two of the three result in bleeding.
- Review the inheritance of different familial disorders.
- Know how the prothrombin time and partial thromboplastin time are done and what each measures. Know when fibrinogen and fibrin degradation products assays should be done.
- Know the most common inherited factor deficiency and how it is treated.
- Know the definition of a hypercoagulable state.
- Understand the paradox of disseminated intravascular coagulation and the rationale for use of heparin in patients with this condition.
- Above all, understand how heparin and warfarin work and how administration of these drugs is controlled.

HISTORY AND PHYSICAL EXAMINATION

A personal history, family history, and physical examination are important parts of the evaluation of a person with bleeding or clotting or a patient going to surgery. If the laboratory work is negative and the history is positive for bleeding or clotting, the history should be believed. From the history, one can often distinguish abnormalities of the vascular/platelet phase from abnormalities of the soluble phase of clotting. Disorders of platelets or blood vessels often cause purpura and mucosal or superficial bleeding; deficiency of a coagulation factor results in a tendency to form soft tissue hematomas or to suffer from repeated hemarthrosis (Fig. 18-1).

In taking a history, it is not enough to simply ask, "Do you or any of your blood relatives bleed abnormally?" You need to also determine how the hemostatic system has been stressed: "Have you had any operations or teeth extractions?" If so, "Did you bleed abnormally or require blood transfusions afterward?" "Are your menstrual periods heavy?" "Are you an active athlete?"

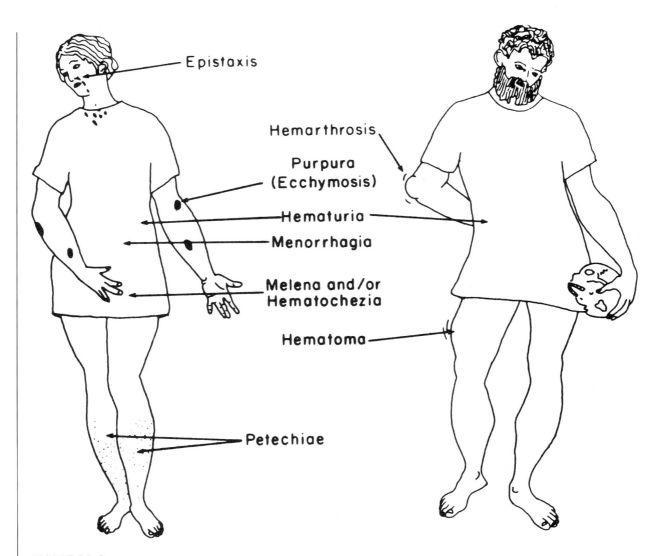

Epistaxis

Hemarthrosis

Purpura
(Ecchymosis)

Hematuria

Menorrhagia

Melena and/or
Hematochezia

Hematoma

Petechiae

FIGURE 18-1.

Patterns of bleeding in thrombocytopenia (*left*) and hemophilia (*right*). Disorders of platelets cause mucosal bleeding and petechiae in the skin. Clotting factor deficiencies cause deep tissue bleeding.

Although severe hemophiliacs with repeated hemarthroses may seem to suffer from spontaneous hemorrhage, patients usually can identify initiating events for bleeding episodes. Drugs and medications should always be listed. The time of onset is also important. A venous thrombosis in a sedentary 75-year-old has less significance than the same event in an otherwise healthy 25-year-old.

A formal family tree indicating how many family members are at risk should be constructed. Family studies are often crucial to the evaluation of a patient. For instance, a random female with a half-normal factor VIII level is probably not a carrier of hemophilia A. However, if the sister of a hemophiliac has a half-normal factor VIII level, the sister has a 95% chance of being a carrier. Therefore, a physician should try to arrange family studies even though the insurance and health care industries may put up financial barriers. The information gathered will help both patient and family members.

The physical examination is equally as important as the history. Purpura directs the observer to platelets and blood vessels. Ecchymosis suggests deficiency of one or more factors. Hemarthrosis is typical of hemophilia (factor VIII or IX deficiency). Thrombosis of a leg vein is most commonly associated with venous insufficiency, whereas thrombosis of an arm vein should be regarded with suspicion of malignancy. The sudden onset of an arterial clot in the leg suggests an embolus, whereas closure of coronary or carotid arteries is most commonly due to atherosclerosis.

The history and physical examination thus lead to the appropriate choice of laboratory tests.

SCREENING TESTS

A simple battery of tests screens for significant abnormalities of blood vessels, platelets, and the coagulation factor network.

Complete Blood Count and Smear

Red cells should be examined for schistocytes, which suggest microangiopathic hemolytic anemia. Platelets should be examined for size and evidence of granules. White cells may show dysplastic changes, suggesting dysfunction.

Platelet count and bleeding time were discussed in Chapter 16.

Partial Thromboplastin Time

The partial thromboplastin time (PTT) screens for deficiencies in the intrinsic clotting system. Contact factors (XII, XI, prekallikrein, and high-molecular-weight kininogen), and factors IX, VIII, X, V, and II are bioassayed along with fibrinogen (see Chapter 17). Practically, PTT is most useful for discovering factor VIII or IX deficiency or a circulating anticoagulant. PTT is the best test to monitor heparinized patients.

PTT is obtained by first exposing plasma to contact with foreign material such as kaolin and then recalcifying in the presence of a standardized amount of a phospholipid reagent (cephaloplastin). The normal PTT is about 20 to 35 seconds.

Prothrombin Time

The prothrombin time (PT) measures the integrity of the extrinsic clotting system, involving factors II, V, VII, and X and fibrinogen. Prolongation occurs when deficiencies of the extrinsic clotting factors occur singly or in combination. *PT is the best test to monitor patients on warfarin therapy* because factor VII has a short half-life and is sensitive to changes in warfarin dose. Prolongation also occurs in the presence of heparin therapy, but the PT is not used to follow up patients on heparin therapy, because it is relatively insensitive to the activity of heparin and because heparin is neutralized to varying degrees by different lots of thromboplastin.

PT is measured by adding an excess of tissue thromboplastin (a source of phospholipid and tissue factor) and an optimum concentration of calcium ions to citrated plasma and the clotting time (normal about 12 seconds) determined under controlled conditions.

Because of laboratory to laboratory variation in the sensitivity of the thromboplastin reagent to the effects of warfarin, PT results are converted to an international normalized ratio (INR). The INR is the ratio of the patient's sample over the normal sampled corrected for the known sensitivity of the reagent. The INR has played a crucial role in large multicenter studies that have determined optimal degree of anticoagulation in a variety of clinical situations.

Thrombin Time

Thrombin time (TT) is a test used to estimate fibrinogen concentrations. It is performed by adding bovine thrombin to citrated plasma. The normal time is adjusted to 12 seconds. If the TT is long, all other tests depending on fibrin formation (e.g., PT, PTT) are abnormal as well.

Urea Clot Solubility Screening for Factor XIII

As described in Chapter 17, factor XIII is the zymogen of a transglutaminase (factor XIIIa) and is activated by thrombin. It acts on polymerized fibrin and introduces covalent amide cross-links among adjacent molecules of fibrin. The resulting cross-linked or stabilized clot is insoluble in 6 M urea. Deficiency of factor XIII causes a bleeding disorder but will not be detected by tests like the PTT and activated PTT, which depend on rate of fibrin formation. Factor XIII deficiency is a rare disease, and the test is not routinely performed.

EVALUATION OF PLATELET/ VASCULAR-TYPE BLEEDING

Much of the understanding of bleeding disorders is based on the bleeding time—time to cessation of bleeding after a standardized cut [Fig. 18-2].

A long bleeding time in a person with a normal platelet count may be due to abnormal blood vessels, abnormally functioning platelets, or lack of von Willebrand factor. Complete lack of circulating fibrinogen (a cofactor for platelet aggregation) also causes a long bleeding time. Lack of one of the other clotting factors usually does not cause a long bleeding time. Specifically, hemophiliacs have a normal bleeding time.

Abnormal blood vessels can cause prolonged bleeding time in congenital connective tissue disorders (e.g., Ehlers-Danlos syndrome) and vasculitis (e.g., Henoch-Shönlein purpura, drug purpura). Such disorders are usually apparent by history and physical examination. Lack of ascorbic acid (scurvy) causes underhydroxylation of collagen and is associated with small perifollicular hemorrhages and a long bleeding time.

There are a number of clinical situations in which the platelet count is satisfactory but platelet function is compromised. Examples include platelets that have been circulating for several hours in a heart-lung oxygenator; platelets of patients with myeloproliferative or myelodysplastic syndromes; and platelets with

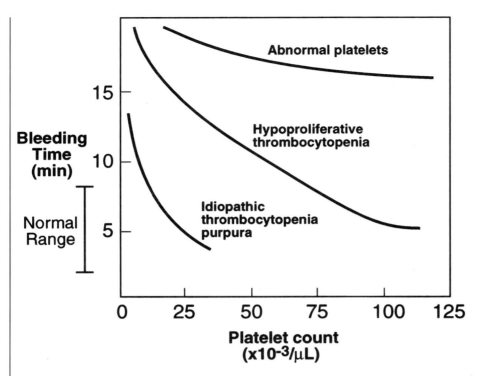

FIGURE 18-2.

Relation between bleeding time and platelet count. Abnormal platelets function poorly even at nearly normal counts, whereas platelets that are newly released from a high turnover condition (idiopathic thrombocytopenic purpura) function well even at low counts. The bleeding time has been largely supplanted by more specific tests of platelet function. (Adapted from Harker LA, Slichter SJ. The bleeding time as a screening test for evaluation of platelet function. *N Engl J Med* 287:155).

genetic disorders (Fig. 18-2). In addition, aspirin and other nonsteroidal anti-inflammatory agents decrease platelet function. Patients with uremia have poor platelet function. Uremic patients also may lose the large multimeric forms of von Willebrand factor in the plasma and have little von Willebrand factor on their platelets.

The diagnostic evaluation of platelet disorders includes a list of tests: platelet aggregation; release of adenosine diphosphate and serotonin, platelet factor 4, and β-thromboglobulin from platelet granules; assay of platelet factor 3 after activation; and electron microscopy. Von Willebrand factor is estimated by immunoassay or crossed immunoelectrophoresis. As shown in Table 16-1, such tests make a firm diagnosis possible.

If platelets are dysfunctional but the platelet count is normal, transfusion of normal platelet concentrations may control bleeding or allow surgical procedures to be done.

EVALUATION OF A LONG PTT OR PT

The first step in evaluating a long PTT or PT is to perform mixing experiments to decide whether the abnormal plasma contains an inhibitor of coagulation or is deficient in a clotting factor. Factor deficiencies are corrected by normal plasma. Inhibitors block normal factors in the added plasma. The "lupus anticoagulant," which is an antibody directed against phospholipid, lengthens the PTT but rarely causes clinical bleeding. Indeed, some patients suffer from repeated episodes of venous and arterial thrombosis. However, inhibitors (antibodies) directed against single factors, especially VIII and IX, can cause serious bleeding. Myeloma proteins at high concentration nonspecifically inhibit clotting.

Hereditary Factor Deficiencies

All the hereditary deficiencies except abnormalities of factors I, VIII, and IX are autosomal recessive. Deficiencies of factors IX and VIII are sex-linked recessive disorders. Certain dysfibrinogenemias are autosomal dominant because abnormalities of half of the molecules can result in altered polymerization of both abnormal and normal fibrin monomer.

Therapy for Hemophilia and Rarer Factor Deficiencies

Factor VIII and IX deficiencies (hemophilias A and B) are sex-linked recessive traits, which were found to be different when plasmas cross-corrected each other. The incidence is about 1 in 10,000 for factor VIII deficiency and 1 in 100,000 for factor IX deficiency. Patients with severe cases of hemophilia A have less than 1% factor VIII and are in constant danger of bleeding into soft tissues, joints, or viscera including brain. Moderate cases have 5% factor VIII, have occasional hemarthrosis, and reach maturity without serious crippling joint deformity. Mild cases (6% to 40% factor VIII) rarely have hemarthrosis and live nearly normal lives.

Because it is impossible to raise factor VIII levels above 10% to 15% with physiologic volumes of plasma, purified concentrates of factor VIII are required for treatment of hemophilia A. The first breakthrough in treatment was the finding that factor VIII can be concentrated by freezing plasma and then thawing it at 4° C. Fibrinogen, fibronectin, and factor VIII/von Willebrand factor remain insoluble and form the so-called "cryoprecipitate." Cryoprecipitate is made from single units of plasma, whereas other preparations of purified VIII concentrate are made from a pool of thousands of units of plasma. In the early days of the AIDS epidemic, cryoprecipitate was therefore much less likely to infect the patient with hepatitis or AIDS. Now, effective methods are used to inactivate viruses in plasma-derived factor VIII; also, factor VIII is produced by recombinant technology.

Because cryoprecipitate is rich in von Willebrand factor, it can be used in von Willebrand's disease to raise levels of both factor VIII (i.e., to normalize the PTT) and von Willebrand factor (i.e., to normalize the bleeding time). Von Willebrand's disease and mild hemophilia also respond to vasopressin, which stimulates the acute release of von Willebrand factor from stores in endothelial cells.

Factor IX concentrates are available for patients with hemophilia B (factor IX deficiency). Bleeding patients are given enough concentrate to raise the plasma level of the deficient factor to 50% to 100% normal, depending on the clinical situation.

After hemophiliacs are educated about their deficiency and learn to treat themselves with factor concentrates at home, they can lead almost normal lives. More than 10%, however, develop antibodies to infused factor VIII or IX and do not respond to factor concentrates. In emergencies, patients with anti-factor VIII or IX antibody can be treated with a concentrate of activated vitamin K-dependent factors (IXa, Xa, VIIa, IIa) that bypass the factor VIII-requiring propagating reaction. Patients with rarer, autosomal recessive factor deficiencies can be treated by administration of plasma.

There are three components to effective hemostasis: the blood vessel, the platelets, and the network of soluble factors. Abnormal bleeding occurs much more frequently when two of the three components are compromised as, for example, in a hemophiliac who suffers trauma (injuring the vessels), a patient on warfarin who takes aspirin (blocking platelet cyclooxygenase), or a patient with thrombocytopenia and peptic ulcer (injuring the gastric mucosa). In the event of an acute episode of bleeding, the second factor, as well as the first should be looked for.

Acquired Factor Deficiencies

The most common cause of a long PTT and PT is deficiency of the vitamin K-dependent clotting factors (II, VII, IX, X). *Deficiency of vitamin K-dependent factors is a second most common clotting problem in medicine* (Table18-1). Rarer causes of acquired deficiencies include selective urinary loss of a clotting factor in nephrotic syndrome and selective adsorption of a clotting factor, especially factor X, to amyloid.

HYPERCOAGULABLE STATES

Clinical indications of the hypercoagulable state are:

- Family history of thrombosis, especially before age 40
- Recurrent thrombosis without precipitating events
- Thrombosis in unusual sites (arm, neck, abdomen)

Patients with one or more of these risk factors should be investigated to decide the need for life-long anticoagulation or other prophylaxis and prevent further damage from abnormal thrombosis. Their diseases fall into two categories: genetic abnormalities of the inhibitor system and acquired disorders of plasma proteins, platelets, other cells, and blood vessels.

Genetic Disorders Leading to a Hypercoagulable State

An important genetic abnormality of the inhibitor system is antithrombin deficiency, which is estimated to affect 1 in 2000 in the general population.

TABLE 18-1. Causes of Deficiency of Vitamin K-Dependent Factors

---

Inadequate supply of vitamin K (green leafy vegetables + gut flora)
    Newborn (hemorrhagic disease of the newborn)
    Intensive care patient on antibiotics with nothing by mouth
Poor absorption of vitamin K (fat malabsorption)
    Biliary obstruction (absence of bile salts) due to:
        Gallstones
        Carcinoma of biliary tract
    Steatorrhea due to:
        Sprue
        Regional ileitis
Poor synthesis of vitamin K-dependent factors
    Liver failure (other factors also affected) due to:
        Alcoholic cirrhosis
        Metastatic carcinoma
Inhibitors of vitamin K
    Coumarins

Protein C deficiency is rarer, but of special interest because the patient may develop skin necrosis when given warfarin. Protein S deficiency and defects in plasminogen or plasminogen activator have been described. Failure to metabolize homocysteine because of an enzymatic defect or folate deficiency is also associated with tendency to thrombosis. The 4% of the general population with factor V polymorphism leading to activated protein C resistance are especially prone to thrombosis when one of the other genetic disorders is present and increases the risk of thrombosis throughout life. However, more than 50% of patients with primary hypercoagulability have no known defect, suggesting that other anticlotting factors have yet to be discovered.

Acquired Disorders

Acquired disorders are a diverse group. The most important disorder is carcinoma. Mucin-secreting adenocarcinomas (stomach, lung, ovary, colon) are especially prone to induce clots in various veins (migratory thrombophlebitis). The mechanism is believed to be the release of thromboplastic materials from tumor emboli. The next most important hypercoagulable state is pregnancy (and pseudo-pregnancy due to oral contraceptives). Late in pregnancy, factors I, VII, VIII, IX, X, and XII double, whereas fibrinolytic activity and antithrombin decline. (This observation suggests that factor concentrations are under hormonal control.) Abnormal platelets are the cause of a hypercoagulable state in polycythemia vera, paroxysmal nocturnal hemoglobinuria, and essential thrombocytosis. Surgery and immobilization increase the risk of thrombosis.

Lupus Anticoagulant

The lupus anticoagulant is an autoantibody against phospholipid that prolongs PTT. It was first described in patients with lupus erythematosus but is also found in patients taking drugs that induce lupus syndrome, as well in patients with no known disease. The lupus anticoagulant is in a family of autoantibodies that includes anticardiolipin (VDRL) and antiplatelet antibody. The phospholipid antibodies are paradoxically associated with thrombosis rather than bleeding, and the patient may present with an arterial clot, a pulmonary embolus, or recurrent spontaneous abortion—all suggestive of a hypercoagulable state.

THROMBOTIC THROMBOCYTOPENIC PURPURA

Thrombotic thrombocytopenic purpura (TTP) is a microangiopathic thrombocytopenia of unknown cause. It is a pentad of microangiopathic hemolytic anemia, thrombopenic bleeding, fever, renal failure, and central nervous system impairment. Diagnostic hallmarks include red cell fragmentation on blood smear and thrombi in the microcirculation of kidney or mucosa. Patients with TTP often respond dramatically to exchange transfusion or plasmapheresis. These procedures appear to replace a factor that normally keeps platelets from aggregating. TTP and a related disorder, hemolytic uremic syndrome, are the most feared complications of the recently publicized epidemics of *Escherichia coli* 0157:H7. Platelet transfusions may make the syndrome worse and should be avoided.

DISSEMINATED INTRAVASCULAR COAGULATION

Disseminated intravascular coagulation (DIC) is an acquired abnormality in which coagulation factors are consumed out of proportion to the normal demands of the body. It is a subset of the hypercoagulable states. DIC can present as four different syndromes, depending on the rate at which fibrin is formed in the circulation:

- Microangiopathic hemolytic anemia
- Migratory thrombophlebitis
- An acquired bleeding disorder
- Defibrination with gross hemorrhage

When fibrin formation is local, as in the case of a patient whose artificial aortic valve is defective, fibrin formation does not disturb the coagulation system because the amount consumed is small. Instead, the red cell shows the abnormality as a hemolytic process (macroangiopathic hemolytic anemia). Usually, red cell fragments are seen in the smear, making the diagnosis clear.

DIC may present as thrombosis. In the case of the mucinous adenocarcinomas, for example, bizarre thrombotic episodes (thrombophlebitis migrans) may precede the recognition of the carcinoma by months or years. However, as the disease advances and the amount of tumor thromboplastic material entering the circulation increases, patients suffer from a decline in platelets, fibrinogen, and factors V and VIII, owing to consumption in clotting. Bleeding then becomes the major problem. Heparin stops the bleeding, paradoxically, by interfering with the intravascular coagulation process, thus allowing the clotting factors to be replenished by synthesis.

DIC accompanies many serious conditions, such as septicemia, obstetric accidents, shock, massive trauma, heat stroke, and snake bite. In most of these situations, a bleeding tendency is observed. Prolonged PT and PTT, low fibrinogen and platelet numbers, and elevated fibrin-split products are expected.

If thrombosis occurs rapidly and intensely, as in premature rupture of the placenta or amniotic fluid embolus, defibrination (consumption of virtually all circulating fibrinogen) with gross hemorrhage is the presenting problem. Thus, some hypercoagulable states may present paradoxically as a bleeding disorder if intravascular coagulation is rapid enough to consume the labile clotting factors I, V, VIII, and platelets. In this case, however, the process usually is self-limited, and replacement with fibrinogen, blood, and platelets restores the blood pressure and stops the bleeding.

SUMMARY POINTS

The diagnosis and treatment of bleeding and clotting disorders reward the clinician who has a detective mind-set. Thoughtful questioning, examination of the patient, and patient pursuit of the laboratory tests are required. Since these diseases are not malignant in themselves, the prognosis is good if the underlying illnesses are effectively treated.

CASE DEVELOPMENT PROBLEMS: CHAPTER 18

Problem I

History: A 38-year-old farmer was admitted to the VA hospital for the first time with a crush injury of 24 hours' duration. One day before admission, a hay-bale conveyor fell on him, pinning his abdomen and legs for several hours. He was admitted to his local hospital with blood pressure of 70/40, a right hip dislocation, and a fracture of the right lateral malleolus. He was hydrated with saline and transferred to this hospital the following day.

Day 1. He had diffuse abdominal tenderness and distention.

Laboratory data on admission: HCT 37%; blood urea nitrogen 37 mg/dL; WBCs 17,700/μL; creatinine 2.5 mg/dL; platelets 196,000/μL; creatine phosphokinase (CPK) 92,000 IU/mL (nL <150); PT 12.5 seconds; PTT 25 seconds.

The patient was taken to the operating room where 500 mL blood were removed from the peritoneal cavity. A small liver laceration was sutured, and his dislocated hip was reduced. He was given intravenous antibiotics because of the risk of infection and kept on gastric suction because of ileus.

Day 2. Oliguria developed, thought to be due to myoglobinuria from the crush injury. (Note CPK, a muscle enzyme above.)

Day 3. The patient was put on every-other-day dialysis for progressive renal failure.

Day 7. While on dialysis, he passed a grossly melanotic stool. His blood pressure fell to 50 systolic, and his hematocrit, which had been 33% that morning, fell to 22%. He subsequently passed three more large stools that looked like blood.

1. What laboratory tests would you order?
2. Consider the following results: platelets 150,000/μL; PT 36 seconds; PTT 59 seconds; bleeding time, not done. Mixing studies demonstrated complete correction of the PT and PTT. (a) What is wrong? (b) Does uremia cause these changes?
3. What should be done? (Your answer will determine whether the patient survives.) Work through the problem as follows:
   - List the most common causes of bleeding in humans.
   - Think of abnormalities of the coagulation system that affect the laboratory tests as listed.
   - Relate these answers to the patient's situation.

Minicase Problems

1. A 12-year-old girl had her first menstrual period. The flow was very heavy and persisted for 2 weeks. Her laboratory tests showed PT 12.5 seconds, PTT 48 seconds, platelet count 250,000/μL, and bleeding time 17 minutes. A mixing study corrected the abnormality.
   (a) What is the most likely diagnosis? (b) Review the pathophysiology of the disorder.
2. A 70-year-old man was admitted for elective surgery. He has no family history and no personal history of abnormal bleeding, and he takes no medicines. Laboratory results are PT 12.5 seconds, PTT 52 seconds, platelet count 267,000/μL, bleeding time 6 minutes, TT 20 seconds. Mixing the patient's plasma with normal plasma did not correct the abnormality.
   (a) What is the probable diagnosis? (b) List the diseases in which one might see this phenomenon.
3. An elderly demented patient entered the hospital from home for routine hernia repair. By the time the intern came to take a history, the family was gone and the patient could say only that he took some unknown medicine. Laboratory results were PT 23 seconds (INR = 2.9), PTT 32 seconds, platelet count 247,000/μL, TT 20 seconds. The mixture of the patient's plasma with normal plasma yielded PT 14 seconds, PTT 26 seconds. What drug was the patient probably taking?
4. A patient entered the hospital with a pulmonary embolus. She was given a loading dose of intravenous heparin and a heparin drip at 1000 units/hour. Predict the results of the following tests taken 1 hour after heparin was

begun: PT, PTT, platelet count, TT, fibrinogen concentration, 1:1 mix with normal plasma, bleeding time, fibrin-split products.

5. A 25-year-old pregnant woman noted small red spots on her ankles and some bleeding of the gums. She did not have an enlarged spleen. She took no medications except vitamins and iron. Lab values: PT 12.5 seconds, PTT 25 seconds, platelet count 5000/μL, WBCs 8000/μL with normal differential.
(a) What was the cause of the bleeding? (b) What is the differential diagnosis? (c) What further tests are needed to establish the diagnosis? (d) What risks does this disease pose for the mother at delivery? (e) What risks does it pose for the newborn?

6. A 65-year-old mechanic developed sepsis after gallbladder surgery. In the intensive care unit, he was noted to be bleeding from his IV sites and to have guaiac-positive stools. Lab values: PT 15 seconds, PTT 50 seconds, platelet count 45,000/μL, fibrinogen 90 mg/dL, fibrin degradation products >80 μg/mL, antithrombin activity 50%, α_2-antiplasmin activity 50%. What was the probable diagnosis?

CASE DEVELOPMENT ANSWERS

Problem I

1. Hematocrit, WBC, platelet count, PT, PTT.
2. (a) The problem involves both limbs of the clotting system. (b) Uremia does not produce these changes.
3. The most common cause of bleeding is thrombocytopenia; the next most common cause is vitamin K deficiency. Vitamin K deficiency affects both the extrinsic and intrinsic limbs of the clotting system because factors VII and IX, as well as X and II, are affected. But why should the patient be vitamin K-deficient? He does not have steatorrhea, or biliary obstruction; he does not have liver disease, and no warfarin has been given. The only remaining possibility is that he has inadequate intake (nothing by mouth for 1 week) plus antibiotics to cover his surgical procedures. The body stores of vitamin K are limited—this is a typical time course for development of profound deficiency.
The treatment is vitamin K, in this case intravenously. Only limited volumes of fresh frozen plasma can be given because the patient's poor renal function would lead to volume overload. On vitamin K, in 24 hours he was markedly improved and PT was normal.

Minicases

1. The girl has a combination of a long bleeding time and a prolonged PTT. She has von Willebrand's disease.
2. (a) Circulating anticoagulant. (b) It could be an inhibitor of a specific protein such as factor VIII, or von Willebrand factor, or an antiphospholipid associated with lupus. Further consultation is necessary.
3. Warfarin. Review its action and indications.
4. PT 14.5 seconds; PTT 40 seconds; platelet count 220,000; TT 12 seconds; fibrinogen 460 mg/dL; 1:1 mix : PTT 38 seconds; bleeding time 8 minutes; fibrin-split products >10 <40.
5. (a) Thrombocytopenia, presumably immune. (b) Drug-induced thrombocytopenia must be considered and also microangiopathy associated with thrombocytopenia. (c) The tests should include an examination of the blood

smear for schistocytes. Idiopathic thrombocytopenic purpura (ITP) is a diagnosis of exclusion. (d) The incidence of spontaneous abortion is also increased. (e) About 50% of babies born to mothers with ITP are also thrombopenic. Cesarean section has been recommended to limit the risk of intracerebral hemorrhage.

6. (a) Disseminated intravascular clotting. DIC. Review the disorder and its management.

Appendix I:
Abnormal Red Cells

Abnormal Red Cell Morphology

Name	Description	Found In
Macrocyte	MCV >100 fL, frequently oval	Megaloblastic anemias, chronic liver disease, reticulocytosis
Microcyte	MCV <80 fL	Iron deficiency, anemia due to inflammation, thalassemia, sideroblastic anemia
Spherocyte	No central pallor	Hereditary spherocytosis, autoimmune hemolytic anemia, traumatic hemolysis, large body burn
Target cell	Central spot of hemoglobin	Liver disease; Hb C, SC, D; thalassemia; splenectomy

Name	Description	Found In
Elliptocyte (ovalocyte)	Elongated	Hereditary elliptocytosis, thalassemia
Stomatocyte	Slit-like central pallor	Alcoholic syndromes, hereditary stomatocytosis
Acanthocyte	Projecting thorns	Hereditary abetalipoproteinemia
Burr or spur cells	Irregular-shaped, thick projections	Uremia, liver disease, intravascular coagulation; may be confused with crenated red cells (artifact)
Schistocyte (helmet cell)	Cell with a "bite" taken out of it	Microangiopathic hemolysis, traumatic hemolysis (burns, chemicals)
Tear-drop cells	Tear- or pear-shaped	Myelofibrosis, pernicious anemia

Abnormal Red Cell Particles

Name	Staining Properties	Biochemical Composition	Significance
Howell-Jolly body	Dark-blue spherule	DNA	Splenic absence or dysfunction
Basophilic stippling	Fine "rash"	Degenerate ribosomes mitochondria	Lead poisoning thalassemia; sideroblastic anemia; 5'-nucleotidase deficiency
Reticulum	Filaments, granules (new methylene blue)	Ribosomes	Increased hematopoiesis especially hemolysis
Siderosome (Pappenheimer body)	Coccoid bodies (Prussian blue)	Hemosiderin	iron overload, splenectomy
Heinz body	Light-blue globule (new methylene blue)	Denatured Hb	Oxidant exposure; G6PD deficiency; thalassemia, unstable Hb

G6PD, glucose-6-phosphate dehydrogenase; Hb, hemoglobin; MCV, mean corpuscular volume.

Appendix II: Normal Laboratory Values

Slide Index

Bilirubin
  Total: 0.6 ± 0.4 mg/dL
  Direct: 0.2 ± 0.1 mg/dL
  Indirect: 0.4 ± 0.3 mg/dL
Bleeding time (template): 1–7 minutes (assuming normal platelet count)
Blood loss effects: 500 mL (10%): no symptoms
                      1500 mL (30%): rapid circulatory collapse
Blood urea nitrogen: 15 ± 5 mg/dL
Blood volume, total
  Males: 68 ± 8 mL/kg
  Females: 63 ± 6 mL/kg
Calcium, serum: 9.5 ± 1.0 mg/dL
Carboxyhemoglobin (CO-Hb)
  Smoker: 3.1 ± 1.0%
  Nonsmoker: <2.3%
Coombs' test, direct and indirect: negative
Fat-to-cell ratio, marrow: 1:1
Ferritin: 50–100 μg/L
Fibrin degradation product (FDP, FSP): <2 μg/mL
Fibrinogen: 200–400 mg/dL
Folic acid, serum: >4 ng/mL
G6PD (erythrocyte): 6.6–8.3 IU/g Hb
G/E ratio, granulocytic-to-erythrocytic precursors: 2:1 to 3:1
G/E ratio response to anemia (e.g., after blood loss)

HCT	45	35	25	15
G/E ratio	2:1 to 3:1	3:2	1:1	1:1 to 1:2

Haptoglobin, serum: 16–200 mg/dL
Hematocrit response to bleeding or a specific hematinic (e.g., iron in an iron-deficient patient):
  0.5–1.0% per day, after a 5- to 7-day lag
Hematocrit response to transfusion of 1 unit of packed cells (250 mL) or whole blood (450 mL):
  3% rise in average adult.
Hemoglobin A_2: 2.8 ± 0.2% (electrophoretic)
Hemoglobin F: <2% (adults) (electrophoretic)
Indices

$$\text{Mean corpuscular volume (MCV)} = \frac{\text{HCT}}{\text{RBC}}$$

e.g., if HCT. is 40%, RBCs are $5 \times 10^6/\mu$L, convert both to liters (L):

$$\frac{0.40 \text{ L/L}}{5 \times 10^{12} \text{ RBCs/L}} = 0.08 \times 10^{-12} \text{ L/RBC} = 80 \times 10^{-15}$$

MCV = 80 fL (normal range: 82–92 fL/RBC)

Mean corpuscular hemoglobin (MCH) $= \dfrac{Hb}{RBC}$

e.g., if Hb = 15 g/dL, RBCs are $5 \times 10^6/\mu L$; convert both to liters:

$$MCH = \dfrac{150 \text{ g/L}}{5 \times 10^{12} \text{ RBCs/L}} = 30 \times 10^{-12} \text{ g/RBC}$$

where MCH = 30 pg/RBC (normal range: 28–32 pg/RBC)

Mean corpuscular hemoglobin concentration (MCHC) $= \dfrac{Hb}{HCT}$

e.g., if Hb = 15 g/dL, HCT is 40%;

$$MCHC = \dfrac{150 \text{ g/L}}{0.40 \text{ L/L}} = 34 \text{ g/dL packed RBCs (normal range: 32–36 g/dL)}$$

Iron: serum: 50–160 μg/dL
Total iron-binding capacity (TIBC): 250–400 μg/dL
Saturation: 15–50%
Megakaryocytes per low-power field of bone marrow: 2–5
Methemoglobin (Fe^{3+}) (spectrophotometric): <1.7%
Osmotic fragility, red blood cell: hemolysis begins at 0.50–0.42% sodium chloride and is complete at 0.30%
Partial thromboplastin time, activated: 22–32 seconds
P_{50}: PO_2 of 27 mm Hg for normal oxyhemoglobin
Plasma volume (^{125}I-labeled albumin):   Males: 40 ± 5 mL/kg
                                              Females: 37 ± 3 mL/kg
Prothrombin time: 11–13 seconds (INR ≤1.2)
Red blood cell life span: metabolic label: 120 days
                                              ^{51}Cr label: $t_{1/2}$ = 28 days
Red blood cell volume (^{51}Cr-labeled red blood cells)
    Males: 29 ± 3 mL/kg
    Females: 26 ± 3 mL/kg
Reticulocyte index (RI): normally, 1% of the red blood cells (i.e., 50,000/μL of 5,000,000/μL are reticulocytes)

$$RI = \{\text{fraction of RBCs that are reticulocyte}\} \times \dfrac{RBC/\mu L}{50,000/\mu L} \times \dfrac{1}{\text{maturation time}}$$

Reticulocyte maturation time

RBCs (millions/L):	5	4	3	2
Maturation time:	1.0 days	1.5 days	2.0 days	2.5 days

Reticulocyte response to anemia (e.g., after blood loss)

HCT:	45	35	25	15
RI:	1	2	3	3–5

Sedimentation rate
    Males: 0–15 Westergren method
    Females: 0–20 Westergren method
Stool guaiac: negative
Total serum protein: 6–8 g/dL
Albumin: 3.5–5.0 g/dL
Albumin/globulin ratio: 1.5–2.7
IgG: 500–1200 mg/dL
IgA: 40–200 mg/dL
IgM: 40–200 mg/mL
Thyroxine, serum: 4–11 μg/dL
Vitamin B$_{12}$, serum: 400 ± 200 pg/mL
(HCT, hematocrit; RBCs, red blood cells

Glossary

acanthocyte—spur cell; a red cell with an irregular shape marked by spine-like projections.

achlorhydria—a pH of gastric juice greater than 6.5 after pharmacologic stimulation.

achylia gastrica—no gastric juice.

agglutination—red cells sticking together in an asymmetric pattern due to antibody attachment; the end point for blood-bank testing.

agranulocytosis—no neutrophils found in a differential count of 200 cells.

alkylating agent—a chemotherapy drug that donates alkyl groups nonspecifically to DNA and other proteins.

allogeneic—cells or tissues from another individual.

anaphylaxis—an immediate immune hypersensitivity reaction characterized by hives, itching, hypotension, and pharyngeal swelling.

anemia—a low hemoglobin (<10 g/dL).

anemia of chronic inflammation—a syndrome in which the hematocrit settles to about 30% and serum iron and iron-binding capacity are low; found in chronic inflammation or cancer.

angina—chest pain due to insufficient oxygen supply to the heart.

anisocytosis—many different sizes of red cells.

anthracyclines—chemotherapy drugs, (daunarubicin, idarubucin, doxorubicin) which attack DNA and topoisomerase and produce DNA breaks.

antibody—an immunoglobulin specific for a given antigen.

antigen—a foreign material capable of stimulating an immune response.

antiglobulin—see *Coombs' (antiglobulin) test.*

antimetabolites—drugs (e.g., methotrexate) that interfere with enzymes or act as false nucleotides (cytosine arabinoside).

aplasia—disappearance of a population of cells from the bone marrow.

aplastic anemia—chronic bone marrow failure, usually involving granulocytes, platelets, and red cells; believed to be an autoimmune disease in at least 40% of cases.

aplastic crisis—precipitous drop in hematocrit of the patient with chronic hemolytic anemia when red cell production is temporarily halted, as in parvovirus B19 infection.

apoferritin—a tissue protein that stores iron; an important regulator of iron absorption by the duodenum.

apoptosis—endonuclease-based self-destruction of the cell.

autocrine—an interleukin that stimulates the cell which secreted it.

autoimmunity—cellular or antibody response against self-antigens.

autologous—related to the self, especially a transfusion or graft of one's own cells.

Bart's hemoglobin—an abnormal hemoglobin of four γ chains found in α-thalassemia.

basophil—a granulocyte with large, irregular blue-black granules.

BFU-E and CFU-E—burst-forming and colony-forming-erythroid; colonies found in culture of unipotent stem cells, which enable further dissection of red cell growth factor requirements and the times required for red cell maturation.

bilirubin—the opened, linear heme porphyrin ring after hemoglobin degradation; a useful indicator of red cell destruction, but also of liver function and bile excretion.

Blackfan-Diamond syndrome—a congenital form of pure red cell aplasia, also called *Diamond-Blackfan syndrome.*

blast cell—an undifferentiated cell whose destiny is determined by its histochemical and antigenic markers.

Bohr effect—low pH causing increased oxygen release from hemoglobin.

bone marrow transplantation—transfusion of stem cell-containing liquid bone marrow to replace lost stem cells.

Burkitt's lymphoma—an extremely aggressive lymphoma of small noncleaved B cells, originally described in African children.

CD—cluster of differentiation antigens; a number classification of cell antigens.

CFU-GEMM—colony-forming units-granulocytic-erythrocytic-monocytic-megakaryocytic; a human pluripotent stem cell capable of generating all four bone marrow cell lines in tissue culture.

CFU-S—colony-forming units spleen; donor mouse stem cells that take root in the spleen after radiation ablation of the recipient mouse's marrow; CFU-S bioassay has been used to study stem cell biology.

coagulation cascade—a chain reaction of enzymes that ultimately converts fibrinogen to fibrin.

cobalamin—vitamin B_{12}

cold agglutinin—an IgM autoantibody that agglutinates red cells in the cold.

cold agglutinin syndrome—pain, numbness, and cyanosis of extremities exposed to cold due to antibody-mediated red cell agglutination.

complement—a set of 18 plasma proteins that are activated in a cascade similar to the clotting system; components are mediators of chemotaxis, clotting, cell lysis, vascular permeability, and phagocytosis.

Coombs' (antiglobulin) test—a test to determine whether an antibody is attached to red cells; anti-immunoglobulin is added in the test cells and agglutination is the positive end point (direct Coombs' test). The indirect Coombs test is done to determine whether an antibody is in the serum that will react with these or other red cells.

Crohn's disease—an inflammatory disease of the bowel usually involving the ileum.

cross-match—determination of the antigenic compatibility of a blood transfusion by mixing the patient's serum with the donor's red cells and checking for agglutination.

cryoglobulin—a serum globulin that precipitates in the cold.

culling—a splenic function, clearing misshapen red cells from the circulation.

cyanocobalamin—a commercially prepared form of vitamin B_{12}.

cytokine—a growth factor such as erythropoietin or an immune modulator such as interleukin-1 (IL-1), and IL-2; subsets are lymphokines, monokines, and interleukins.

cytotoxic cells—cells that kill other cells.

dactylitis—an attack of pain and swelling of hands and fingers found especially in young children with sickle cell disease.

deformability—the property that permits cells to change shape under pressure, especially red cells passing through the capillaries.

Diamond-Blackfan syndrome—see Blackfan-Diamond syndrome.

diapedesis—emigration of cells through intact endothelium.

disseminated intravascular coagulation (DIC)—a complex disorder of inappropriate fibrin formation, clotting factor depletion, and activation of fibrinolysis, most commonly occurring in patients with severe infection, cancer, or obstetrical disaster.

differential—the percent distribution of the various categories of white cells found in peripheral blood or bone marrow (also spinal fluid, pleural, peritoneal, or joint fluid).

Döhle body—a blue cytoplasmic inclusion body of RNA found in neutrophils released during severe infection or inflammation.

ecchymosis—a small hemorrhage, larger than a petechia, smaller than a hematoma.

EDTA (ethylenediaminetetra-acetic acid)—a cation chelator in soft drinks and prepared foods; a powerful antagonist of cation absorption; used in fresh blood, to prevent clotting by binding calcium.

electrophoresis—separation of plasma proteins in an electric field based on charge.

endothelial cells—the single cell layer that lines blood vessels.

eosinophil—a granulocyte distinguished by large, uniform, orange-red granules.

eosinophilia—an absolute eosinophil count greater than $600/\mu L$

Epstein-Barr virus—a herpesvirus that causes infectious mononucleosis, nasopharyngeal carcinoma, and African Burkitt's lymphoma.

erythroblastosis fetalis—hemolytic disease of the newborn characterized by large numbers of nucleated red cells in circulation.

erythrocyte—a red blood cell.

erythrocytosis—an increase in red cells above 5.4 million/μL.

erythrokinetics—a set of tests that enables analysis of anemia in terms of red cell production and destruction.

erythropoiesis—the production of red blood cells.

erythropoietin—a richly glycosylated α-globulin, which is made in the mesangial cells of the kidney and required for erythroid cell maturation.

favism—acute hemolytic anemia on exposure to fava beans in some persons with glucose-6-phosphate deficiency.

ferritin—a spherical iron storage protein, (mol wt 440,000); visible only on electron microscopy. Serum ferritin is a good index of storage iron.

fibrin—the insoluble polymer derived from fibrinogen acted upon by thrombin.

fibronectin—an adhesive glycoprotein involved in platelet, connective tissue, and cell binding.

fibrinolysis—breakdown of fibrin by plasmin or other proteolytic enzyme.

folic acid—pteroylglutamic acid, folate; an essential vitamin found in yeast and leafy vegetables, which is involved in methyl transfer reactions.

glucocorticoids—also called corticosteroids or steroids, they are adrenocortical hormones widely used to suppress inflammation or kill malignant lymphoid cells.

glucose-6-phosphate dehydrogenase deficiency (G6PD)—the most common red cell enzyme deficiency predisposing the red cell to oxidant injury.

glycoprotein—a protein containing carbohydrate conjugates.

graft-versus-host disease (GVHD)—a variety of organ-system injuries induced by grafting allogeneic immunocompetent cells, usually as passengers in the intended graft.

granulocyte—a leukocyte containing specific granules in its cytoplasm, such as neutrophilic, eosinophilic, or basophilic.

granulocyte-to-erythrocyte (G/E) ratio—the percent of developing neutrophils divided by the nucleated red cells in the bone marrow.

haptoglobin—an α_2-globulin that binds free intravascular hemoglobin.

HDN—see hemolytic disease of the newborn.

Heinz body—a round, membrane-based, red cell particle composed of denatured hemoglobin; requires a supravital stain (new methylene blue) for visualization.

hematocrit—the fractional volume of blood occupied by red cells.

hematoma—blood in the tissues large enough to form a palpable mass.

hematopoiesis—production of red cells, granulocytes, platelets, monocytes and lymphocytes in the bone marrow.

hematuria—red blood cells in the urine.

heme—protoporphyrin IX with a central iron atom.

hemochromatosis—recessively inherited iron storage disease. The excess iron leads to oxidant injury of pituitary, heart, pancreas, liver, and joints.

hemoconcentration—lowering of the plasma volume caused by loss of water and plasma components from the intravascular space, leading to an increased hematocrit.

hemodilution—increase in plasma volume leading to a decreased hematocrit.

hemoglobin—a tetramer of two α-globin and two β-globin chains and their four heme moieties, which reversibly binds four oxygen molecules.

hemoglobin H—a tetramer of four β chains found in α-thalassemia

hemoglobinopathy—a genetic abnormality of hemoglobin due to amino acid substitution in the globin chain.

hemoglobinuria—free hemoglobin in the urine, usually indicating intravascular hemolysis.

hemolysis—an erythrocyte survival time less than 100 days.

hemolytic anemia—anemia due to increased destruction of red cells in the blood, exceeding the marrow's ability to compensate.

hemolytic disease of the newborn (HDN)—see *erythroblastosis fetalis.*

hemolytic uremic syndrome (HUS)—hemolytic anemia, thrombocytopenia and renal failure usually occurring in children after hemorrhagic colitis from *Escherichia coli* 0157:H7. It is a variant of thrombotic thrombocytopenic purpura.

hemopexin—a plasma glycoprotein that binds free heme in a 1:1 ratio.

hemosiderin—an iron storage protein composed of partially degraded apoferritin molecules with excess iron; visible on light microscopy as yellow granular material, staining blue with Prussian blue.

hemostasis—stopping the bleeding.

heparin—a naturally occurring, highly sulfated mucopolysaccharide, which can be used to prevent clotting in vivo and in vitro.

hereditary elliptocytosis—a mild hemolytic disease characterized by cigar-shaped red cells.

hereditary spherocytosis (HS)—a hemolytic disorder characterized by spherical red cells.

hereditary stomatocytosis—a hemolytic disorder characterized by red cells with a central "slot."

Hodgkin's disease—a lymphoma characterized by large binucleate cells with prominent nucleoli (Reed-Sternberg cells).

homeostasis—a balance between physiologic forces.

homocysteine—a sulfur-containing amino acid derived from the demethylation of methionine.

Howell-Jolly body—a round, blue, red cell particle composed of retained DNA; found in the setting of splenectomy, megaloblastosis, or hemolytic anemia.

hydrops fetalis—a grossly edematous, usually dead newborn with severe anemia and liver and heart failure.

hyperplasia—an increase in nonmalignant cells.

hyperviscosity—decreased fluidity of blood due to high hematocrit or increased serum protein.

hyperviscosity syndrome—abnormalities of central nervous system (confusion, coma), heart (congestive failure), and coagulation (bleeding) due to a high serum protein or high hematocrit.

hypoproliferative anemia—anemia due to decreased production of red cells.

immune thrombocytopenic purpura (ITP)—a low platelet count due to autoantibodies to platelet glycoproteins IIb-IIIa or Ib-IX. The platelet-antibody combination is recognized by the spleen and phagocytized, destroying the platelets and increasing the risk of bleeding.

immunoglobulin—an antibody molecule, any of classes A-E.

inclusion bodies—foreign particles in cells, usually the result of metabolic disorders.

ineffective erythropoiesis—anemia due to increased destruction of red cells in the bone marrow.

infectious mononucleosis—see *mononucleosis.*

interleukin—a cytokine that stimulates or inhibits cell function.

intrinsin factor—a glycoprotein secreted by gastric parietal cells, which binds to vitamin B_{12} and greatly facilitates its absorption.

kernicterus—bile staining of the poorly myelinated basal ganglia and cerebellum of the newborn with severe hemolysis or liver disease.

kinetic classification of anemia—a method of analyzing anemia by measurements of red cell production and destruction; erythrokinetics.

Kupffer's cells—macrophages of the liver sinusoids.

lactic dehydrogenase (LDH)—a useful serum enzyme that indicates cell breakdown; elevated in hemolysis and high-grade lymphomas with large cell turnover.

lactoferrin—an iron-binding protein found in neutrophil granules, which has antibacterial properties.

leukemia—"white blood"; a group of malignant diseases of circulating blood cells, which may be chronic or acute and may involve any of the hemopoietic cells.

leukemoid reaction—white cell count higher than $50,000\mu L$, seen occasionally in infection or inflammation, which may lead to the erroneous impression of leukemia.

leukocyte—white blood cell, so called because of its lack of pigment.

lymphoblast—a lymphocyte in cell cycle; not necessarily malignant.

lymphokine—a glycoprotein secreted by lymphocytes, which directs activities of other cells; term includes interleukins and cytokines.

lymphoma—a malignancy of lymphoid tissue.

lymphopenia—an absolute lymphocyte count less than $800/\mu L$.

lymphoproliferative disease—a disorder of the lymphocytic system characterized by increased cell numbers; both benign and malignant processes are included.

lyonization—normal random inactivation of one X chromosome in females.

macrocyte—a red cell larger than 100 fL.

macrophage—a family of large phagocytes, most of which originate from the bone marrow monocyte.

mean corpuscular hemoglobin (MCH)—the average amount of hemoglobin per red cell, expressed in picrograms (pg).

mean corpuscular hemoglobin concentration (MCHC)—the average concentration of hemoglobin found in red cells, expressed as percent.

mean corpuscular volume (MCV)—the average volume of a red cell, expressed in femtoliters (fL) or cubic microns

megaloblast—a nucleated red cell with cytoplasm showing good hemoglobin formation but with a nucleus that appears immature, that is, nucleocytoplasmic dissociation.

mesangial cells—renal parenchymal source of erythropoietin.

methemalbumin—ferriheme bound to albumin; a sign of intravascular hemolysis.

methemoglobin—hemoglobin with iron in the ferric $(^{+3})$ form.

methylmalonate (MMA)—a product of intermediary metabolism that accumulates in vitamin B_{12} deficiency.

microcyte—a red cell smaller than 85 fL.

mitosis—cell division that divides DNA equally between two daughter cells.

monocyte—an immature phagocyte that circulates on its way to becoming a fixed macrophage in the tissue.

mononucleosis, infectious—a common infectious disease of young people characterized by lymphadenopathy, fever, pharyngitis, splenomegaly, and increased CD8 atypical lymphocytes in the blood; caused by Epstein-Barr virus or rarely by cytomegalovirus.

myelodysplasia—a preleukemic marrow stem cell disorder characterized by poorly made red cells, platelets, and granulocytes.

myelofibrosis—a chronic myeloproliferative disorder characterized by wasting, hepatosplenomegaly, anemia, and variable leukopenia or thrombopenia. Fibrosis of the marrow is the pathologic criterion.

myelophthisis—replacement of the marrow by fibrous tissue or other pathologic cells.

natural killer lymphocytes (NK)— (CD3⁻CD4⁻CD8⁻CD16⁺CD56⁺) do not require previous exposure to kill foreign cells; distinct from T lymphocytes.

neutropenia—fewer than 1500 neutrophils/μL on a peripheral blood differential count.

neutrophil—a multilobed granulocyte with very small flesh-colored granules; the first line of defense against bacterial invaders.

neutrophilia—a differential count that yields more than 3000 neutrophils/μL.

non-Hodgkin's lymphoma—one of a large group of lymphoid malignancies (excluding Hodgkin's disease).

normoblast—a nucleated red cell.

ovalocytosis—see *hereditary elliptocytosis.*

P₅₀—the PO₂ at which hemoglobin is 50% saturated with oxygen.

painful crises—recurring episodes of abdominal, musculoskeletal, and chest pain, which plague sickle cell anemia patients.

pancytopenia—decreased red cell, platelet, and granulocyte numbers in circulation.

paracrine—an interleukin function that acts at short range, the distance of a few cells.

paroxysmal nocturnal hemoglobinuria (PNH)—an acquired somatic mutation that renders red cell membranes susceptible to complement attack, leading to intravascular hemolysis, a thrombotic tendency and marrow failure.

Pelger-Huët anomaly—a benign congenital abnormality of the neutrophil nucleus, which remains unilobular or bilobed throughout its circulation time; mimicked by some myeloproliferative malignancies (pseudo-Pelger-Huët anomaly).

peripheral blood—venous blood that can be sampled from an arm vein.

pernicious anemia—anemia caused by vitamin B₁₂ deficiency due to autoimmune or idiopathic gastric atrophy with loss of intrinsic factor.

petechia—a dot-like hemorrhage due to leakage of a small number of red cells from an intact capillary when platelets are very low.

phagocyte—a cell that ingests particles such as bacteria.

Philadelphia chromosome—a reciprocal translocation of chromosome 9 with chromosome 22, which results in a hybrid gene (c-*abl-bcr*) with altered tyrosine kinase activity; pathognomonic of chronic myelogenous leukemia.

pica—a taste for unusual substances such as clay, laundry starch, ice, or rubber; found in persons with iron deficiency and disappears promptly with iron replacement.

pitting—a splenic function, removing foreign particles such as DNA, iron, and denatured hemoglobin from red cells.

plasma cell—a mononuclear cell of B-lymphocyte origin with royal blue cytoplasm, a round eccentrically placed nucleus and a perinuclear halo; synthesizes and secretes immunoglobulin.

plasmin—a proteolytic enzyme that digests fibrin.

plasminogen activator—one of a group of enzymes that cleaves plasminogen to plasmin and activates its proteolytic properties.

platelet—a non-nucleated sponge-like fragment of megakaryocyte, which initiates the first stage of clotting.

poikilocytosis—nonspecific variation in red cell shape.

polychromatophilic macrocytes—or "shift cells"; bluish-stained red cells on ordinary Wright-Giemsa stains; reticulocytes.

polycythemia vera—(many cells in blood) a chronic myeloproliferative disorder with excess production of red cells, granulocytes, and platelets. (The term is incorrectly used to indicate a high hematocrit.)

priapism—unremitting engorgement of the penis due to vascular obstruction, most often found in sickle cell disease; a medical emergency.

progenitor cell—a generic term for a stem cell.

promyelocyte—a granulocyte precursor that shows only primary granules and is not yet visibly committed to one of the three granulocyte lineages.

pronormoblast—a young red cell precursor with a nucleolus and no visible hemoglobin formation.

prostacylin I₂—a prostaglandin synthesized by endothelial cells that inhibits platelet aggregation.

prostaglandin—one of a family of arachadonic acid derivatives that mediate various physiologic responses.

prothrombin—the inactive circulating precursor of thrombin.

pure red cell aplasia—a severe chronic anemia due to selective failure of red cell production.

purpura—visible bleeding beneath the skin.

pyruvate kinase (PK) deficiency—the most common hereditary enzyme deficiency of the glycolytic pathway of the red cell. It results in a hemolytic anemia.

R binders—transcobalamins I, III; vitamin B₁₂ transport proteins, so called because of their rapid electrophoretic mobility (i.e., more rapid than transcobalamin II). They are active in the upper gastrointestinal tract and may serve to bind false cobalamins.

Raynaud's phenomenon—an attack of pain and pallor of the extremities followed by redness on exposure to cold; cryoproteins may be causal agents.

red blood cell—see *erythrocyte.*

Reed-Sternberg cell—a large binucleate cell with prominent nucleoli ("owl's eyes"), which is characteristic but not diagnostic of Hodgkin's disease.

reticulocyte—a newly made, non-nucleated erythrocyte with a residual collection of RNA-rich mitochondria and ribosomes that are visible when stained by supravital dyes, such as new methylene blue.

reticulocyte index—the percent reticulocytes multiplied by the number of red cells and divided by the maturation time; an accurate measure of effective red cell production.

rouleaux—red cells arranged in stacks like coins due to altered surface charge, usually from high protein in the plasma, as in multiple myeloma.

Schilling test—a vitamin B₁₂ oral absorption test.

schistocytes—a red cell fragmented in the circulation when it passes over roughened surfaces layered with fibrin.

secretor—normal person who secretes ABH antigens in body fluids.

segs—see *neutrophil.*

Sézary's syndrome—a variant of CD4 helper-cell lymphoma (mycosis fungoides) in which the malignant cells circulate in the blood.

sickle cell—a red cell distorted into the shape of a banana or sickle by the polymerization of its S hemoglobin.

sideroblast—a nucleated red cell containing visible coccoid bodies (Pappenheimer bodies) of nonhemoglobin iron.

spherocyte—a red cell that looks more like a ball than a disc; has no central pallor on the blood smear.

spoon nails—fingernails that are concave rather than convex, owing to iron deficiency.

spur cell anemia—a hemolytic anemia usually seen in severe liver disease, characterized by irregular spiculated red cells (spur cells, acanthyocytes).

stem cells—undifferentiated precursors which can sustain their own numbers as well as differentiate into functioning cells. *Totipotent* stem cells can make all known cells of the bone marrow. *Pluripotent* or *unipotent* stem cells can make one to four lineages.

stromal cell—a supporting cell especially of the bone marrow, which may be important for stem cell homing and nurture.

sulfhemoglobin—a green hemoglobin derivative produced by sulfation of heme that participates in Heinz body formation.

suppressor cell—a lymphocyte that inhibits other lymphocytes or hemopoietic cells.

thalassemia—a genetic disorder in which hemoglobin synthesis is impaired. Thalassemia minor patients are heterozygous; thalassemia major patients are homozygous.

thrombin—an enzyme that cleaves fibrinogen to fibrin, generating a clot.

thrombocythemia—a platelet count higher than $400,000/\mu L$.

thromboplastin—a complex of phospholipid, calcium, accessory proteins, and enzymes that catalyzes the formation of thrombin from prothrombin.

thrombopoietin—a glycosylated protein that promotes megakaryocyte growth and differentiation.

thrombotic thrombocytopenic purpura (TTP)—a pentad of microangiopathic hemolytic anemia, fever, thrombocytopenia, and disorders of brain and kidney, which is due to widespread intravascular platelet aggregation.

thromboxane A_2—an arachadonic acid derivative that induces platelet aggregation.

thymoma—a malignant tumor of the thymus sometimes associated with pure red cell aplasia or aplastic anemia (as well as myasthenia gravis).

transcobalamin II—a B_{12}-transport plasma protein that picks up the vitamin from the ileum and delivers it to the liver for storage or to other cells for various synthetic functions.

transferrin—a serum β-globulin that binds and transports iron.

transfusion reaction—one of several kinds of unwanted physiologic responses to transfused blood.

transplantation—see *bone marrow transplantation*.

urticaria—hives.

vinca alkyloids—chemotherapy drugs (vincristine, vinblastine) derived from plants, which arrest cells in mitosis by binding to tubulin.

vitamin B_{12}—an essential vitamin found in animal tissues; a cobalamin involved in the transfer of methyl groups.

von Willebrand's disease— genetic bleeding disorders due to defects in the amount and molecular configuration of von Willebrand factor.

von Willebrand factor—a large multimeric adhesive protein that carries factor VIII and aids binding of platelets to subendothelium.

white blood cell—see *leukocyte*.

zeta potential—the electrostatic charge that repels red cells from each other.

Index

Anticonvulsants, 30
Antigens
    defined, 323
    granulocyte, 151
    human leukocyte, 151
    plasma proteins, 152
    platelet, 151
    red cell, 144–151
    Rh system, 148, 152
Antiglobulin
    defined, 323
    screening technique, 155–157
Antimetabolites, 323
Antithrombin, 313
Antithymocyte globuline, 201
Antithyroid drugs, 192, 202
Aplasias, 15
    Blackfan-Diamond syndrome, 323
    defined, 201, 323
    pure red cell, 64–65, 326
Aplastic anemia, xvii, 64–65, 143,
        201–202
    defined, 323
Aplastic crisis, xvii, 82, 89, 119
    defined, 323
Apoferritin, 323
Apoptosis, 233
    defined, 323
    factors impairing, 266–267
    failure, 241, 246
Arsenic poisoning, 30, 86, 202
Arterial thrombosis, 310
Arthralgias, 236
Ascites. See Hydrops fetalis
Aspirin, 310
Asthma, 196
Atherosclerosis, 220
    platelets and, 283
Atopic dermatitis, 196
ATPase deficiency, 86
Autoantibodies, 86
Autoimmune hemolytic anemia,
        171–178, 318
    cold, 173
    cold agglutinin syndrome, 173–174
    drug-induced hymolytic anemia,
        174–177
    etiologic classification, 171–172
    incidence, 171
    membrane modification, 176
    paroxysmal cold hemoglobinuria,
        174
    treatment, 177–178
    true, 176
    warm, 172–173
Autoimmune neutropenia, 151, 193
Autoimmunity, 237
    defined, 323
Autologous transplantation, 13, 262
    defined, 323
AZT. See Zidovudine

B cells, 151, 227–231
    differentiating factor, 13
    stimulating factor, 13
Bacterial toxins, 86
Bart's hemoglobin, 111
    defined, 323

Basophilia, 197
Basophilic normoblast, 17–19
Basophilic stippling, 320
Basophils, 196–197
    defined, 184
BCNU, 248
Bence Jones proteins, 256
Benzene, 201–202
Bernard Soulier disease, 282
BFU-E, 323
Bilirubin, 84, 89, 95–97, 169
    defined, 323
    normal lab value, 321
Bismuth subnitrate, 136
Bisphosphanate, 262
Blackfan-Diamond syndrome, 65
    defined, 323
Blast cells, 211
    defined, 343
Blast logs, 211–213
Bleomycin, 248
Blind loop syndrome, 49
Blood banking, 139–179
    2,3–BPG, 134
    immune hemolysis, 166–179
    transfusion, 141–165
Blood count, 308 volume
    normal lab value, 321
Blood groups, xvii, 144–152
    ABO system, 144–147
    granulocyte antigens, 151
    human leukocyte antigens, 151
    plasma protein antigens, 152
    platelet antigens, 151
    red cell antigen systems, 144–151
    Rh system, 147–149
Blood loss effects
    anemia, 26–27, 69–71
    normal lab value, 321
Blood transfusion, 134, 141–165
    ABO typing, 152
    antibody screening, 153–157
    aplastic crisis, 82
    autoimmune hemolytic anemia, 178
    blood components, 142–144
    blood groups, 144–152
    cross-match procedures, 153–157
    defined, 327
    HDN, 170–171
    history, 142
    immune reactions, 158–162
    infections, 157–158
    PNH treatment, 95
    reactions, 157–162
    reactions, 86
    Rho(D) typing, 152
    standard pretesting, 152–153
    thalassemia, 116
Blood urea nitrogen
    normal lab value, 321
Blundell, J., 142
Bohr effect, 132–133, 137
    defined, 323
Bone formation, 220
Bone marrow, 221
    acute leukemias, 208–213
    anatomy, 14–15
    aplastic anemias, 201–202

damage, 65
    defined, 5
    differentiated cells, 15
    granulocyte production, 184–187
    myelodysplasia, 202–203
    myeloproliferative syndromes,
        203–207
    production disorders, 200–215
    response to anemia, 16, 23–25
    response to hemolysis, 81–82
    sampling methods, 14
    stem cell growth, 8–9
    transplantation, 323
Bradykinin, 297
Bubonic plague, 247
Burkitt's lymphoma, 228, 235–236,
        239–240
    defined, 323
    translocations, 241
    variant chromosomes, 240
Burns, 86, 318, 319
Burr cells, 319

C(hr') antigen, 149–150
Cachexia, 224
Calcium, serum
    normal lab value, 321
Cancer cells, 15, 172, 193, 237, 312–313
Carbimazole, 202
Carbon dioxide, 133
Carbon monoxide, 134–136
Carboxyhemoglobin, 134–136
    normal lab value, 321
Carcinomas. See Cancers
Cardiac arrhythmias, 261
Cardiac valvular abnormalities, 86
Cardiovascular drugs, 175
Cartilage-hair hypoplasia, 193
Cascade effect, 297
Castle, William, 32
Cat-scratch disease, 247
Cell markers, 227–228
Cephalosporins, 172, 175
Ceramide trihexoside, 224
Ceroid, 224
CFU-E, 323
CFU-GEMM, 205
    defined, 323
CFU-GM, 184, 189, 217
CFU-S, 323
Chédiak-Higashi syndrome, 195
Chemotaxis, 189–190
    abnormal, 194–195
Chemotherapy, 30, 193–194, 202, 208,
        266
    anthracyclines, 323
    Hodgkin's disease treatment, 246
    leukemia treatment, 209–213
    multiple myeloma treatment,
        261–262
Chloramphenicol, 192–193, 202
Chlordiazepoxide, 202
Chlorinated hydrocarbons, 175
Chlorpromazine, 175, 202
Cholecystitis, 89, 95
Chonic renal failure, 60–61, 64
Chromium-51 survival, 84–85
Chromosome translocation, 239–241, 266

Slide Index

1. Myeloblast. Although by definition it contains no granules, a prominent nucleolus, and blue cytoplasm, cells often show the first primary granules indicating commitment to the myeloid line.
2. Promyelocyte (*upper, left*) is slightly larger than the myeloblast and is characteristically covered with red primary granules. The cytoplasm has expanded, and the nucleolus is still prominent.
3. Myelocyte. This is the first cell to show specific (in this case neutrophilic) granules. Primary granules persist as well. The nucleus is condensing; the nucleolus is fading.
4. Neutrophilic metamyelocyte. It has an indented or kidney-shaped nucleus.
5. Neutrophilic band has a horseshoe-shaped nucleus. There is a metamyelocyte in the field.
6. Neutrophilic segmented or polymorphonuclear cell has thin filaments separating nuclear lobes.
7. Basophil. This granulocyte is distinguished from the neutrophil by its large, irregular magenta granules.
8. Eosinophil has large orange-red granules that are refractile under the light microscope.
9. Monocyte is distinguished from the neutrophil by its gray cytoplasm, fine reddish granules, and occasional vacuoles. Its nucleus is often indented, and its chromatin is delicate.
10. The small lymphocyte typically has a round, dense, and thin ring of cytoplasm with few granules.
11. Plasma cell. Although the progeny of the lymphocyte, it is rarely seen in the peripheral blood. Its eccentric, spoke-like nucleus, royal blue cytoplasm, and perinuclear Golgi apparatus make it quite distinctive.
12. Pronormoblast resembles the myeloblast except for its wider rim of dark blue cytoplasm and a single pale area representing the Golgi apparatus. Its nucleus is irregularly dense and centrally placed, and the nucleolus is still visible.
13. Basophilic normoblast has a dense and spoke-like nucleus and dark blue cytoplasm. The nucleolus is no longer visible and the cell diameter is smaller.
14. Polychromatophilic normoblast has a mixture of blue and pink cytoplasm as hemoglobin synthesis increases and RNA fades.
15. Orthochromatic normoblast has pyknotic nuclei and pink cytoplasm.
16. Hypochromic microcytic erythrocytes have thin rims of hemoglobin. Size must be judged by other criteria, such as ocular micrometer or a normal reference slide.
17. Macrocytes with polychromatophilia. The cells are large and many have bluish color, indicating RNA. They will stain as reticulocytes with supravital dyes.
18. Siderocytes are red cells with hemosiderin granules. The granules are often coccoid-shaped and are called Pappenheimer bodies. They stain specifically with Prussian blue.
19. Sideroblasts are nucleated red cells with visible hemosiderin granules. Ringed sideroblasts (illustrated here) are pathologic cells in which the iron in mitochondria makes a partial or complete circle around the nucleus.
20. Iron stained with Prussian blue in the dense part of the marrow particle. Individual macrophages can be seen with dark blue cytoplasm and pink nuclei.
21. Megaloblastic bone marrow. Polychromatophilic cells with immature nuclei are mixed with other cells that are maturing normally.
22. Megaloblastic bone marrow.
23. Megaloblastic bone marrow.

24. Hypersegmented polymorphonuclear leukocytes are found in disorders of DNA synthesis. Since vitamin B_{12} and folate deficiencies are associated with leukopenia, these cells are probably from a patient with leukemia.
25. Ovalocytes.
26. Spherocytes.
27. Burr cells.
28. Acanthocytes or spur cells.
29. Stomatocytes.
30. Fragments, target cells, spherocytes in microangiopathic hemolytic anemia.
31. Reticulocytes stained with new methylene blue.
32. Howell-Jolly bodies.
33. Hemoglobin crystals (*central, left upper*) in hemoglobin C disease. Target cells are also prominent.
34. Target cells.
35. Sickle cell disease.
36. Wet sickle cell preparation.
37. Thalassemia major. This is a hypochromic, microcytic anemia in which targets, teardrops, and fragments are frequent.
38. Basophilic stippling (*top center*).
39. Hemoglobin SC disease with a mixture of sickle and target cells.
40. Red cells stained with new methylene blue showing both reticulum (reticulocytes) and Heinz bodies (round single blue spots).
41. Demonstration of random inactivation of X-linked genes. A female heterozygous for glucose-6-phosphate dehydrogenase shows that half of the cells are normal, and half are affected using the methemoglobin elution method.
42. Red cell agglutination. Note the irregular clumping.
43. Red cell rouleaux. Note the regular stacking.
44. Spherocytes in acquired hemolytic anemia.
45. Platelets, normal size and shape.
46. Large platelet.
47. Young megakaryocyte. The nucleus has two to four lobes; the cytoplasm is just beginning to show red granules.
48. Increased megakaryocytes. At least six are visible in this field.
49. Megakaryocyte shedding platelets.
50. Dohle body and toxic (coarse, dark) granulations in a neutrophil of a patient with inflammation. The Dohle body is the crescentic blue structure on the left side of the cytoplasm.
51. Alder-Reilly anomaly. Prominent red granules in a lymphocyte. Similar granules may be seen in other leukocytes.
52. Pelger-Huët anomaly. The neutrophils are bilobed and have a "pince-nez" appearance.
53. May-Hegglin anomaly. Dohle body (*gray discoloration on right upper part of the neutrophil*) is a hallmark of this disease.
54. The lupus erythematosus cell is a neutrophil (*right center*) (the nucleus is flattened over the top of the cell) that has ingested a nucleus denatured by anti-DNA antibody.
55. Skin window. After sterile abrasion to expose capillaries, a sterile coverslip is taped to the site. In 1 hour, the neutrophils can be seen attached to the slide.
56. Skin window. At 6 hours, nuclear debris (pus) predominates.
57. Skin window. At 12 hours, there is a dense infiltrate of mononuclears.
58. Skin window. At 24 hours, neutrophils are largely gone. Some eosinophils have migrated in.
59. Myeloblast with Auer rod.
60. Atypical lymphocytes. A polygonal nucleus with pale blue cytoplasm, darker where it is compressed by red cells.
61. Atypical lymphocyte.
62. Atypical lymphocyte, plasmacytoid type, with eccentric nucleus and prominent Golgi.
63. Small lymphocytes, chronic lymphocyte leukemia. Note smudges.
64. Small lymphocytes, chronic lymphocyte leukemia. These cells have more cytoplasm.
65. Lymphoblasts, acute lymphocytic leukemia. In contrast to previous two frames, these cells have fine chromatin in the nucleus and more prominent nucleoli.
66. Young plasma cells, multiple myeloma.
67. Plasma cells, multiple myeloma.
68. Plasma cells, multiple myeloma.
69. Pathologic fracture of the humerus, multiple myeloma.
70. Lytic lesions of the ischium, multiple myeloma.
71. Lytic lesions of the calvarium, multiple myeloma.
72. Monocyte.
73. Malignant histiocytes.
74. Histoplasma capsulatum cysts in macrophage.
75. Gaucher cell.
76. Acute leukemia (myelocytic).
77. Acute leukemia (myelocytic).

78. Acute leukemia (monocytic).
79. Hairy cell leukemia.
80. Chronic myelogenous leukemia: Variety of cells is typical.
81. Scanning view of normal bone marrow smear.
82. Normal bone marrow smear, × 10.
83. Normal bone marrow smear, × 10.
84. Normal bone marrow smear, × 40.
85. Hypocellular bone marrow biopsy, × 40. No bone seen.
86. Normal bone marrow biopsy, × 40. No bone seen.
87. Aplastic bone marrow smear, × 10.
88. Normal bone marrow smear, × 40.
89. Myeloid hyperplasia, × 40. Prominent megakaryocyte.
90. Bone marrow smear, × 40; RBC aplasia.
91. Bone marrow biopsy × 40, with myelofibrosis, bony trabecula.
92. Bone marrow smear, × 40. Myeloid hyperplasia with excess megakayocytes.
93. Bone marrow smear, × 40. Myeloid hyperplasia with excess megakaryocytes.
94. Normal bone marrow smear, × 40.
95. Lymphocytosis in bone marrow, × 10.
96. Erythroid cluster in bone marrow, × 10.
97. Erythroid cluster in bone marrow, × 10.
98. Breast cancer cells in bone marrow, × 40.
99. Acute myelocytic leukemia, × 40.
100. Acute myelocytic leukemia, × 40.
101. Bone marrow, × 10. Acute myelocytic leukemia. Rare segmented neutrophils are seen.
102. Neutrophils, × 40. Chédiak-Higashi syndrome.
103. Large granular lymphocyte, × 40.
104. Excess platelets, × 10. Megakaryocyte fragment in blood.
105. Large granular lymphocyte, × 40.
106. Expansion of maxillary bone in sickle cell disease.
107. "Sea fans"; peripheral retinal infarctions in sickle cell disease.
108. Enlarged heart and pneumonitis in sickle cell disease.
109. Gallstones in sickle cell disease. Bone infarcts in sickle cell disease.
110. Osteomyelitis in sickle cell disease.
111. Dactylitis in baby with sickle cell disease.
112. Aseptic necrosis of femoral head with pseudoarthrosis in sickle cell disease.
113. Leg ulcers in sicklemia.
114. Priapism in sickle cell disease.
115. Chronic lymphocytic leukemia lymph node, low-power view.
116. Chronic lymphocytic leukemia, lymph node, × 40.
117. Follicular lymphoma.
118. T-cell lymphoma crowding out B-cell follicles at the periphery of the lymph node.
119. Lymphadenopathy in neck of a child.
120. Lymphoid mass removed from mediastinum. Nodular sclerosing Hodgkin's disease.
121. Nodular sclerosis Hodgkin's disease. Arrows indicate fibrous band and lymphoid tissue.
122. Reed-Sternberg cell.